Geometrical and Visual Optics

Geometrical and Visual Optics

A Clinical Introduction

SECOND EDITION

Steven H. Schwartz, OD, PhD
Professor
Department of Biological and Vision Sciences
College of Optometry
State University of New York
New York, New York

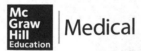

New York   Chicago   San Francisco   Athens   London   Madrid
Mexico City   Milan   New Delhi   Singapore   Sydney   Toronto

Geometrical and Visual Optics: A Clinical Introduction, Second Edition

Copyright © 2013 by McGraw-Hill Education. All rights reserved. Printed in the United States of America. Except as permitted under the United States Copyright Act of 1976, no part of this publication may be reproduced or distributed in any form or by any means, or stored in a data base or retrieval system, without the prior written permission of the publisher.

Previous edition copyright © 2002 by The McGraw-Hill Companies, Inc.

3 4 5 6 7 8 9 0   DOC/DOC   18 17 16

ISBN 978-0-07-179082-6
MHID 0-07-179082-9

This book was set in Janson Text by Thomson Digital.
The editors were Andrew Moyer and Robert Pancotti.
The production supervisor was Catherine H. Saggese.
Project Management was provided by Shaminder Pal Singh, Thomson Digital.
The text designer was Eve Siegel; the cover designer was LaShae V. Ortiz.
Cover photograph credit: BSIP/Science Source.
RR Donnelley was printer and binder.

This book was printed on acid-free paper.

Library of Congress Cataloging-in-Publication Data

Schwartz, Steven H., author.
  Geometrical and visual optics : a clinical introduction / Steven H. Schwartz. —
Second edition.
    p. ; cm.
  Includes bibliographical references and index.
  ISBN 978-0-07-179082-6 (paperback : alk. paper)—ISBN 0-07-179082-9
(paperback : alk. paper)
  I. Title.
  [DNLM: 1. Optics and Photonics—Problems and Exercises. 2. Lenses—Problems and Exercises. 3. Refraction, Ocular—Problems and Exercises. 4. Vision, Ocular—Problems and Exercises. WW 18.2]
  617.7'5076—dc23
                                                                        2012048759

McGraw-Hill Education books are available at special quantity discounts to use as premiums and sales promotions or for use in corporate training programs. To contact a representative, please visit the Contact Us pages at www.mhprofessional.com.

Contents

Preface

...I strove that not one hour
Should idly pass. My eyes and mind took pride
In sacred Optics.[1]

Jan Vredeman De Vries
1527–c.1604

This book is intended as an approachable and appropriately rigorous introduction to geometrical and visual optics. It is meant to be a concise and learner-friendly resource for clinicians as they study optics for the first time and as they subsequently prepare for licensing examinations. The emphasis is on those optical concepts and problem-solving skills that underlie contemporary clinical eye care.

Because of its clinical utility, a vergence approach is stressed. While formulae are an inevitable part of optics, an attempt has been made to keep these to a minimum by emphasizing underlying concepts. Plentiful schematic figures and clinical examples are used to engage reader interest and foster understanding. Every effort is made to provide the reader with an intuitive and clinical sense of optics that will allow him or her to effectively care for patients.

To develop facility in geometrical and visual optics, it is necessary to solve problems. Each chapter includes self-assessment problems of varying complexity with detailed worked-out solutions given at the end of the book. These problems are an integral part of the text.

The second edition has several new features intended to improve student learning. Figures have been upgraded and are now in color. Summaries, sample problems, and tables within chapters are color highlighted. At the conclusion of each chapter, there is a brief summary and list of formulae. New self-assessment problems have been added to many chapters. To meet student demand for additional self-assessment tools, two comprehensive practice examinations (with answers) are

---

1. Vredeman De Vries, Jan (1604). *Studies in Perspective*. Republished in 2010 by Dover Publications, Inc.

included. Throughout the book, sections have been rewritten and reorganized to make the material less intimidating and more comprehensible.

It was my good fortune to be able to call upon knowledgeable and generous colleagues to review all or portions of earlier drafts of the second edition. The thoughtful input of Drs. Kathy Aquilante, Ian Bailey, Cliff Brooks, Jay Cohen, Geoffrey Goodfellow, Ralph Gundel, John Mark Jackson, Phil Kruger, Cristina Llerena Law, Jeff Rabin, Alan Reizman, Jie (Jason) Shen, and Frank Spors is greatly appreciated. Any shortcomings of the book are, of course, entirely my responsibility.

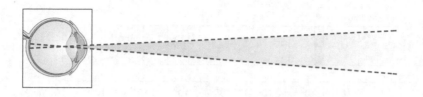

Basic Terms and Concepts

While we may think we're aware of what's going on around us, we're missing out on quite a bit. Our eyes are continuously bombarded by electromagnetic (EM) radiation, but as illustrated in Figure 1-1, we see only a small fraction of it. The remainder of the EM spectrum, including x-rays, ultraviolet (UV) and infrared radiation, and radar and radio waves, is invisible.

EM radiation is specified by its wavelength. As can be seen in Figure 1-2, wavelength and frequency are inversely proportional—as the wavelength increases, frequency decreases (and vice versa).[1] They are related to each other as follows:

$$f = \frac{v}{\lambda}$$

where f is the frequency of the EM radiation, v is the speed of the EM radiation, and λ is the wavelength of the EM radiation.

Visible radiation—light—ranges from about 380 to 700 nm.[2] This region of the spectrum is absorbed by the retinal photopigments, setting in motion a complex chain of events that result in vision.[3]

EM radiation is emitted in discrete packages of energy referred to as **photons** or **quanta**. The amount of energy in a photon is given by

$$E = hf$$

where E is the amount of energy per photon and h is Planck's constant.

---

1. As light travels from a less dense material, such as air, to a more dense material, such as water, its frequency does not change, but its speed and wavelength decrease.
2. One nanometer is equal to 10^{-9} m.
3. For a basic introduction to visual processes see Schwartz SH. *Visual Perception: A Clinical Orientation.* 4th ed. New York: McGraw-Hill; 2010.

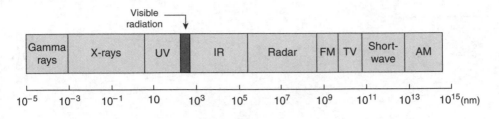

Figure 1-1. Light (visible radiation), a small portion of the EM spectrum, ranges from about 380 to 700 nm. UV radiation, which because of its high energy contributes to the development of various ocular and skin conditions, can be classified as UVA, UVB or UVC. (*Reproduced with permission from Schwartz SH.* Visual Perception: A Clinical Orientation. *4th ed. http://www.accessmedicine.com. Copyright © 2010 McGraw-Hill Education. All rights reserved.*)

By substitution, we have:

$$E = \frac{hv}{\lambda}$$

As the wavelength decreases, the amount of energy per photon increases. For this reason, the absorption of short-wavelength radiation by body tissues is typically more damaging than the absorption of longer-wavelength radiation. The

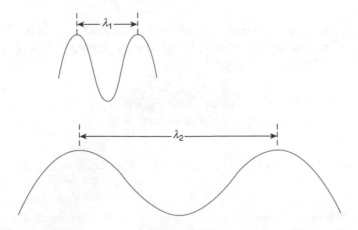

Figure 1-2. Wavelength (λ) and frequency are inversely proportional to each other. (*Adapted with permission from Schwartz SH.* Visual Perception: A Clinical Orientation. *4th ed. http://www.accessmedicine.com. Copyright © 2010 McGraw-Hill Education. All rights reserved.*)

development of skin cancer, pinguecula, pterygium, photokeratitis, cataracts, and age-related macular degeneration has been linked to exposure to short-wavelength, high-energy UV radiation. Ocular exposure can be minimized by use of spectacles that block these rays and headgear (hats, visors) that protect the eye and its adnexa.

Longer-wavelength UV radiation may be categorized as either UVB, which ranges from 280 to 320 nm, or UVA (320–400 nm). UVB is absorbed by the skin epidermis resulting in sunburns. This radiation is most abundant during the summer months. In comparison, UVA, which penetrates deeper into the skin and is absorbed by the dermis, is present all year long. Accumulated damage to the dermis results in wrinkling of the skin and is responsible for commuter aging—wrinkling in areas that are exposed to sunlight (e.g., neck and back of hands) while driving to work. Both UVB and UVA have been associated with skin cancer.

SOURCES, LIGHT RAYS, AND PENCILS

For the study of geometrical and visual optics, we are interested primarily in the wave nature of light rather than its quantal nature. Figure 1-3 shows that a **point source**[4] of light, such as a star, emits concentric waves of light in much the same

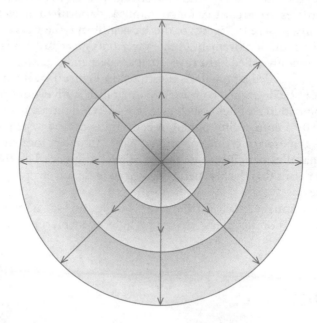

Figure 1-3. A point source of light emits concentric waves of light in much the same way a pebble dropped into a quiet pond of water produces waves of water. Light rays, represented by arrows, are perpendicular to the wavefronts.

---

4. The size of a point source approaches zero—it is infinitely small.

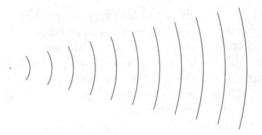

Figure 1-4. The curvature of wavefronts becomes less as the distance from the point source increases. They are arcs of a circle whose center is the point source. At infinity, the wavefronts are flat.

way that a pebble dropped into a quiet pond of water generates waves of water. The peaks of the waves are called wavefronts. Think of them as circles with radii equal to the distance from the point source.

Let's look at this in more detail. Figure 1-4 shows wavefronts traveling from left to right. Consider these to be arcs of a circle whose center is the point source. As you can see, the curvature of these wavefronts decreases as the distance from the source increases. An arc with a longer radius is flatter than one with a shorter radius. At infinity (where the radius of the arc is infinity), the wavefronts are flat.

Note that direction of movement of the wavefronts in Figure 1-3 is represented by arrows—commonly called **light rays**—that are perpendicular to the wavefronts. A bundle of rays is called a **pencil**. As illustrated in Figure 1-5, the light rays that form a pencil can be diverging, converging, or parallel. A **diverging pencil** is produced by a point source of light, such as a star. When light rays are focused at a point, they create a **converging pencil**. A converging optical system (e.g., a magnifying lens) is required to create converging light. An object located infinitely far away forms a **parallel pencil** because, as we've seen in Figure 1-4, the wavefronts are flat (which means that the rays perpendicular to these wavefronts must be parallel to each other).

An **extended source**, such as the arrow in Figure 1-6, is composed of an infinite number of point sources. Diverging light rays emerge from each of the point sources.

VERGENCE

When it comes to understanding and solving clinical optical problems, the concept of vergence goes a long way. At this point, I'll provide some working definitions that will get you going. Once we start looking at optical problems in subsequent chapters, vergence will become second nature to you (I hope!).

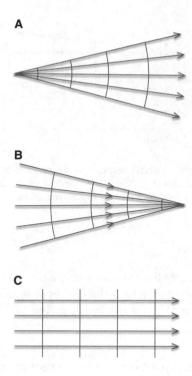

Figure 1-5. A. A diverging pencil of light rays emerges from a point source. **B.** A converging pencil of light rays is focused at a point. **C.** An object located at infinity produces a parallel pencil of light rays. Note that the light rays are perpendicular to the wavefronts.

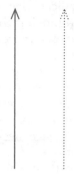

Figure 1-6. An extended object, such as an arrow, may be considered to consist of an infinite number of point sources. Each point emits diverging light rays.

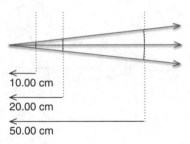

10.00 cm

20.00 cm

50.00 cm

Figure 1-7. Diverging light rays have negative vergence. At distances of 10.00, 20.00, and 50.00 cm, the vergence is −10.00, −5.00, and −2.00 D, respectively. The magnitude of the vergence (ignoring the sign) *decreases* as the distance to the source *increases*.

Vergence is a way to quantify the curvature of a wavefront. For point sources, curvature is greatest near the source and diminishes with distance from the source. The more curved a wavefront is, the greater its vergence. Likewise, the less curved it is, the less its vergence.

When solving optical problems, the vergence of diverging light is always—yes, *always*—labeled with a negative sign. The amount of divergence is quantified by taking the reciprocal of the distance *to* a point source. To arrive at the correct units for vergence—diopters (D)—the distance must be in meters. This may sound more difficult than it is. Figure 1-7, which gives vergence at three distances from a point source, should help. At 10.00 cm the vergence is −10.00 D, at 20.00 cm it is −5.00 D, and at 50 cm it is −2.00 D. In each case, we convert the distance to meters, take the reciprocal, and then label the vergence as negative to indicate that the light is diverging.[5] **Note that the magnitude of the vergence (ignoring the sign) is greatest close to the source and diminishes as the distance increases.**

As we mentioned previously, not all light is diverging. An optical system, such as a magnifying lens, can produce converging light. **To solve optical problems, the vergence of converging light is always—yes, *always*—labeled with a plus sign. It is quantified by taking the reciprocal of the distance (in meters) *to* the point where the light is focused.** Consider Figure 1-8, which shows light converging to a point focus. The vergence measured at distances of 10.00, 20.00, and 50.00 cm from this focus point is +10.00, +5.00, and +2.00 D, respectively. **Note that the vergence is greatest close to the focus point and decreases as the distance increases.**

---

5. In Chapter 3, we'll learn that when light rays are in a substance other than air, the vergence is increased. We'll talk more about this later.

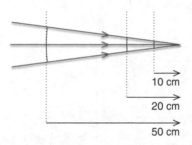

Figure 1-8. Converging light rays have positive vergence. At the distances of 10.00, 20.00, and 50.00 cm, the vergence is +10.00, +5.00, and +2.00 D, respectively. As the distance to the point of focus *increases*, convergence *decreases*.

What is the vergence of a light source located infinitely far away? The wavefronts are flat—they have no curvature—making the vergence equal to zero. Thinking of it in quantitative terms, the reciprocal of the distance to the object (infinity) is zero. Or think of it this way: since the light rays are neither diverging nor converging, the vergence is zero. For clinical purposes, we normally consider distances equal to or greater than 20 ft (or 6 m) as infinitely far away.

REFRACTION AND SNELL'S LAW

The velocity of light depends on the medium in which it is traveling. Light travels more slowly in an optically dense medium, such as glass, than it does in a less dense medium, such as air. The degree to which an optical medium slows the velocity of light is given by its refractive index, which is the ratio of the speed of light in a vacuum to its speed in the medium. Refractive indices of materials commonly encountered in clinical practice are given in Table 1-1.

TABLE 1-1. REFRACTIVE INDICES OF COMMON MATERIALS

Material	Refractive Index
Air	1.000
Water	1.333
Ophthalmic plastic (CR39)	1.498
Crown glass	1.523
Trivex	1.532
Polycarbonate	1.586
Essilor Airwear (plastic)	1.59
Essilor Thin & Lite (plastic)	1.67 or 1.74

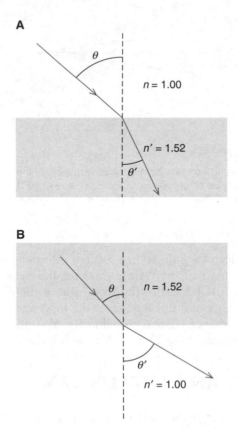

Figure 1-9. A. A light ray entering a denser medium is refracted *toward* the normal. **B.** A ray entering a rarer medium is refracted *away* from the normal.

The change in velocity that occurs as light travels from one optical medium into another may cause a light ray to deviate from its original direction, a phenomenon referred to as **refraction**. Figure 1-9A illustrates the refraction that occurs when light traveling in air strikes a glass surface at an angle, θ, as measured with respect to the normal to the surface. The decrease in velocity causes the ray to change its direction. In this case, the light ray is refracted so that the angle made with the normal to the surface is decreased to θ'.

This illustrates a general rule that you should memorize—when a light ray traveling in a material with a low index of refraction (an optically rarefied medium) enters a material with a higher index of refraction (an optically denser medium), the light ray is refracted *toward* (i.e., bent toward) the normal to the surface.

What occurs when light traveling in an optically dense medium enters one that is less dense? As can be seen in Figure 1-9B, the increase in velocity causes the light ray to be deviated away from the normal. Again, this is a handy fact to memorize.

It can be useful to quantify the refraction that occurs as light travels from one medium, which we'll call the **primary medium**, into another medium, which is called the **secondary medium**. Snell's law, which is given below, allows us to do so:

$$n(sin\,\theta) = n'(sin\,\theta')$$

where n is the index of refraction of the primary medium, n' is the index of refraction of the secondary medium, θ is the angle of incidence (with respect to the normal), and θ' is the angle of refraction (with respect to the normal).

Let's do a problem. *For a light ray traveling from air to crown glass, the angle of incidence is 20.00 degrees. What is the angle of refraction?*

In this and almost all optical problems, it's a very good idea to draw a diagram. Figure 1-10 shows a light ray striking the glass surface such that it makes an angle of 20 degrees with the normal to the surface. Before doing the calculation, we know that the light ray is refracted toward the normal. How do we know this?

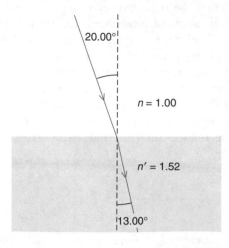

Figure 1-10. For a light ray that strikes a crown glass surface at an angle of 20.00 degrees, the angle of refraction is 13.00 degrees.

As we mentioned earlier, when a light ray travels into a material with a higher index of refraction, it is deviated toward the normal. Snell's law allows us to determine the angle of refraction as follows:

$$n(\sin \theta) = n'(\sin \theta')$$

$$(1.00)(\sin 20.00°) = (1.52)(\sin \theta')$$

$$\theta' = 13.00°$$

Let us look at another example. *A light ray travels from a diamond (n = 2.42) into air. What is the angle of refraction if the angle of incidence is 5.00 degrees?*

Because the light ray is entering a medium with a lower index of refraction, we know that it is refracted away from the normal, as illustrated in Figure 1-11A. The angle of refraction is calculated using Snell's law:

$$n(\sin \theta) = n'(\sin \theta')$$

$$(2.42)(\sin 5.00°) = (1.00)(\sin \theta')$$

$$\theta' = 12.18°$$

An interesting situation occurs when the angle of incidence for the light ray traveling from diamond to air is increased to 24.40 degrees. According to Snell's law:

$$n(\sin \theta) = n'(\sin \theta')$$

$$(2.42)(\sin 24.40°) = (1.00)(\sin \theta')$$

$$\theta' \approx 90°$$

Figure 1-11B shows that the refracted ray is approximately parallel to the surface. What happens if the angle of incidence is further increased? As can be seen in Figure 1-11C, when the angle of incidence exceeds 24.40 degrees, which is referred to as the **critical angle**, the light ray does not emerge from the material—it undergoes a phenomenon referred to as **total internal reflection**.

Total internal reflection prevents the clinician from seeing the structures that constitute the angle of the eye—structures that must be assessed in glaucoma and other diseases—unless a special instrument called a goniolens is used. Figure 1-12 shows that the goniolens reduces total internal reflection, allowing the angle of the eye to be visualized.

SUMMARY

A bundle of light rays—commonly referred to as a pencil—can be diverging, converging, or parallel. The amount of divergence or convergence, which we call vergence, can be quantified by taking the reciprocal of the distance (in meters) to the

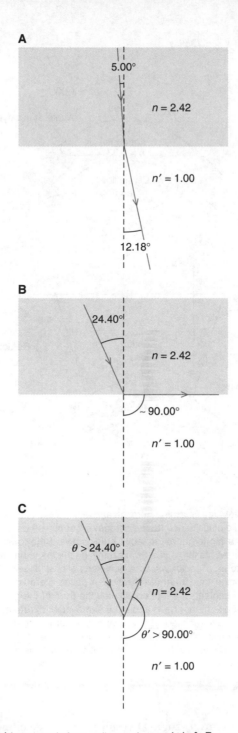

Figure 1-11. A light ray travels from a diamond toward air. **A.** For an angle of incidence of 5.00 degrees, the angle of refraction is 12.18 degrees. **B.** If the angle of incidence is 24.40 degrees, the angle of refraction is about 90.00 degrees. The refracted ray is approximately parallel to the surface. **C.** When the angle of incidence exceeds the critical angle (~24.40 degrees), the light ray undergoes total internal reflection.

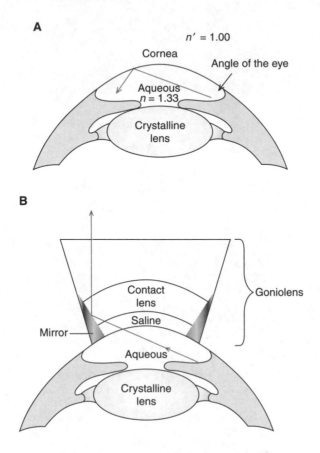

Figure 1-12. A. A light ray emerging from the angle of the eye undergoes total internal reflection if the angle of incidence (at the cornea) exceeds ~49 degrees. (The light ray is traveling from the higher index aqueous humor toward the lower index air.) Total internal reflection prevents the doctor from examining the angle unless he or she uses a device referred to as a *goniolens*. **B.** A goniolens allows visualization of the angle of the eye by reducing total internal reflection. A saline-like fluid is placed between the cornea and the contact lens that constitutes the front of the goniolens. Since the saline and the aqueous humor have about the same index of refraction, total internal reflection is substantially reduced. This allows rays emerging from the angle to pass out of the eye. They are reflected by a mirror in the goniolens that the doctor looks into, allowing him or her to see the structures that constitute the angle. (This diagram is a simplification.)

point of divergence or convergence. Diverging light is specified with a minus sign and converging light with a plus sign.

The direction of a light ray can change when it travels from one medium to another. The magnitude of this change is given by Snell's law, which is probably the most fundamental law of geometrical optics.

KEY FORMULA

Snell's law:

$n(\sin \theta) = n'(\sin \theta')$

SELF-ASSESSMENT PROBLEMS

1. A ray of light emerges from a pond of water at an angle of 45 degrees to the normal. What angle did the incident ray make with the normal?

2. A ray of light is incident upon a pond of water that is 2.0 m deep. If the angle of incidence is 25 degrees, by how many centimeters is the ray deviated as it travels through the pond?

3. A crown glass slab, 75.00 cm thick, is surrounded by air. A ray of light makes an angle of 30 degrees to the normal at the front surface of the slab. At what angle (to the normal) does the ray emerge from the slab?

4. What is the smallest angle of incidence that will result in total internal reflection for a light ray traveling from a high-index glass (index of 1.72) to air?

5. What is the critical angle for a diamond surrounded by water?

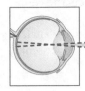

Refraction at Spherical Surfaces

CONVERGING AND DIVERGING SPHERICAL SURFACES

In clinical practice, we are concerned mostly with lenses, not surfaces. But lenses have surfaces, and this is where the action—in our case, refraction—occurs. This chapter will help you understand how light is refracted by surfaces to form images. It will give you a foundation for understanding lenses used in clinical practice.

Refraction does not always occur when light travels from one optical medium to another. Figure 2-1A shows parallel light rays striking a plane (flat) glass surface. Although there is a change in the index of refraction as the light rays travel from the primary medium (air) to the optically denser secondary medium (glass), the angle of incidence is zero and refraction does not occur (Snell's law). As illustrated in Figure 2-1B, the same holds true when light rays are directed toward the **center of curvature** (C) of the spherical surface of a glass rod; rays strike perpendicular to the surface and are not refracted.

Now, consider parallel light rays (originating from an object located at infinity) that are incident upon a spherical convex front surface of a crown glass rod. These are drawn as solid lines in Figure 2-2. The dotted lines in this figure are radii that originate at the sphere's center of curvature. The radii are normal (perpendicular) to the sphere's surface. Rays 1, 2, 4, and 5 are each refracted toward the normal to the surface. The amount of refraction, as given by Snell's law, is greater for those rays that have a larger angle of incidence. Hence, ray 1 is refracted more than ray 2, and ray 5 is refracted more than ray 4. Ray 3 is not refracted at all (it is not deviated) because it is normal to the glass surface and has an angle of incidence of zero degrees. This ray travels along the surface's **optical axis**, which connects the center of curvature and the surface's focal points (defined below).

The crown glass surface illustrated in Figure 2-2 converges light. Such a surface is often called **positive** or **plus** because it adds positive vergence (i.e., convergence) to rays of light.

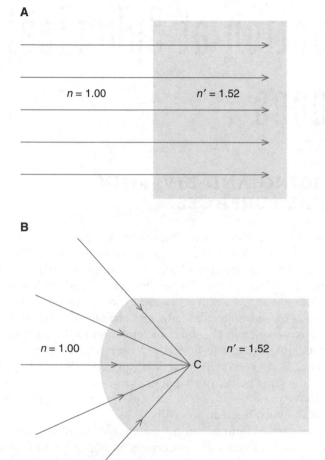

Figure 2-1. A. Parallel light rays that strike a plane (i.e., flat) glass surface perpendicular to its surface are not deviated. **B.** Similarly, rays headed toward the center of curvature (C) of a spherical glass surface strike the surface perpendicular to its surface and are not deviated. A spherical surface is a section of a sphere. Its radius, which is frequently referred to as the radius of curvature, is the distance from the surface to the center of curvature.

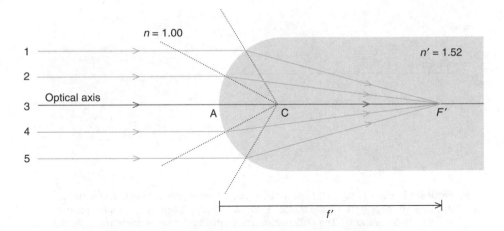

Figure 2-2. Parallel light rays that are incident upon a converging spherical glass surface are focused at F', the surface's *secondary* focal point. The dotted lines are normal to the spherical surface. As a ray travels from air to glass, it is refracted toward the normal. The optical axis connects the center of curvature and the secondary focal point. The distance from the apex of the surface, A, to the secondary focal point is the secondary focal length, f'. All material to the right of the surface is assumed to be glass.

How do we specify how powerful a refractive surface is? We do so by determining its effect on light rays that originate from infinity. These light rays, which are parallel to each other, travel from the primary medium (index of n) into the secondary medium (index of n'). After being refracted at the surface, they converge at a point, F', which is defined as the **secondary focal point of the surface** (Fig. 2-2).[1] The distance from the surface apex (A) to the secondary focal point is the **secondary focal length**, f'. The **dioptric power**, also called **refractive power**, of the surface is calculated by multiplying the reciprocal of the secondary focal length (in meters) by the index of refraction of the secondary medium (n')—the medium in which the refracted rays exist. This is expressed as

$$F = \left| \frac{n'}{f'} \right|$$

Note that this formula gives us the *absolute* value of the surface's dioptric power. For example, if the secondary focal length of the convex surface in Figure 2-2 is 20.00 cm, the surface power is calculated as

$$F = \left| \frac{1.52}{0.20 \text{ m}} \right|$$

---

1. In case you're wondering, we'll talk about *primary* focal points later in this chapter.

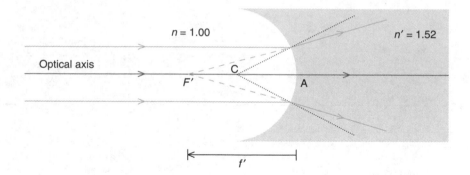

Figure 2-3. Parallel rays that are incident upon a diverging spherical glass surface appear to diverge from *F'*, the surface's *secondary* focal point. Dashed lines connect the refracted rays to *F'*. The dotted lines are normal to the spherical surface. As the rays travel from air to glass, they are refracted toward the normal. All material to the right of the surface is assumed to be glass.

Since the surface converges light, its power is designated with a plus sign, as indicated below:

$$F = +7.60 \ D$$

The power of an optical system must always be preceded by a plus or minus sign. Converging systems are designated by a plus sign, and diverging systems with a minus sign.

Next, consider the spherical surface of the glass rod in Figure 2-3. Parallel light rays traveling in the primary medium and incident upon the denser secondary surface are bent toward the normals (the dashed radii of curvature). Because of the concave curvature of the glass, the light rays diverge. **This is a negative (or minus surface) because it increases the divergence (i.e., negative vergence) of the light rays.**

When parallel light rays are refracted by this minus surface, they diverge in the secondary medium (*n'*), and *appear* to originate from what we define as the surface's secondary focal point (*F'*). As is the case with a converging surface, the surface power is given by the following relationship:

$$F = \left| \frac{n'}{f'} \right|$$

If the secondary focal point for the spherical surface in Figure 2-3 is 20.00 cm to the left of the surface, then

$$F = \left| \frac{1.52}{0.20 \ m} \right|$$

Since this is a diverging surface, we must designate its power with a minus sign, as follows:

$$F = -7.60 \text{ D}$$

An important take-home point from this section is that we can determine whether a surface is plus (converging) or minus (diverging) by drawing normals (i.e., radii originating at the center of curvature) to the surface and applying Snell's law. Self-Assessment Problem 1 at the end of this chapter will give you the opportunity to apply this concept.

A WORD ON SIGN CONVENTIONS

In the following chapter, we'll learn in detail how a linear sign convention can be useful in solving optical problems. **In this sign convention, light is assumed to travel from left to right. Distances to the right of a surface are positive and those to the left are negative.**

How can we apply this sign convention to what we have learned so far? Consider the surface in Figure 2-2, which has its secondary focal point 20.00 cm to its right. Since the secondary focal point is to the right, it is labeled as a positive distance. We can now calculate the surface power as

$$F = \frac{n'}{f'}$$

$$F = \frac{1.52}{+0.20 \text{ m}} = +7.60 \text{ D}$$

Note that we did not determine the absolute power of the surface. Instead, by using the linear sign convention, we calculate both the magnitude and sign of the power.

Next, consider the surface in Figure 2-3, which has its secondary focal point to its left. Since this is a negative distance, the surface power is calculated as

$$F = \frac{n'}{f'}$$

$$F = \frac{1.52}{-0.20 \text{ m}} = -7.60 \text{ D}$$

PRIMARY AND SECONDARY FOCAL POINTS

Light rays can, of course, travel from left to right, right to left, or in any direction. For consistency in working out problems in this book, we'll assume that light travels from left to right. As we've discussed, the first medium in which light exists

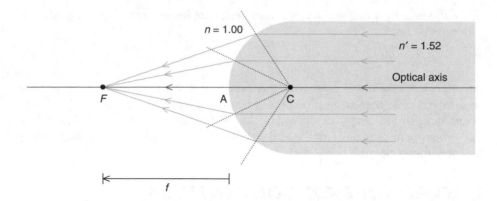

Figure 2-4. The *primary* focal point of this converging spherical surface, *F*, is located by reversing the direction of light rays so that they travel from the secondary medium (crown glass) to the primary medium (air). The primary focal point is associated with refraction that occurs as light enters the primary medium. Since the rays travel from a more optically dense medium (glass) to a less dense medium (air), they are refracted away from the normal. All material to the right of the surface is assumed to be glass.

is called the primary medium; after refraction, light rays exist in the secondary medium. When parallel light rays travel from the primary medium to the secondary medium, the **secondary focal point (F′)** is (1) the point to which the light converges (see plus surface in Fig. 2-2) or (2) the point from which the light appears to diverge (see minus surface in Fig. 2-3).[2] **The secondary focal point is associated with the refraction that occurs as light enters the secondary medium.**

A refracting surface also has a primary focal point (*F*), which is located by reversing the direction of the light rays.[3] When parallel light travels from the secondary medium to the primary medium, the **primary focal point** is (1) the point to which the light converges (plus surfaces) or (2) the point from which the light appears to diverge (minus surfaces). **The primary focal point is associated with the refraction that occurs as light enters the primary medium.**

Where is the primary focal point for the converging surface in Figure 2-4? To locate *F*, we reverse the direction of the light rays so that they travel from the secondary to the primary medium (rather than from the primary to secondary medium, as we have discussed up to now). These rays are bent away from the normal as they enter the primary medium and converge at the primary focal point *F*. The distance from the apex of the surface (*A*) to the primary focal point is the **primary focal length (f)**.

Although a spherical refracting surface has the same power regardless of the direction of the rays (e.g., left to right or right to left), the primary focal

---

2. *F′* is sometimes called F_2.
3. *F* is sometimes called F_1.

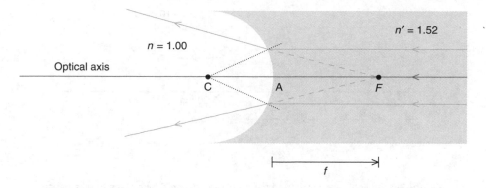

Figure 2-5. The *primary* focal point of this diverging spherical surface, *F*, is located by sending rays from the secondary medium (crown glass) to the primary medium (air). The primary focal point is associated with refraction that occurs when light enters the primary medium. As the rays travel from glass to air, they are refracted away from the normal, appearing to come from *F*. All material to the right of the surface is assumed to be glass.

length does not equal the secondary focal length.[4] The relationship between the surface power and primary focal length is as follows:

$$F = \frac{-n}{f}$$

The minus sign is necessary because we reverse the direction of the light rays to locate *F*.[5]

The location of the primary focal point for a diverging surface is illustrated in Figure 2-5. Light rays travel in a reverse direction, from the secondary medium to the primary medium. Refraction occurs as the rays enter the primary medium; the focal point associated with this refraction is *F*.

A VERY HANDY FORMULA

A spherical surface is by definition derived from a sphere, allowing us to determine its dioptric power when we know its radius of curvature and refractive index. The following is one of the handiest optical formulae that you'll learn[6]:

$$F = \left| \frac{n' - n}{r} \right|$$

---

4. As we will learn in Chapter 4, the primary and secondary focal lengths for thin lenses are equal when the lens has the same medium on both sides.

5. For the surfaces in Figures 2-2 and 2-3, the primary focal lengths are −13.16 and +13.16 cm, respectively.

6. This is the first term of the Lensmaker's formula, which gives the power of a thin lens when its refractive index and the radii of curvature of both surfaces are known.

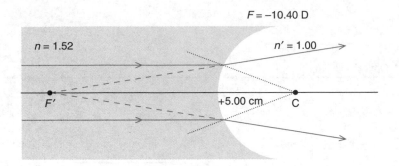

Figure 2-6. As light rays travel from more optically dense crown glass to less dense air, they are refracted away from the surface. Because of its shape, the surface is diverging. As discussed in the text, the surface's radius of curvature and refractive index can be used to determine its power. All material to the left of the surface is assumed to be glass. You can think of this as the back surface of a lens.

where r is the surface's radius of curvature in meters, n' is the index of refraction of secondary medium, and n is the index of refraction of the primary medium.

There are three things you should note about this formula. First, it gives us the absolute power of the surface. It doesn't tell us if the surface is plus (converging) or minus (diverging). We should be able to figure that out by tracing rays as we did, for example, in Figures 2-2 and 2-3. Second, it tells us that radius of curvature and dioptric power are inversely related—the more curved a surface (or the shorter its radius), the greater its power. Finally, the greater the difference between the primary and secondary media, the greater the surface's dioptric power.

Let's apply this formula to the spherical surface in Figure 2-6. Light rays are traveling from glass to air, as with the back surface of a lens. *If the radius of curvature is 5.00 cm, what is the surface's power?*

The first step is to determine if the surface is converging or diverging. Drawing normals to the surface and tracing light rays that are refracted away from the normal when they enter the less dense medium tells us that the surface diverges light.[7] Its power is calculated as follows:

$$F = \left| \frac{n' - n}{r} \right|$$

$$F = \left| \frac{1.00 - 1.52}{0.05} \right|$$

---

7. Be sure to compare this surface with that in Figure 2-2, which has the same shape but is converging.

Since the surface is diverging, we designate its power with a negative sign:

$$F = -10.40 \text{ D}$$

Calculating the absolute power of a surface and then designating its sign based on ray tracing is a great way to learn about surfaces, but not always practical. We can also solve this problem using our linear sign convention. Since the center of curvature is located to the right of the surface, it is a positive distance, meaning that $r = +5.00$ cm. We can calculate the surface power as follows:

$$F = \frac{n' - n}{r}$$

$$F = \frac{1.00 - 1.52}{0.05 \text{ m}}$$

$$F = -10.40 \text{ D}$$

Note that this form of the formula gives us both the power and sign of the surface.

Let's try one more problem. *What is the power of the polycarbonate surface in Figure 2-7 that has a radius of curvature of 10.00 cm?*

Like the previous example, light rays are traveling from an optically denser material into air, as with the back surface of a lens. Let's first solve this problem by determining the absolute surface power. Before plugging numbers into the formula, we'd be wise to first determine if the surface is converging or diverging. Since

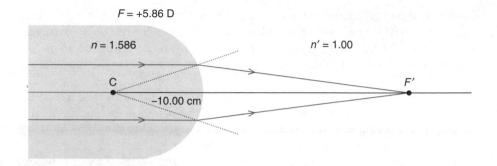

Figure 2-7. As light rays travel from more optically dense polycarbonate to less dense air, they are refracted away from the surface. Because of its shape, the surface is converging. As discussed in the text, the surface's radius of curvature and refractive index can be used to determine its power. All material to the left of the surface is assumed to be glass. You can think of this as the back surface of a lens.

rays travel from a higher to a lower index, they are refracted away from the normal. Because of the shape of the surface, it is converging.[8] Now that we've got the hard work out of the way, we can calculate the surface's power as follows:

$$F = \left| \frac{n' - n}{r} \right|$$

$$F = \left| \frac{1.000 - 1.586}{0.1} \right|$$

Since the surface is converging, we designate its power as positive:

$$F = +5.86 \text{ D}$$

Alternatively, we can solve this problem using our linear sign convention. Because the surface's center of curvature is to its left, $r = -10.00$ cm. Substituting, we find

$$F = \frac{n' - n}{r}$$

$$F = \frac{1.000 - 1.586}{-0.10 \text{ m}}$$

$$F = +5.86 \text{ D}$$

IMAGE FORMATION BY SPHERICAL SURFACES

The images formed by optical systems can be either real or virtual. In this section, we'll use ray tracing to help us understand the differences between these two types of images.

Real Images

Figure 2-8 shows an extended light source, which serves as an object for the converging spherical surface of a crown glass rod. Light rays diverge from each point on the object. Three specific rays, which originate from the tip of the arrow and travel from the primary to the secondary index, allow us to locate the image of the arrow's tip.

To simplify drawing Figure 2-8 (and Fig. 2-9), we'll make the incorrect, but helpful, assumption that all refraction occurs in the plane of the surface's apex. We'll represent this plane by a vertical line that is tangential to the apex. All material to the right of this plane is the secondary medium.

Ray 1 originates from the object, travels parallel to the optical axis in the primary medium, and after refraction is deviated through F'. Passing though F, ray 2 is refracted at the surface so that it is parallel to the optical axis in the secondary

---

8. Be sure to compare this surface with that in Figure 2-3, which has the same shape but is diverging.

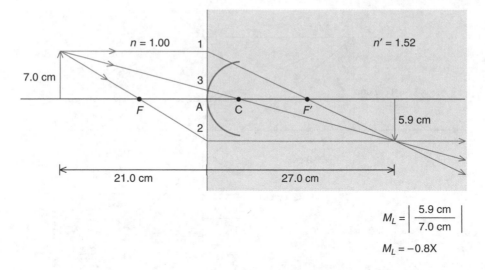

$$M_L = \left| \frac{5.9 \text{ cm}}{7.0 \text{ cm}} \right|$$

$$M_L = -0.8X$$

Figure 2-8. Ray tracing can be used to locate an image and determine its size. To make the diagram easier to draw and understand, we'll assume that all refraction takes place at the vertical plane that is tangential to the surface apex. All distances are measured from this vertical plane. Air is to the left and glass is to the right of the plane. When an object is outside of the primary focal length of a converging surface, the image is real and minified. The lateral magnification (M_L) produced by the surface is the ratio of the image height to the object height. Since the image is inverted, the magnification is designated with a minus sign. This diagram is drawn to scale.

medium. Since ray 3 is perpendicular to the spherical surface (it is headed toward the surface's center of curvature), it is not deviated. The point where all three rays intersect is the *image* of the arrow's tip. We have traced only three rays, but all rays that originate from the tip of the arrow—and there are an infinite number of such rays—are focused here.

By definition, objects and images are **conjugate**. This means that if we were to reverse the direction of the light rays so that they travel from right to left and place an object in the location of the original image, an image would be formed at the location of the original object. Another way of saying this is that the path taken by a light ray does not change when we reverse its direction.

Because the diagram is drawn to scale, we can locate the image with respect to the surface. By comparing the sizes of the object and image (using a ruler), we can also determine the **lateral magnification** (M_L) produced by the surface. Figures 2-8 and 2-9 are drawn to scale, with the object and image distances and sizes given along with the magnification.

The image is labeled as real because it is formed by converging light rays. If a screen were placed in the plane of the image, the arrow would

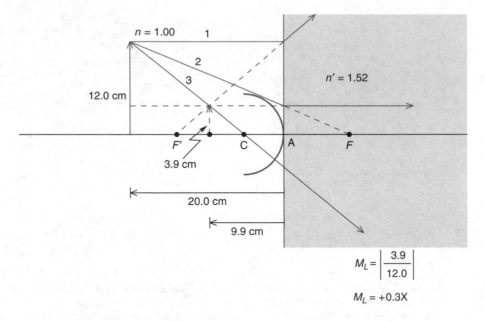

$$M_L = \left| \frac{3.9}{12.0} \right|$$

$$M_L = +0.3X$$

Figure 2-9. Ray tracing can be used to locate the virtual image produced by a diverging surface. The virtual image is erect and minified. All distances are measured from the plane of the surface's apex, which is indicated by the vertical line. (For illustrative purposes, the object is drawn larger than the surface.) Since the image is erect, its magnification is designated with a positive sign.

be focused on this screen. Note that the arrow is *inverted*. An inverted image is designated by a minus sign preceding the magnification. **Real images are always inverted.**

Virtual Images

Consider the arrow that is imaged by the diverging crown glass spherical surface in Figure 2-9. Ray 1 originates parallel to the optical axis in the primary medium and diverges at the surface so that it appears to emerge from F'. Ray 2 is headed toward F and is refracted so that it is parallel to the optical axis in the secondary medium. Finally, ray 3 travels through the glass surface's center of curvature, striking the surface perpendicular to its surface (and is undeviated).

The light rays that *exist* in the secondary medium *appear* to emerge from a single point located in the primary medium. *Dashed lines* connect the diverging light rays in the secondary medium to the image from which they appear to come. All rays that are emitted from the arrow's tip *appear* to emerge from this image. Since the

TABLE 2-1. BASIC PROPERTIES OF REAL AND VIRTUAL IMAGES

	Vergence of Rays	Focusable on a Screen	Orientation
Real	Converging	Yes	Inverted
Virtual	Diverging	No	Erect

rays appear to come from the image and are not actually focused in the plane of the image, the image is *virtual*. Dashed lines are used to draw a virtual image.

Virtual images are formed by diverging light rays. A virtual image cannot be focused on a screen because it is not formed by converging light rays. The image is, however, visible. If you could place your eye into the glass material and view the diverging light rays, you would see a virtual image of the arrow. Note that the arrow is erect; when an image is erect, its magnification is designated by a plus sign. **Virtual images are always erect.** Basic properties of real and virtual images are summarized in Table 2-1.

SUMMARY

Due to their shape (i.e., convex or concave) and refractive index, spherical surfaces refract light. Light rays from an infinitely distant object are focused at the secondary focal point of a converging surface, but appear to diverge from the secondary focal point of a diverging surface. The power of a surface can be calculated from its refractive index and radius of curvature.

The image formed by a spherical surface may be located through ray tracing. If an image is formed by converging rays, it is real, but if formed by diverging rays, it is virtual. Real images are inverted and can be focused on a screen. Virtual images are erect and, although visible, they cannot be focused on a screen.

KEY FORMULAE

Relationship between surface power and secondary focal length:

$$F = \frac{n'}{f'}$$

Relationship between surface power and primary focal length:

$$F = \frac{-n}{f}$$

Relationship between refractive index, radius of curvature, and surface power:

$$F = \frac{n' - n}{r}$$

SELF-ASSESSMENT PROBLEMS

1. (a) Is the crown glass spherical surface drawn below converging or diverging? (b) What is its power if its radius of curvature is 15.00 cm? (c) Locate and label F'.

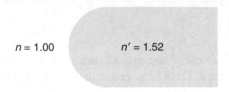

$n = 1.00$ $n' = 1.52$

2. For the crown glass spherical surface below, answer the questions in Problem 1. The radius of curvature is 200.00 mm.

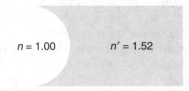

$n = 1.00$ $n' = 1.52$

3. Label each of the following refracting surfaces as plus or minus.

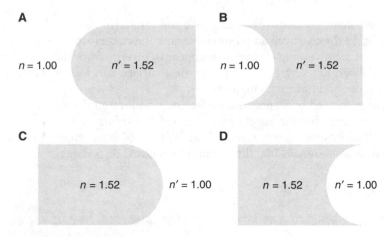

A

$n = 1.00$ $n' = 1.52$

B

$n = 1.00$ $n' = 1.52$

C

$n = 1.52$ $n' = 1.00$

D

$n = 1.52$ $n' = 1.00$

4. An object, 3.0 cm in height, is located in air. It is 9.0 cm in front of a −10.00 D crown glass surface. (a) On a diagram drawn to scale, label the primary and secondary focal points and radius of curvature. (b) Use ray tracing to determine the image distance from the apex of the surface and the size of the image. (c) What is the magnification of the image? (d) Is the image erect or inverted? Is it real or virtual? Explain.

5. Answer the questions in Problem 4 for a 2.0-cm-high object located 20 cm in front of a +10.00 D crown glass surface.

6. A rock sits on the bottom of a pond 3.0 m deep. (a) Does the rock appear to be 3.0 m from the upper surface of the pond? Explain with a diagram. (b) Is the image of the rock real or virtual?

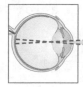

The Vergence Relationship

As we learned in the previous chapter, ray diagrams can be used to determine the location and size of an image. Drawing diagrams, however, can be time-consuming and inconvenient, so we generally use the **vergence relationship**, sometimes referred to as the **paraxial relationship**, to locate images and determine magnification.[1] Before we introduce this relationship and show you how to use it, however, we need to talk a bit more about vergence and linear sign conventions. After these short detours, we'll jump into the vergence relationship and see how useful it can be.

MORE ON VERGENCE

We learned some important things about vergence in Chapter 1, but not the whole story. Let's review and expand upon this. Recall that the vergence of light rays emitted from an object that is located in air is the reciprocal of the distance (in meters) to the object. We'll designate this distance as l. The absolute value of the object vergence is given by

$$L = \left| \frac{1.00}{l} \right|$$

For the object in Figure 3-1A, the vergence is

$$L = \left| \frac{1.00}{0.33 \text{ m}} \right|$$

---

1. This relationship applies only to paraxial rays—those light rays that are in relatively close proximity to the optical axis of the surface. For these rays, the angle of incidence, θ (in radians), approximates $\sin \theta$. Most basic optical problems can be solved by assuming that the rays are paraxial. See Appendix E for a derivation of the paraxial equation.

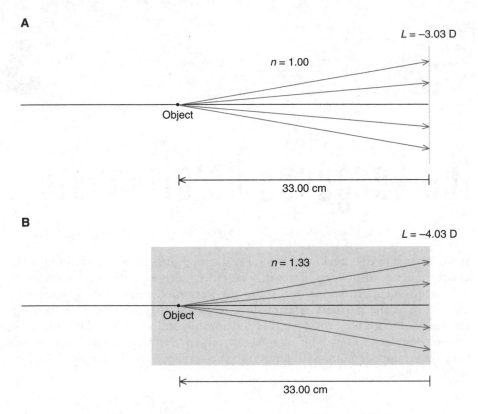

Figure 3-1. Object vergence is influenced by the medium in which the object exists. **A.** For an object in air at a distance of 33.00 cm, the vergence is –3.03 D. **B.** For the same distance, the vergence is –4.03 D when the object is located in water.

Since the light rays are diverging, the object vergence is designated with a minus sign, giving

$$L = -3.03 \text{ D}$$

When the object is located in a primary medium other than air, the medium's refractive index increases the absolute value of the vergence. For an object located in a medium n, the absolute value of the vergence is given by the following relationship:

$$L = \left| \frac{n}{l} \right|$$

What is the vergence for the object in Figure 3-1B that is located in water rather than air?

$$L = \left| \frac{n}{l} \right|$$

$$L = \left| \frac{1.33}{0.33 \text{ m}} \right|$$

Since the rays are diverging, we have

$$L = -4.03 \text{ D}$$

It is often more convenient to keep the distance in centimeters and compensate by placing a factor of 100 in the numerator as follows[2]:

$$L = \left| \frac{(100)(1.33)}{33.00 \text{ cm}} \right|$$

$$L = -4.03 \text{ D}$$

How do we calculate the vergence of light rays that form an image? Consider the real image formed by the converging spherical glass surface in Figure 3-2A. The image, which is formed by light rays that exist in crown glass, is 40.00 cm from the surface. Image vergence (absolute value) is given by

$$L' = \left| \frac{n'}{l'} \right|$$

where l' is the distance from the refracting surface to the image[3] and n' is the index of the medium in which the rays that form the image are located (i.e., secondary medium).

Substituting into this relationship, we have

$$L' = \left| \frac{n'}{l'} \right|$$

$$L' = \left| \frac{1.52}{0.40 \text{ m}} \right|$$

Since the rays that form the real image are converging, the vergence is designated with a plus sign as indicated below:

$$L' = +3.80 \text{ D}$$

It bears repeating that the index is 1.52 because the light rays that form the image exist in glass. While this may be obvious in this case of a real image, it's not so obvious, as we'll see, in the case of virtual images.

---

2. If the distance were in millimeters, we could enter a factor of 1000 in the numerator and keep the distance in millimeters (rather than converting to meters).

3. All sorts of symbols are used to represent object and image distances. Do not let these confuse you. For example, u is sometimes used to represent object distance and v to represent image distance. The concepts are important, not the symbols!

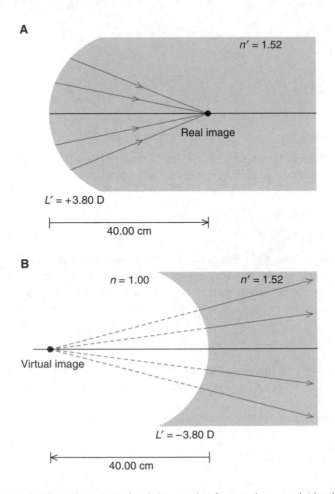

Figure 3-2. A. When the converging light rays that form an image exist in glass, the refractive index of glass is used to calculate the image vergence. **B.** Since the diverging light rays that form the virtual image exist in glass, the refractive index of glass is used to determine the image vergence.

What is the vergence of the rays forming the virtual image in Figure 3-2B?

The key is to recognize that the rays forming the image exist in the secondary medium, glass. They *appear* to emerge from a point in the primary medium (air), but "live" in glass. Therefore, the image vergence is calculated as

$$L' = \left| \frac{n'}{l'} \right|$$

$$L' = \left| \frac{1.52}{0.40 \text{ m}} \right|$$

Since the rays that form a virtual image are diverging, their vergence must be designated with a minus sign as follows:

$$L' = -3.80 \text{ D}$$

LINEAR SIGN CONVENTION

Up to now, we've calculated the absolute value of the vergence and then assigned this vergence a sign depending on whether the light rays are diverging or converging. Although this approach works just fine, most students prefer not to calculate absolute values and to instead use a linear sign convention that labels distances as negative or positive. A linear sign convention provides convenience in solving optical problems, but it can also undermine an understanding of what is happening and lead to errors.

To minimize these problems, it's a good idea to draw a diagram—it doesn't need to be anything fancy—so that you understand what is happening to the light rays. If you keep in mind a few things that we've emphasized up to now—in particular, that converging light rays have plus vergence and diverging light rays have negative vergence—you should be in good shape when using a linear sign convention.

In this text, we use a linear sign convention with the following rules:

1. Light is assumed to travel from the left to the right.
2. Object and image distances are measured *from* the refracting, reflecting, or lens surface.
3. Object and image heights are measured *from* the optical axis.
4. Distances to the left of the surface are designated as negative and those to the right as positive.
5. Heights above the optical axis are designated as positive and those below the optical axis as negative.

These rules are summarized in Figure 3-3. Note that when a distance is measured in the same direction that light travels, it is positive. Distances measured in the opposite direction are negative.

Let's use this sign convention to calculate the vergence for the object in Figure 3-1A. Since the object is located to the left of the surface, the linear distance is −33.00 cm. The object vergence is calculated as follows:

$$L = \frac{n}{l}$$

$$L = \frac{1.00}{-0.33 \text{ m}} = -3.03 \text{ D}$$

Likewise, the vergence for object in Figure 3-1B, which sits in water, is

$$L = \frac{1.33}{-0.33 \text{ m}} = -4.03 \text{ D}$$

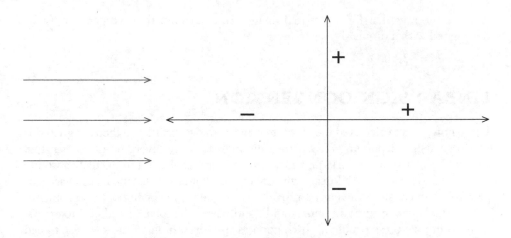

Figure 3-3. For the linear sign convention used in this book, light is assumed to travel from left to right. Object and image distances are measured *from* the refractive surface with distances to the right labeled positive and those to the left labeled negative. Object and image sizes are measured *from* the horizontal axis. Distances above the axis are positive and those below are negative.

For the real image in Figure 3-2A, which is formed by rays that exist in glass, we have an image distance of $+40.00$ cm. The image vergence is

$$L' = \frac{n'}{l'}$$

$$L' = \frac{1.52}{0.40 \text{ m}} = +3.80 \text{ D}$$

And for the virtual image in Figure 3-2B, which is located 40.00 cm to the left of the surface and formed by rays that exist in glass, the image vergence is

$$L' = \frac{n'}{l'}$$

$$L' = \frac{1.52}{-0.40 \text{ m}} = -3.80 \text{ D}$$

VERGENCE RELATIONSHIP

Now we're ready to introduce the vergence relationship, probably the most used relationship in geometrical optics. Figure 3-4 shows an object emitting diverging light rays that are incident upon a spherical refracting surface. After being refracted by the surface, the lights rays converge to form a real image. As we have learned,

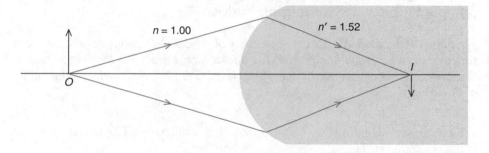

Figure 3-4. Light rays diverging from an object (*O*) are converged by a plus spherical refracting surface to form a real image (*I*).

the amount of divergence or convergence of light rays can be quantified. This is the basis for the vergence relationship. The vergence of the object rays is added to the dioptric power of the refractive surface to give us the vergence of the image rays. This can be expressed as:

object vergence + surface power = image vergence

Designating the object vergence as *L*, the surface power as *F*, and the image vergence as *L'*, we have[4]

$$L + F = L'$$

or

$$L' = L + F$$

The sign of the image vergence tells us whether the image is real or virtual. If the rays are converging (i.e., positive vergence), the image is real. When the rays are diverging (negative vergence), the image is virtual.

SAMPLE PROBLEMS

Although the intuitive understanding of optics that we use to help our patients is often qualitative—not quantitative—in nature, we can't get to this level of understanding without solving optical problems. In a certain sense, when it comes to optics, solving problems is where the rubber meets the road. In this spirit, let's see how the vergence relationship can be used to solve some basic problems involving spherical refracting surfaces. In the next chapter, we'll work with lenses.

---

4. Unfortunately, a plethora of symbols are used to represent object vergence and image vergence. For example, *U* is sometimes used to represent object vergence and *V* to represent image vergence. Do not let this confuse you. Just think in terms of object vergence and image vergence rather than memorizing symbols.

Sample Problem 1: Converging Surface

An object is located 50.00 cm to the left of a +5.00 D spherical crown glass surface. How far is the image from the apex of the surface? Is the image real or virtual? Is it erect or inverted? If the object is 3.00 cm in height, what is the height of the image?

First, draw a diagram (Fig. 3-5). (Always draw a diagram!) The object vergence at the refracting surface is

$$L = \frac{n}{l}$$

$$L = \frac{1.00}{-0.50 \text{ m}} = -2.00 \text{ D}$$

or

$$L = \frac{(100)(1.00)}{-50.00 \text{ cm}} = -2.00 \text{ D}$$

Light with a vergence of −2.00 D is incident upon a surface whose power is +5.00 D. What is the vergence of the light rays after they are refracted? According

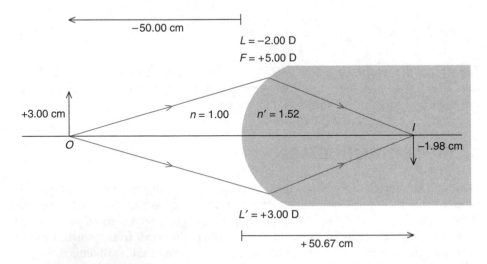

Figure 3-5. Rays diverging from an object, *O*, are converged by the plus surface to form a real image, *I*. The diagram shows rays emerging from the base of the object, at the point where it intersects the optical axis. Object vergence and surface power are given above the surface, and image vergence is given below the surface; we will follow this convention throughout this book. *This diagram and others in this chapter are not drawn to scale.*

to the vergence relationship, the vergence of the light rays that form the image is the sum of the incident vergence and the surface power:

$$L' = L + F$$

$$L' = -2.00 \text{ D} + (+5.00 \text{ D}) = +3.00 \text{ D}$$

Be sure to note that in Figure 3-5 and subsequent figures where we solve optical problems, the object vergence and surface power are indicated above the surface. In this case, L is −2.00 D and F is +5.00 D. The sum of these, the image vergence, L', which is +3.00 D, is given below the refracting element. It's a good idea to get into the habit of labeling your diagrams like this.

Since converging light rays form the image, it is real. Where is it located? The rays that form the image have an image vergence of +3.00 D. *These rays exist in the secondary medium* (glass), which has an index of refraction of 1.52. Therefore, to calculate the distance at which the image rays converge, we use the secondary index of refraction as follows:

$$L' = \frac{n'}{l'}$$

or

$$l' = \frac{n'}{L'}$$

$$l' = \frac{1.52}{+3.00 \text{ D}} = +0.5067 \text{ m, or } +50.67 \text{ cm}$$

Alternatively, the image distance in centimeters may be calculated by placing a factor of 100 in the numerator[5]:

$$l' = \frac{(100)(1.52)}{+3.00} = +50.67 \text{ cm}$$

The image is located 50.67 cm from the surface. Is it to the left (as is the object) or right? Since the value is positive, our linear sign convention tells us that the image is located 50.67 cm to the right of the surface. (But we really shouldn't need to rely on our linear sign convention to tell us this since we know that an image formed by converging light rays must be located to the right of the surface.)

It is helpful to visualize the light rays in terms of their vergence. In the current example, diverging light rays (−2.00 D) are incident upon a converging surface (+5.00 D). Upon refraction they converge (+3.00 D) to form a real image.

To calculate the image size, we need to know the lateral magnification (M_L) produced by the surface, which we defined in Chapter 2 as the ratio of the image

---

5. If a factor of 1000 is placed in the numerator, the calculated distance would be in millimeters.

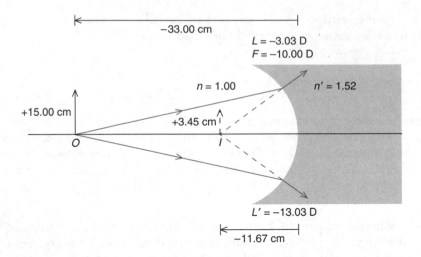

Figure 3-6. A negative surface produces a virtual image.

size to the object size. It is equal to the ratio of the object vergence to the image vergence[6] as indicated below:

$$M_L = \frac{\text{image size}}{\text{object size}} = \frac{\text{object vergence}}{\text{image vergence}}$$

or simply

$$M_L = \frac{L}{L'}$$

In our sample problem, we have

$$M_L = \frac{-2.00 \text{ D}}{+3.00 \text{ D}} = -0.66\times$$

Because the magnification is less than 1.00×, the real image is smaller than the object—it is minified. Negative magnification tells us that the image is inverted. Since the object height is 3.00 cm, the image height is

$$(-0.66)(3.00 \text{ cm}) = -1.98 \text{ cm}$$

Sample Problem 2: Diverging Surface

An object 15.00 cm in height is located 33.00 cm to the left of a spherical crown glass surface that has a power of −10.00 D. Locate the image and specify its magnification. Is the image real or virtual? Is it erect or inverted?

As always, first draw a diagram (Fig. 3-6). Since the surface has negative power, we know that the diverging rays emitted by the object are further diverged by the

---

6. Lateral magnification is sometimes called *transverse magnification* or *linear magnification*.

surface. Therefore, before we do any calculations we know that the image is (1) virtual (because it is formed by diverging rays), (2) on the same side of the surface as the object (because the rays that form it *appear* to diverge from this side of the lens), and (3) erect (since virtual images are erect).

To use the vergence relationship, we must first determine the object vergence. Since the object rays exist in air, the object vergence is

$$L = \frac{n}{l}$$

$$L = \frac{(100)(1.00)}{-33.00 \text{ cm}} = -3.03 \text{ D}$$

This -3.03 D of vergence is incident upon a surface whose power is -10.00 D, resulting in an image vergence of -13.03 D. Or, stated another way,

$$L' = L + F$$

$$L' = -3.03 \text{ D} + (-10.00 \text{ D}) = -13.03 \text{ D}$$

The object vergence and surface power are given above the surface in Figure 3-6, and the image vergence is below. Because the vergence is negative, the image must be virtual (and erect). The refracted image rays exist in glass; therefore, to determine the image distance, we use the index of refraction of crown glass (the secondary medium):

$$L' = \frac{n'}{l'}$$

or

$$l' = \frac{n'}{L'}$$

$$l' = \frac{(100)(1.52)}{-13.03 \text{ D}} = -11.67 \text{ cm}$$

The image is located 11.67 cm to the left of the surface.

The magnification produced by the surface is given by the ratio of the object vergence to the image vergence:

$$M_{\text{L}} = \frac{L}{L'}$$

$$M_{\text{L}} = \frac{-3.03 \text{ D}}{-13.03 \text{ D}} = +0.23\times$$

The positive magnification confirms what we should have known all along—the image is erect. Since the magnification is less than one, the image is minified. Its size is

$$(+0.23)(+15.00 \text{ cm}) = +3.45 \text{ cm}$$

Sample Problem 3: Locating the Object

A virtual image is located 12.00 cm to the left of a 5.00 D crown glass diverging spherical surface situated in air. The image is 4.00 cm in height. Locate the object and give its height.

First, draw a diagram that shows a diverging surface forming a virtual image (Fig. 3-7). The figure helps us to understand that the diverging rays forming the virtual image exist in glass. Since the image is to the left of the surface, its distance is designated with a minus sign. Thus, the image vergence is

$$L' = \frac{n'}{l'}$$

$$L' = \frac{(100)(1.52)}{-12.00 \text{ cm}} = -12.67 \text{ D}$$

The object vergence is given by the vergence relationship as follows:

$$L' = L + F$$

$$-12.67 \text{ D} = L + (-5.00 \text{ D})$$

$$L = -7.67 \text{ D}$$

The light rays that emerge from the *object* have a vergence of −7.67 D. From Figure 3-7, we see that these light rays exist in air (n = 1.00). The object distance is therefore

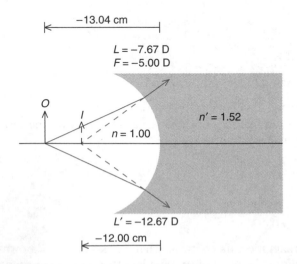

Figure 3-7. Given the location of the image, the vergence relationship can be used to locate the object.

$$L = \frac{n}{l}$$

$$l = \frac{n}{l}$$

$$l = \frac{(100)(1.00)}{-7.67 \text{ D}} = -13.04 \text{ cm}$$

The object is on the same side of the surface as the image (both are to the left of the surface) but further from the surface than the image. This shouldn't be surprising—by examining Figure 3-7, you can see that the diverging rays emitted by the object are further diverged by the negative surface to form a virtual image that is closer to the surface.

The lateral magnification is

$$M_L = \frac{L}{L'}$$

$$M_L = \frac{-7.67 \text{ D}}{-12.67 \text{ D}} = +0.61\times$$

The object and image have the same orientation, and the image is smaller. The object size is calculated as follows:

$$+4.00 \text{ cm} = (+0.61)(\text{object height})$$

$$\text{object height} = +6.56 \text{ cm}$$

Sample Problem 4: A Flat (Plane) Refracting Surface

A quarter is located at the bottom of an aquarium 38.00 cm from the surface of the water. In looking down into the aquarium, how far does the quarter appear to be from the surface? Is it magnified or minified?

If we draw the diagram correctly, as in Figure 3-8, we see that light travels upward. This is a problem for our linear sign convention, which assumes that light travels from left to right. There are two ways to get around this and solve the problem. One solution is to *not* use the linear sign convention and to rely on our understanding of vergence. The second solution is to turn the aquarium on its side, pretend that light is traveling from left to right, and then use our linear sign convention. I'll show you how to use both approaches, and you can decide which works better for you.

First, let's look at the vergence approach. As can be seen in Figure 3-8, the light rays coming from the quarter travel in water (the primary medium) and are refracted at the water–air interface. By drawing normals to the surface and applying Snell's law, we can see that the rays are refracted away from the normals—they diverge. These

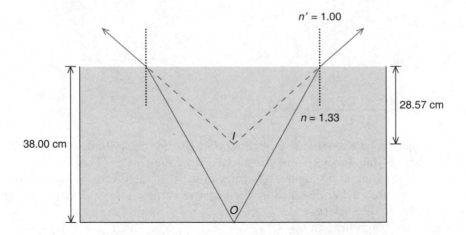

$n' = 1.00$

$n = 1.33$

28.57 cm

38.00 cm

Figure 3-8. An object located at the bottom of an aquarium appears closer to the surface than it actually is. Looking into the aquarium from above, the viewer sees a virtual image of the coin. The surface refracts light even though it has a dioptric power of zero. The vertical dotted lines are normal to the surface.

diverging rays, which exist in air (the secondary medium), appear to come from a virtual image that is closer to the surface than to the true location of the quarter.

If we can determine the object vergence and surface's dioptric power, we'll be able to use the vergence formula to determine the location of the virtual image. Since we won't be using our linear sign convention, we need to calculate the absolute value of the object vergence. Keeping in mind that (1) the object "lives" in water and (2) its vergence must be labeled with a minus sign since the rays are diverging, we have

$$L = \left| \frac{n}{l} \right|$$

$$L = \left| \frac{1.33}{0.38 \text{ m}} \right|$$

$$L = -3.50 \text{ D}$$

What is the power of the surface? Since it is flat and has an infinite radius of curvature, it has zero dioptric power.[7] Applying the vergence relationship, we have

$$L' = L + F$$

$$L' = -3.50 \text{ D} + 0.00 \text{ D}$$

$$L' = -3.50 \text{ D}$$

---

7. Although the flat surface refracts light, it has zero dioptric power. Only spherical refracting surfaces, which change the vergence of incident light, have dioptric power. Another way to think about this is that a surface with dioptric power has a finite radius of curvature (not an infinite radius of curvature as does a flat surface).

The negative image vergence confirms that the image is virtual. It is formed by diverging rays that exist in air, and its distance is calculated as follows:

$$L' = \left| \frac{n'}{l'} \right|$$

or

$$l' = \left| \frac{n'}{L'} \right|$$

$$l' = \left| \frac{1.00}{3.50 \text{ D}} \right|$$

$$l' = 0.2857 \text{ m, or } 28.57 \text{ cm}$$

Since this virtual image is located 28.57 cm below the surface, the quarter *appears* closer to the surface than it really is. The lateral magnification is

$$M_L = \frac{L}{L'}$$

$$M_L = \frac{-3.50 \text{ D}}{-3.50 \text{ D}}$$

$$M_L = +1.00\times$$

The *image* of the quarter is of the same size and orientation as a quarter itself.[8]

The alternative solution to this problem, in which we use linear sign conventions, is illustrated in Figure 3-9. The aquarium is tilted so that it stands on its side. Now, we can assume that light travels from left to right. The only tricky thing is to keep straight which indices should be used to calculate object and image vergences. Since the object "lives" in water, the object vergence is

$$L = \frac{n}{l}$$

$$L = \frac{1.33}{-0.38 \text{ m}}$$

$$L = -3.50 \text{ D}$$

As is the case for other surfaces we discussed in this chapter, the object vergence in Figure 3-9 is given above the surface, as is the surface power of zero. The image vergence, which is given below the surface, is determined with the vergence relationship as follows:

$$L' = L + F$$

$$L' = -3.50 \text{ D} + 0.00 \text{ D}$$

$$L' = -3.50 \text{ D}$$

---

8. Although the image of the quarter is the same size as the quarter, it appears larger because it is closer to the surface. This is referred to as angular magnification (discussed in Chapter 12).

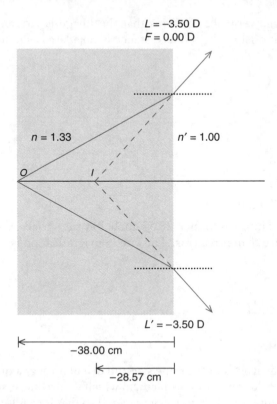

Figure 3-9. By turning the aquarium on its side, we can use our linear sign convention to locate the image. As with other diagrams in this chapter, object vergence and surface power are given above the surface, while image vergence is given below. The horizontal dotted lines are normal to the surface.

The diverging rays that form the virtual image exist in air. Consequently, the image distance is

$$-3.50 \text{ D} = \frac{(100)(1.00)}{l'}$$

$$l' = -28.57 \text{ cm}$$

The minus sign tells us that the image is located 28.57 cm to the left of the surface.

SUMMARY

A refractive surface changes the vergence of light incident upon it. This changed vergence can be determined with the vergence relationship, which states that the sum of object vergence and surface power is equal to image vergence. By knowing the image vergence and the refractive index of the medium in which the image rays exist, we can calculate the image distance. Magnification is given by the ratio of the object vergence to the image vergence.

KEY FORMULAE

Vergence relationship:

$L' = L + F$

Relationship between object distance and object vergence:

$L = \dfrac{n}{l}$

Relationship between image distance and image vergence:

$L' = \dfrac{n'}{l'}$

Lateral magnification produced by a spherical surface (or lens):

$M_L = \dfrac{L}{L'}$

SELF-ASSESSMENT PROBLEMS

1. A polycarbonate spherical surface has a power of −10.00 D. (a) What is the surface's radius of curvature? (b) What is the secondary focal length?

2. A plastic spherical surface has a power of +20.00 D. (a) What is the surface's radius of curvature? (b) What is the *primary* focal length?

3. A crown glass spherical surface has a radius of curvature of +15.00 cm. (a) What is the dioptric power of the surface? (b) What is the secondary focal length?

4. A polycarbonate spherical surface has a radius of curvature of −125.00 mm. What is the dioptric power of the surface?

5. An object 6.00 mm in height is located 20.00 cm from a crown glass spherical surface whose power is −10.00 D. (a) Using the vergence relationship, locate the image and determine its size. (b) Is the image real or virtual? (c) Is the image erect or inverted?

6. An object 10.00 mm in height is located 20.00 cm from a crown glass spherical surface whose power is +10.00 D. (a) Using the vergence relationship, locate the image and determine its size. (b) Is the image real or virtual? (c) Is the image erect or inverted?

7. Answer the questions in Problem 6 if the object is located 5.00 cm from the surface.

8. A virtual image is located 5.00 cm from a +15.00 D crown glass spherical surface. How far is the object from the surface?

9. A real image is located 20.00 cm from a +15.00 D crown glass spherical surface. How far is the object from the surface?

10. A rock sits on the bottom of a pond of water that is 3.00 m deep. How far does the rock appear to be from the surface of the pond?

11. The pupil is located 3.60 mm from the cornea. Assume that the cornea is a surface with a radius of curvature of 7.80 mm that separates air and aqueous humor, which has an index of refraction of 1.333. How far does the pupil appear to be from the cornea?

12. If the diameter of the pupil in Problem 11 is 4.00 mm, what does the diameter appear to be?

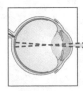

4

Thin Lenses

A lens is made up of two surfaces, both of which are often, but not always, spherical.[1] The back surface of an **ophthalmic lens**—the term we use to designate lenses used in clinical practice—is sometimes referred to as the ocular surface. Common lens forms are given in Figure 4-1. Most ophthalmic lenses have a meniscus shape, which tends to minimize aberrations that can reduce vision.

As illustrated in Figure 4-2, each surface may contribute to the lens's total dioptric power. The thickness of the lens also contributes to its power, but in many ophthalmic applications we can ignore lens thickness because its contribution to lens power is very small. When we ignore the effect of thickness, we call the simplified lens a **thin lens**. (Chapters 5 and 6 provide a detailed discussion of lens thickness.)

Since we are ignoring thickness, the power of a thin lens is simply the sum of the powers of the front and back (ocular) surfaces. We refer to this as the lens's **nominal or approximate power**. Expressed as an equation, we have

$$F_T = F_1 + F_2$$

where F_T is the nominal (or approximate) power, F_1 is the power of the front surface, and F_2 is the power of the back (ocular) surface.

As illustrated in Figure 4-3, thin lenses are represented as vertical lines. Figures 4-4 and 4-5 show that the secondary (F') and primary (F) focal points are located in the same manner as for a spherical refracting surface (Chapter 2). When parallel light rays travel from left to right, the secondary focal point is (1) the point to which the light rays converge for a plus lens or (2) the point from which they appear to originate for a minus lens (Fig. 4-4). The primary focal point is located by reversing the

---

1. Certain ophthalmic lenses have aspheric surfaces that are intended to reduce aberrations, and in the case of plus lenses, to also decrease center thickness.

Plus lenses

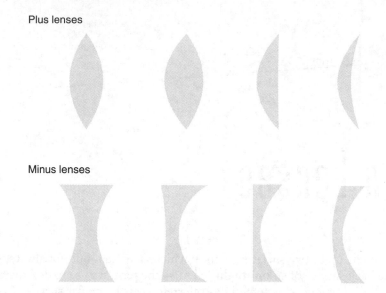

Minus lenses

Figure 4-1. Common lens forms. The plus lenses (from left to right) are equiconvex, biconvex, plano-convex, and plus meniscus. The minus lenses (from left to right) are equiconcave, biconcave, plano-concave, and minus meniscus. Meniscus lenses have a positive front-surface and a minus back-surface power. In a plus meniscus lens, the front surface is stronger, while in a minus meniscus, the back surface is stronger.

direction of light so that the parallel rays travel from right to left (Fig. 4-5). **When the medium on both sides of a thin lens is the same, which is almost always the case in clinical applications, the primary and secondary focal points are equidistant from the lens.**

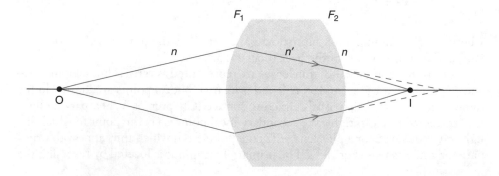

Figure 4-2. A lens is formed by two spherical surfaces. Refraction occurs at each of the two surfaces. If treated as a thin lens, the total power (F_T) is the sum of the powers of the front surface (F_1) and back surface (F_2) of the lens.

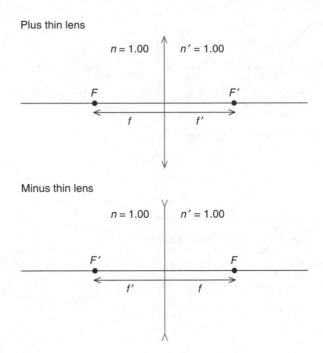

Figure 4-3. Schematic representations of a thin plus lens (top) and a thin minus lens. The front and back surfaces are collapsed to a single plane—a vertical line—where all refraction is assumed to occur. When the medium on both sides of a lens is the same (as for these lenses, which are in air) the secondary and primary focal lengths are equal.

RAY TRACING

The same principles that we learned for ray tracing with spherical surfaces apply to thin lenses. The following three key rays, which each emanate from the object, can be used to locate the image and determine its size (and magnification):

- Ray 1 passes undeviated through the lens's optical center (which is the intersection of the lens and its optical axis).
- Ray 2 travels parallel to the optical axis and after refraction passes through the lens's secondary focal point (plus lens) or appears to emerge from the secondary focal point (minus lens).
- Ray 3 passes through (plus lens) or is headed toward (minus lens) the primary focal point and after refraction is parallel to the optical axis.

Figures 4-6 through 4-9 show how these rays can be used to locate the images formed by converging and diverging lenses.

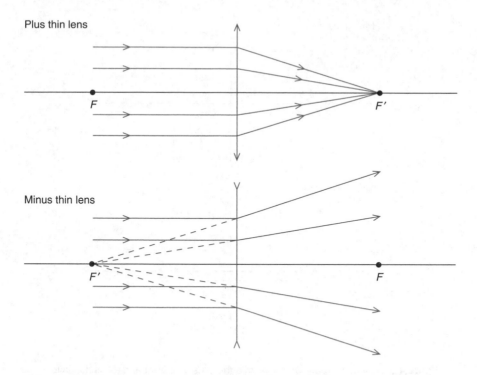

Plus thin lens

Minus thin lens

Figure 4-4. Determination of the secondary focal points for a plus and minus lens.

A converging lens may form either a real or virtual image. When the object is located farther from the lens than its focal point, as in Figure 4-6, the image is always located on the other side of the lens, real and inverted. It is real because the rays are converging after refraction. Is this image smaller or larger than the object? As can be seen in Figure 4-7, the magnification depends on the object distance. When the object is at twice the focal length, the real image is the same size as the object (and also twice the focal length from the lens), but when the object is farther than this distance, the image is minified (and located farther than the focal length, but less than twice the focal length from the lens). In comparison, if the object is located closer than twice the focal length (but farther than the focal length), the image is larger than the object (and located farther than twice the focal length from the lens).

As illustrated in Figure 4-8, the situation is very different when the object is located *closer* than the focal point of a plus lens. **In this case, the rays remain divergent after refraction necessarily making the image virtual, enlarged, and erect. It is located on the same side of the lens as the object and farther than the focal length from the lens.** The image is larger than the object because the rays that form the image are diverging less than those that emerge from the object. (You may need to think about this a bit!)

Plus thin lens

Minus thin lens

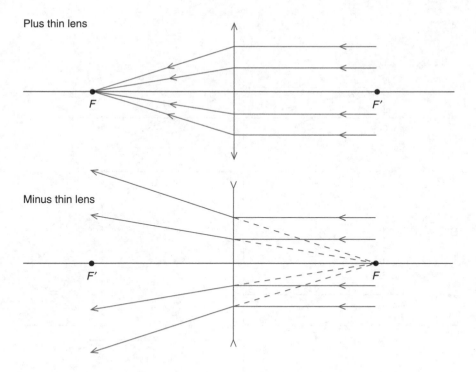

Figure 4-5. The primary focal points for a plus and a minus lens are determined by reversing the direction of light.

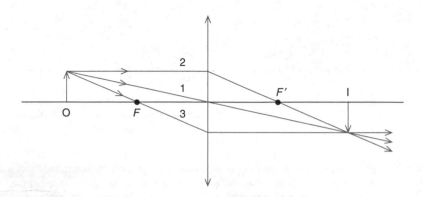

Figure 4-6. Ray tracing can be used to locate the image formed by a lens. In this case, the object is farther from a plus lens than the focal length. Rays 1, 2, and 3 are described in the text.

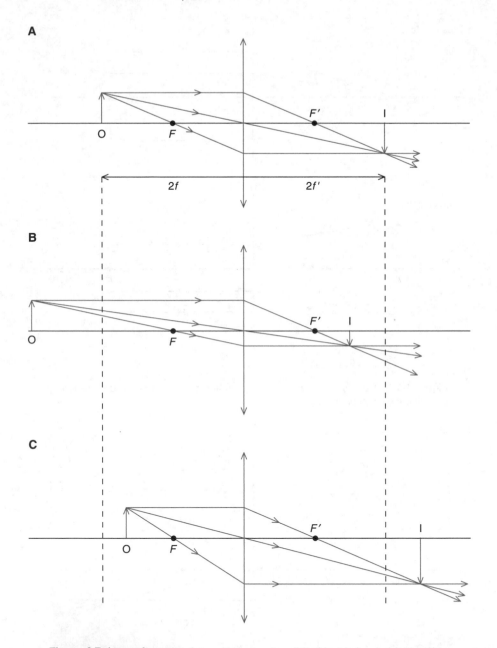

Figure 4-7. Image formation for a plus lens when the object is located farther than the focal length. **A.** When the object is at a distance of 2*f*, the image is located at a distance of 2*f'* and is the same size as the object. **B.** If the object is farther than 2*f* from the lens, the image is minified and located at a distance greater than *f'* but less than 2*f'* from the lens. **C.** Positioning the object at a distance that is less than 2*f*, but greater than *f*, results in an image that is magnified and located at a distance greater than 2*f'* from the lens.

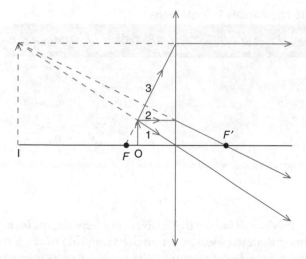

Figure 4-8. When an object is located within the focal length of a plus lens, the image is located on the same side of the lens as the object (and farther from the lens than the object), virtual, enlarged, and erect. Rays 1, 2, and 3 are described in the text.

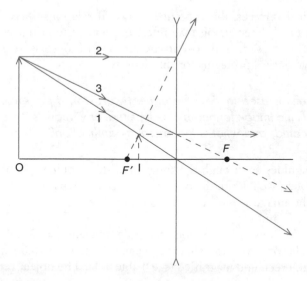

Figure 4-9. A minus lens creates a virtual, minified, and erect image on the same side of the lens as the object (and closer to the lens than the object). Rays 1, 2, and 3 are described in the text.

TABLE 4-1. IMAGE FORMATION BY THIN LENSES

	Object Distance	Image Location*	Image Distance	Nature of Image	Image Orientation	Image Size
Plus lens	2f	Positive	2f'	Real	Inverted	Equal to object
Plus lens	>2f	Positive	>f' but <2f'	Real	Inverted	<Object
Plus lens	>f but <2f	Positive	>2f'	Real	Inverted	>Object
Plus lens	<f	Negative	>l	Virtual	Erect	>Object
Minus lens	Anywhere	Negative	<l	Virtual	Erect	<Object

*A positive location means the image is to the right of the lens and a negative location means it is to the left.

By examining Figure 4-9, we see that **a diverging lens always forms a virtual and erect image closer than the focal point on the same side of the lens as the object because the light rays become more divergent after refraction. The image formed by these more divergent rays is necessarily closer to the lens than the object and smaller.** Image formation by thin lenses is summarized in Table 4-1.

VERGENCE RELATIONSHIP

As with spherical surfaces, the vergence (paraxial) relationship is convenient for locating images and determining magnification. Since the primary and secondary media are usually the same—almost always air ($n = 1.00$)—it is generally straightforward to solve optical problems for thin lenses.

A +10.00 D lens is used to view the printed words on a page located 9.00 cm from the lens. Is the image formed by the lens real or virtual? Is it erect or inverted? Where is it located, and what is the lateral magnification?

Figure 4-10 guides us through the solution of this problem. Similar to spherical refracting surfaces, we'll write the object vergence and lens power at the top of the diagram and the image vergence at the bottom. We won't, however, continue to label these as L, F, and L'.

The object is located within the focal length of the lens ($f = -10.00$ cm), so before doing any calculations, we know that the image is more than 10.00 cm to the left of the lens, virtual, erect, and magnified (see Table 4-1). The object vergence is

$$L = \frac{n}{l}$$

$$L = \frac{(100)(1.00)}{-9.00 \text{ cm}}$$

$$L = -11.11 \text{ D}$$

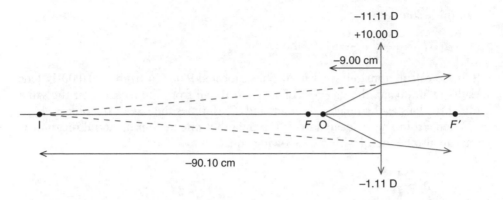

Figure 4-10. The vergence relationship can be used to locate the image formed by a thin lens. At the top of the lens are the object vergence (L) and lens power (F_T), respectively. Below the lens is the image vergence (L'). Since the object is within the focal length, the converging lens forms a virtual image.

The paraxial relationship gives us

$$L' = L + F$$

$$L' = -11.11 \text{ D} + 10.00 \text{ D}$$

$$L' = -1.11 \text{ D}$$

The negative image vergence tells us that although the light rays' divergence is diminished subsequent to their refraction by the plus lens, they continue to diverge, thereby forming a virtual image.[2] Since the lens is surrounded by air ($n = n' = 1.00$), the image distance is

$$L' = \frac{n'}{l'}$$

$$l' = \frac{(100)(1.00)}{-1.11 \text{ D}}$$

$$l' = -90.10 \text{ cm}$$

The virtual image is located 90.10 cm to the left of the thin lens.

As with a spherical surface, the lateral magnification is given by

$$M_L = \frac{L}{L'}$$

---

2. As we learned in Chapter 3, an image formed by rays with negative vergence (i.e., diverging rays) is always virtual, and an image formed by rays with positive vergence (converging rays) is always real.

In this example,

$$M_L = \frac{-11.11\ D}{-1.11\ D} = +10.00\times$$

These calculations tell us that an object located 9.00 cm from a +10.00 D lens results in an image, that is (1) virtual, (2) 90.10 cm from the lens, (3) on the same side of the lens as the object, (4) erect, and (5) 10 times the size of the object.

When a thin lens is located in air (or any other one medium), lateral magnification can also be found with the following equation:

$$\boldsymbol{M_L = \frac{l'}{l}}$$

It bears repeating that this relationship is valid only when the medium is the same on both sides of a thin lens.

A 7.00 mm high object is located 8.00 cm from a +15.00 D lens. Is the image real or virtual? Is it erect or inverted? Where is it located, and what is its size?

A +15.00 D lens has a focal length of 6.67 cm, so the object is located at a distance greater than f, but less than $2f$, from this converging lens. This tells us that the image is located more than twice the focal length to the right of the lens, real, inverted, and larger than the object (Table 4-1).

Figure 14-11 illustrates this problem. First, we calculate the object vergence

$$L = \frac{n}{l}$$

$$L = \frac{(100)(1.00)}{-8.00\ cm}$$

$$L = -12.50\ D$$

To determine the image vergence, we used the vergence relationship

$$L' = L + F$$

$$L' = -12.50\ D + 15.00\ D$$

$$L' = +2.50\ D$$

Since the vergence is positive, we know that the image is located to the right of the lens, real, and inverted. Its location is

$$L' = \frac{n'}{l'}$$

$$l' = \frac{(100)(1.00)}{(+2.50\ D)}$$

$$l' = +40.00\ cm$$

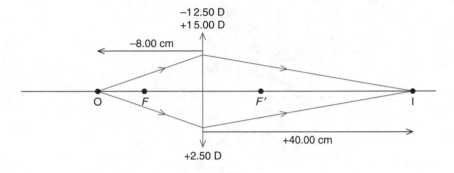

Figure 4-11. Formation of a real image by a converging lens.

The magnification is

$$M = \frac{l'}{l}$$

$$M = \frac{40.00 \text{ cm}}{-8.00 \text{ cm}}$$

$$M = -5.00\times$$

The object height is 7.00 mm, making the image height

$$(-5.00)(7.00 \text{ mm}) = -35.00 \text{ mm}$$

The minus sign reminds us that the magnified image is inverted.

Before moving on, let's try one more example. A 5 mm high object is located 10.00 cm from a –5.00 D lens. Is the image real or virtual? Is it erect or inverted? Where is it located, and what is its size?

Because the lens is diverging, we know that the image is located on the same side of the lens as the object, closer to the lens than the object, virtual, erect, and mini-fied (Table 4-1). The solution is diagramed in Figure 14-12. First, we determine the object vergence

$$L = \frac{n}{l}$$

$$L = \frac{(100)(1.00)}{-10.00 \text{ cm}}$$

$$L = -10.00 \text{ D}$$

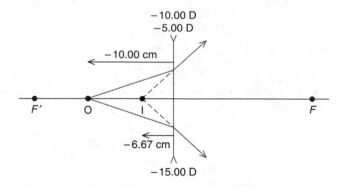

Figure 4-12. Formation of a virtual image by a diverging lens.

Substituting into the vergence relationship, we have

$$L' = L + F$$

$$L' = -10.00 \text{ D} + (-5.00 \text{ D})$$

$$L' = -15.00 \text{ D}$$

Since the image vergence is negative, we know that the image is located to the left of the lens, virtual, and erect. Its location is

$$L' = \frac{n'}{l'}$$

$$l' = \frac{(100)(1.00)}{-15.00 \text{ D}}$$

$$l' = -6.67 \text{ cm}$$

The magnification is

$$M = \frac{l'}{l}$$

$$M = \frac{-6.67 \text{ cm}}{-10.00 \text{ cm}}$$

$$M = +0.67\times$$

The object height is 5.00 mm, making the image height

$$(+0.67)(5.00 \text{ mm}) = +3.35 \text{ mm}$$

This confirms that the virtual image is minified and erect.

NEWTON'S RELATION

As we have learned, when a thin lens is located in air (or any other single medium), the primary and secondary focal lengths are equidistant from the lens. This is the basis for Newton's relation, which can be used to locate the object and image with respect to the focal points of a plus lens. Other than its application in the lensometer, the device used to determine the back vertex power (defined in Chapter 6) of a patient's corrective lenses, this relation isn't used much, but it is generally included in courses on geometrical optics, so you should know about it. In Figure 4-13, an object is located at the distance x from the primary focal point of a plus thin lens and the image is located at a distance x' from the secondary focal point. Newton's relation tells us that

$$\mathbf{xx' = f^2}$$

In this book, we'll designate the distances x and x'—sometimes referred to as **extra-focal distances**—as positive.

Let's take an example. An object located 10.00 cm to the left of the primary focal point of a lens results in an image that is 40.00 cm to the right of the secondary focal point. What is the power of the lens? Assume the lens is in air.

Using Newton's relationship, we find that

$$xx' = f^2$$
$$(+10.00\ \text{cm})(+40.00\ \text{cm}) = f^2$$
$$f = +20.00\ \text{cm}$$

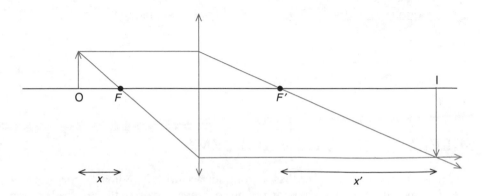

Figure 4-13. The extrafocal distances, x and x', are designated as positive when substituting into Newton's relation.

Since the lens is in air, its power is simply the reciprocal of the focal length:

$$F = \frac{n}{f}$$

$$F = \frac{1.00}{+0.20 \text{ m}}$$

$$F = +5.00 \text{ D}$$

SUMMARY

In reality, the thickness of a lens always contributes to its power, but for clinical applications, it is sometimes acceptable to treat a lens as if its thickness is insignificant. The power for such a lens, which is called a thin lens, is simply the sum of its front and back surface powers.

A plus lens forms a real image when the object distance is greater than the focal length and a virtual image when the object is located closer than the focal length. Minus lenses always produce a minified virtual image.

The vergence relationship is useful for locating the images formed by thin lenses. Object and image distances are measured from the plane of the lens. If the lens is located in air, the primary and secondary media have a refractive index of 1.00.

KEY FORMULAE

Nominal (approximate) power of a thin lens:

$F_T = F_1 + F_2$

Lateral magnification produced by a surface or lens:

$M_L = \dfrac{L}{L'}$

Lateral magnification for a thin lens when there is one medium:

$M_L = \dfrac{l'}{l}$

Newton's relation for extrafocal distances

$xx' = f^2$

SELF-ASSESSMENT PROBLEMS

1. A lens made of crown glass has a front surface with a radius of curvature of +8.00 cm and a back surface with a radius of curvature of –6.00 cm. (a) Treating this lens as a thin lens, what is its power? (b) Calculate the secondary and primary focal lengths. (c) What is the lens form?

2. An object that is 13.00 mm in height is located 15.00 cm from a +20.00 D lens. (a) Using the vergence relationship, locate the image and determine its size. (b) Is the image real or virtual? (c) Is the image erect or inverted?

3. An object that is 30.00 mm in height is located 5.00 cm from a +10.00 D lens. Answer the questions in Problem 2.

4. An object that is 30.00 mm in height is located 10.00 cm from a −30.00 D lens. Answer the questions in Problem 2.

5. A real image is located 50.00 cm from a +25.00 D lens. Locate the object.

6. A virtual image is located 50.00 cm from a +25.00 D lens. Locate the object.

7. A virtual image is located 10.00 cm from a −5.00 D lens. Locate the object.

8. A object that is located 25.00 cm from the primary focal point of a plus lens results in a real image that is 40.00 cm from the secondary focal point. What is the power of the lens?

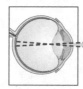

Optical Systems with Multiple Surfaces

Up to now, we have worked with optical systems where refraction occurs (or can be considered to occur) at a single surface. Many optical systems, however, consist of more than one refracting surface. The two thin lenses at the top of Figure 5-1 and the thick lens at the bottom are both examples of optical systems with multiple refracting surfaces.

This chapter brings together many of the concepts in the previous four chapters, and the examples that we work through will help you to firm up what you have learned. Spending time on these examples will be a good investment of your time!

MULTIPLE THIN LENS SYSTEMS

The simplest multiple-surface optical system is a series of thin lenses that are assumed to have no significant separation between them, as illustrated in Figure 5-2. The total power of such a system is the sum of the power of the various lenses.

In actuality, of course, there may be a physical gap between thin lenses; this separation can have a substantial effect on the refractive properties of the lens system.

Let's consider an example. *A −5.00 D thin lens is positioned 2.00 cm to the left of a +15.00 D thin lens. An object is located 15.00 cm to the left of the −5.00 D lens. Locate the image with respect to the +15.00 D lens. If the object is 7.00 mm in height, what is the image's size? Is the image real or virtual? Is it erect or inverted? (Assume that the optical system is in air.)*

With this type of problem, it is more important than ever to draw a diagram (Fig. 5-3). We approach the optical system lens by lens, one thin lens at a time,

A

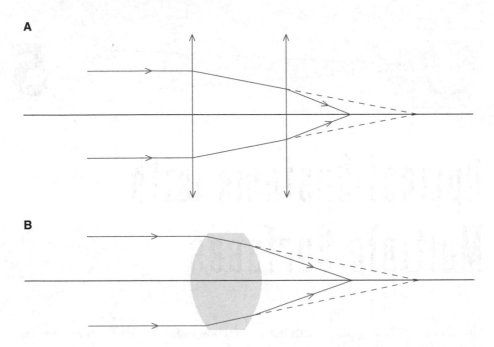

B

Figure 5-1. A. A series of thin lenses is an example of an optical system with multiple refracting surfaces. **B.** A thick lens is another example.

writing the object vergence and power above each lens and the image vergence below it. The first surface is the −5.00 D thin lens. To locate the image produced by this thin lens, we use the vergence relationship. First, we determine the object vergence[1]:

$$L = \frac{n}{l}$$

$$L = \frac{(100)(1.00)}{-15.00 \text{ cm}} = -6.67 \text{ D}$$

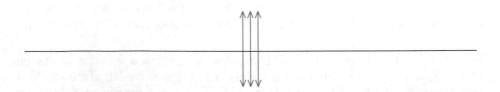

Figure 5-2. When there is no significant distance between thin lenses, the total power is the sum of powers of the individual thin lenses.

---

1. As in previous chapters, when the distances are given in centimeters, a factor of 100 is placed in the numerator of the object and image vergence equations. Alternatively, we could convert the distances to meters.

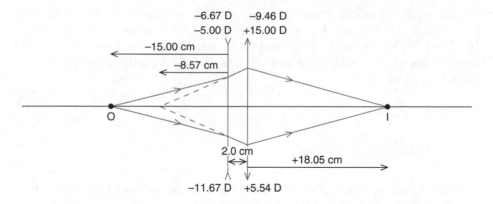

Figure 5-3. This optical system, which consists of a thin minus lens followed by a thin plus lens, forms a real image. The object vergence and lens power are given, respectively, at the top of each thin lens and the image vergence at the bottom of each thin lens.

Substituting into the vergence relationship, we have

$$L' = L + F$$

$$L' = -6.67 \text{ D} + (-5.00 \text{ D})$$

$$L' = -11.67 \text{ D}$$

The negative vergence tells us that the image is virtual and must be located to the left of the first lens. The image distance is

$$L' = \frac{n'}{l'}$$

$$l' = \frac{n'}{L'}$$

$$l' = \frac{(100)(1.00)}{-11.67 \text{ D}} = -8.57 \text{ cm}$$

What is the lateral magnification produced by the first lens?[2]

$$M_\text{L} = \frac{L}{L'}$$

$$M_\text{L} = \frac{-6.67 \text{ D}}{-11.67 \text{ D}} = +0.57\times$$

Therefore, the image size is

$$(+0.57)(7.00 \text{ mm}) = +3.99 \text{ mm}$$

---

2. Since we are working with a thin lens in air, we could also determine the lateral magnification using the following formula: $M_\text{L} = \frac{l'}{l}$.

This erect and minified virtual image serves as an object for the second lens (i.e., the +15.00 D lens). Light rays diverge from this image, which is located 10.57 cm (8.57 + 2.00 cm = 10.57 cm) to the left of the second lens. (You should confirm this by examining the diagram.) At the second lens, these rays produce an *object vergence* of

$$L = \frac{n}{l}$$

$$L = \frac{(100)(1.00)}{-10.57 \text{ cm}} = -9.46 \text{ D}$$

This vergence is written above the second lens. To locate the image produced by this lens, we use the vergence relationship as follows:

$$L' = L + F$$

$$L' = -9.46 \text{ D} + (+15.00 \text{ D}) = +5.54 \text{ D}$$

This value is written below the second lens.

Since the rays that emerge from the lens are converging—they have positive vergence–the image is real. How far is it from the second lens?

$$L' = \frac{n'}{l'}$$

$$l' = \frac{n'}{L'}$$

$$l' = \frac{(100)(1.00)}{+5.54} = +18.05 \text{ cm}$$

The final image is located 18.05 cm to the right of the +15.00 D lens.

The lateral magnification produced by the second lens is

$$M_L = \frac{L}{L'}$$

$$M_L = \frac{-9.46 \text{ D}}{+5.54 \text{ D}} = -1.71\times$$

Since the object for this lens (i.e., the image formed by the first lens) is +3.99 mm in height, the final image's height is

$$(-1.71)(+3.99 \text{ mm}) = -6.8 \text{ mm}$$

The (real) image produced by this optical system is inverted and minified relative to the initial object (which is 7.00 mm in height).

Another way to determine the final image size is to calculate the lateral magnification for the system as a whole and multiply this total magnification times the initial object size. The lateral magnification for the system is the product of the two lenses' magnifications:

Total lateral magnification = (M_L for first lens)(M_L for second lens)

Total lateral magnification = (+0.57) (−1.71) = −0.97×

Therefore, the final image size is

(−0.97)(7.00 mm) = −6.8 mm

This is the same image size we calculated previously.

Let's consider another example. *An object is located 33.33 cm to the left of a +10.00 D thin lens that is located 50.00 cm to the left of a −2.00 D thin lens. Locate the image, and calculate the magnification.*

We won't go through all the calculations, but you should confirm that they are correct. Viewing Figure 5-4, we see that an object vergence of −3.00 D is incident upon the first lens, resulting in an image vergence of +7.00 D. (The image vergence is obtained by adding together the object vergence and lens power.) The image is real (therefore inverted) and located 14.29 cm to the right of the first lens or 35.71 cm in front of the second lens.

The real image formed by the first lens serves as an object for the second lens. This object emits diverging light rays that are incident upon the second lens with an object vergence of −2.80 D. The image vergence of the rays leaving the second lens is −4.80 D. The image formed by this lens, which is virtual, is located 20.83 cm to its left.

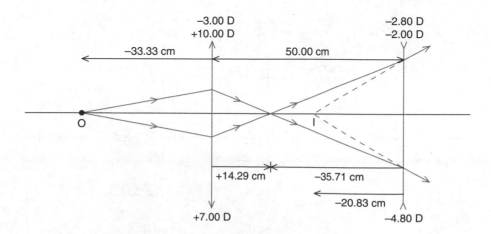

Figure 5-4. The real image formed by the plus lens serves as an object for the minus lens. A virtual image is formed by this optical system.

The total image magnification is

$$\text{Total lateral magnification} = (M_L \text{ for first lens})(M_L \text{ for second lens})$$

$$\text{Total lateral magnification} = \left(\frac{-3.00 \text{ D}}{+7.00 \text{ D}}\right)\left(\frac{-2.80 \text{ D}}{-4.80 \text{ D}}\right) = -0.25\times$$

This tells us that the final image is inverted (indicated by the minus sign) and minified (the magnification is less than 1.00). Think of it this way: the real inverted image produced by the first lens is not inverted again by the second lens (which is minus).

VIRTUAL OBJECTS

A surefire way to elicit sighs of exasperation from clinicians is to mention virtual objects. Although the term may sound complicated, it isn't all that bad. The best way to understand virtual objects is to solve a problem.

Figure 5-5 shows a two-lens optical system consisting of a +4.00 D thin lens followed by a –2.00 D thin lens. The lenses are separated by 28.00 cm. An object 10.00 mm in height is located 66.67 cm to the left of the first lens. Locate the final image, calculate its size, and determine if it is real or virtual and erect or inverted.

The object vergence at the first thin lens is

$$L = \frac{n}{l}$$

$$L = \frac{(100)(1.00)}{-66.67 \text{ cm}} = -1.50 \text{ D}$$

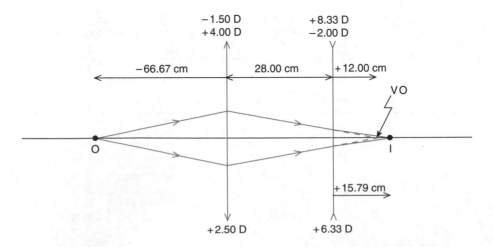

Figure 5-5. The image formed by the first lens serves as a virtual object (VO) for the second lens.

The image vergence for the first lens is calculated as

$$L' = L + F$$

$$L' = -1.50 \text{ D} + (+4.00 \text{ D}) = +2.50 \text{ D}$$

Therefore, the image location is

$$L' = \frac{n'}{l'}$$

$$l' = \frac{n'}{L'}$$

$$l' = \frac{(100)(1.00)}{+2.50 \text{ D}} = +40.00 \text{ cm}$$

This real (therefore, inverted) image *would* be located 40.00 cm to the right of the first lens. The image is not actually formed, however, because the rays that would form it pass through the second lens and are refracted. The image that *would* have been formed 12.00 cm to the right of the second lens (40.00 − 28.00 cm = 12.00 cm) is considered a virtual object for the second lens. You can think of a **virtual object** as the real image that would have been formed by the first lens *if* the second lens did not get in the way. A virtual object always has positive vergence and can be formed only by a converging surface or lens.

What is the *object* vergence that is incident on the second lens? Since the rays would have been focused 12.00 cm to the right of the second lens, the object vergence at the second lens is

$$L = \frac{n}{l}$$

$$L = \frac{(100)(1.00)}{+12.00 \text{ cm}} = +8.33 \text{ D}$$

The *image* vergence produced by the second lens is

$$L' = L + F$$

$$L' = 8.33 \text{ D} + (-2.00 \text{ D}) = +6.33 \text{ D}$$

Since the vergence is positive, the final image is real and to the right of the second lens. Its distance from the lens is

$$L' = \frac{n'}{l'}$$

$$l' = \frac{n'}{L'}$$

$$l' = \frac{(100)(1.00)}{+6.33 \text{ D}} = +15.79 \text{ cm}$$

To determine the size of the final image, we'll first calculate the total lateral magnification as follows:

$$\text{Total lateral magnification} = \left(\frac{-1.50\ \text{D}}{+2.50\ \text{D}}\right)\left(\frac{+8.33\ \text{D}}{+6.33\ \text{D}}\right) = -0.79\times$$

Therefore, the final image height is

$$(-0.79)(10.00\ \text{mm}) = -7.90\ \text{mm}$$

The minus sign tells us that *relative to the original object*, the final image is inverted.

THICK LENSES

The multiple-surface optical systems that we have considered thus far consist of multiple thin lenses. A lens, as illustrated in Figure 5-6, also has multiple surfaces—it has a front and back (sometimes called ocular) surface. As we learned in Chapter 4, it is sometimes acceptable to ignore a lens's thickness and simply add together the surface powers to arrive at what is called the nominal (or approximate) power. When we ignore the refractive effect of the thickness, we refer to the lens as a thin lens.

We could use the nominal power to determine image location, but a more accurate answer can be obtained by taking into account the lens thickness. When we do so, the lens is, unsurprisingly, referred to as a **thick lens**. To locate the image produced by a thick lens, we apply the vergence relationship at each of the surfaces. (In the next chapter, we'll learn an alternative approach to solving thick lens problems.)

Let's look at an example. *An object is located 25.00 cm in front of a biconvex crown glass lens that has a front surface radius of curvature of 10.00 cm and a*

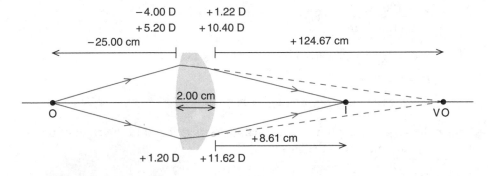

Figure 5-6. The image formed by the first surface of this thick lens serves as a virtual object for the second surface. After refraction by the first surface, the light rays exist in glass; therefore, the image vergence for the first surface and object vergence for the second are calculated using a refractive index of 1.52. The object vergence and surface power are given, respectively, at the top of each surface and the image vergence at the bottom of each surface.

back surface radius of curvature of –5.00 cm (Fig. 5-6). The lens has a thickness of 20.00 mm. Treating the lens as a thick lens, locate the image with respect to the back surface and calculate the magnification produced by the lens. Is the image real or virtual? Is it erect or inverted?

The first step is to calculate the powers of the surfaces. We'll use our linear sign convention keeping in mind that when the center of curvature is to the right of the surface, the radius is positive and when it is to the left of the surface, the radius is negative. For the front surface,

$$F = \frac{n' - n}{r}$$

$$F = \frac{1.52 - 1.00}{+0.10 \text{ m}}$$

$$F = +5.20 \text{ D}$$

And for the back surface,

$$F = \frac{n' - n}{r}$$

$$F = \frac{1.00 - 1.52}{-0.05 \text{ m}}$$

$$F = +10.40 \text{ D}$$

Powers are given above each surface in Figure 5-6. Now we can determine the image location. The object vergence at the first surface is:

$$L = \frac{n}{l}$$

$$L = \frac{(100)(1.00)}{-25.00 \text{ cm}} = -4.00 \text{ D}$$

The image vergence produced by the first surface is

$$L' = L + F$$

$$L' = -4.00 \text{ D} + (+5.20 \text{ D}) = +1.20 \text{ D}$$

The positive vergence tells us that the image is real. Where is it located? **Since the refracted rays exist in glass, we use the index of refraction of glass to locate the image as follows[3]:**

$$L' = \frac{n'}{l'}$$

---

3. Prior to refraction by a surface, light rays are said to exist in **object space**. After refraction by the surface, the rays exist in **image space**. For a thick lens, the image space of the first surface is the object space for the second surface.

$$l' = \frac{n'}{L'}$$

$$l' = \frac{(100)(1.52)}{+1.20 \text{ D}} = +126.67 \text{ cm}$$

If the back surface did not exist, a real image would be located 126.67 cm to the right of the front surface (and situated in glass). However, this image is never formed—it serves as a virtual object for the back surface. What is the object vergence at the back surface? Taking into account the thickness of the lens, we calculate that the virtual object is located 124.67 cm to the right of the back surface (126.67 − 2.00 cm = 124.67 cm). **The rays that form this virtual object exist in glass.** Therefore the object vergence at the back surface is

$$L = \frac{n}{l}$$

$$L = \frac{(100)(1.52)}{+124.67 \text{ cm}} = +1.22 \text{ D}$$

The vergence relationship is used to calculate the image vergence produced by the back surface:

$$L' = L + F$$

$$L' = +1.22 \text{ D} + (+10.40 \text{ D}) = +11.62 \text{ D}$$

Since the rays are converging, the image is real. Where is it located? **The light rays that form the image live (i.e., exist) in air; therefore, we use the index of refraction of air to locate the image:**

$$L' = \frac{n'}{l'}$$

$$l' = \frac{n'}{L'}$$

$$l' = \frac{(100)(1.00)}{+11.62 \text{ D}} = +8.61 \text{ cm}$$

The final image is located 8.61 cm to the right of the second surface.

The total lateral magnification of the thick lens is calculated by multiplying the lateral magnification produced by the first surface by the lateral magnification produced by the second surface:

Total lateral magnification = (M_L for first surface)(M_L for second surface)

$$\text{Total lateral magnification} = \left(\frac{-4.00 \text{ D}}{+1.20 \text{ D}}\right)\left(\frac{+1.22 \text{ D}}{+11.62 \text{ D}}\right) = -0.35\times$$

The final image is inverted and minified.

In summary, after refraction by the positive first surface of the thick lens, the light rays converge. These rays, which exist in glass, are incident on the lens's positive back surface, which converges them even more.

Before we finish this chapter, let's look at one more thick-lens example. A 3.00 cm thick polycarbonate lens has front and back surface powers of +2.00 and −10.00 D, respectively. An object, 15.00 mm in height, is located 20.00 cm from the lens front surface. Locate the image and give its size. Is the image real or virtual? Is it erect or inverted?

The solution to this problem is illustrated in Figure 5-7. The object vergence at the first surface is:

$$L = \frac{n}{l}$$

$$L = \frac{(100)(1.00)}{-20.00 \text{ cm}} = -5.00 \text{ D}$$

The image vergence produced by the first surface is

$$L' = L + F$$

$$L' = -5.00 \text{ D} + 2.00 \text{ D} = -3.00 \text{ D}$$

The negative vergence tells us that the image is virtual and located to the left of the surface. How far is it from the surface? **Since the refracted rays exist in**

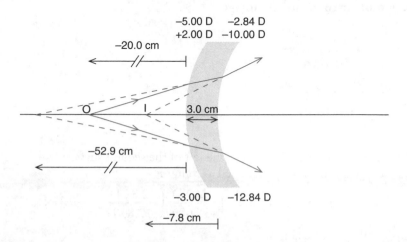

Figure 5-7. The front surface of this thick lens forms a virtual image that serves as an object for the minus back surface, which further diverges the light rays, forming a virtual image.

polycarbonate, we use the index of refraction of polycarbonate to locate the image as follows:

$$L' = \frac{n'}{l'}$$

$$l' = \frac{n'}{L'}$$

$$l' = \frac{(100)(\mathbf{1.586})}{-3.00 \text{ D}} = -52.87 \text{ cm}$$

Because the image is 52.87 cm to the left of the first surface, it must be 55.87 cm to the left of the second surface (52.87 + 3.00 cm = 55.87 cm). The rays that form this image exist in polycarbonate. Therefore, the object vergence at the back surface is

$$L = \frac{n}{l}$$

$$L = \frac{(100)(\mathbf{1.586})}{-55.87 \text{ cm}} = -2.84 \text{ D}$$

The vergence relationship is used to calculate the image vergence produced by the back surface:

$$L' = L + F$$

$$L' = -2.84 \text{ D} + (-10.00 \text{ D}) = -12.84 \text{ D}$$

Since the rays are diverging, the image is virtual. Where is it located? **The light rays that form the image live (i.e., exist) in air; therefore, we use the index of refraction of air to locate the image:**

$$L' = \frac{n'}{l'}$$

$$l' = \frac{n'}{L'}$$

$$l' = \frac{(100)(\mathbf{1.00})}{-12.84 \text{ D}} = -7.78 \text{ cm}$$

The final image is located 7.78 cm to the left of the second surface.

The total magnification is calculated as follows:

$$\text{Total lateral magnification} = \left(\frac{-5.00 \text{ D}}{-3.00 \text{ D}}\right)\left(\frac{-2.84 \text{ D}}{-12.84 \text{ D}}\right) = +0.37\times$$

Therefore, the image size is

$$(+0.37)(15.00 \text{ mm}) = +5.55 \text{ mm}$$

The plus sign tells us that the final minified image is erect.

To summarize this problem, the object is within the focal length of the positive first surface, resulting in a virtual image. This virtual image serves as the object for the minus second surface, which also creates a virtual image.

The problems we just solved are about as complicated as any you'll see. As always, drawing a diagram is invaluable. Of particular importance is to know where the object and image rays exist.

SUMMARY

A series of thin lenses and thick lenses are examples of optical systems with more than one surface. Image location is determined by applying the vergence relationship sequentially to each surface. When calculating the object and image vergence, we must use the refractive index of the material in which the light rays exist.

Virtual objects occur when a refracting surface prevents incident light rays from forming an object. The vergence of the virtual object is determined with the refractive index of the material in which these rays exist.

KEY FORMULAE

Lateral magnification for optical system with two lenses:

Total lateral magnification = (M_L for first lens)(M_L for second lens)

Lateral magnification for optical system with two surfaces:

Total lateral magnification = (M_L for first surface)(M_L for second surface)

SELF-ASSESSMENT PROBLEMS

1. A real object, which is 30.00 mm in height, is located 25.00 cm from a crown glass lens that is 30.00 mm thick. The front surface of the lens has a radius of curvature of +5.00 cm and the back surface has a radius of curvature of −2.50 cm. (a) How far is the image from the back surface of the lens? (b) What is the height of the image? (c) Is the image real or virtual? (d) Is the image erect or inverted? (e) What is the lens form?

2. A real object, which is 30.00 mm in height, is located 3.00 cm from a crown glass lens that is 25.00 mm thick. The front surface of the lens has a radius of curvature of +12.00 cm and the back surface a radius of curvature of −7.00 cm. Answer the questions in Problem 1.

3. A real object, which is 30.00 mm in height, is located 40.00 cm from a crown glass lens that is 30.00 mm thick. The front surface of the lens has a radius

of curvature of +15.00 cm and the back surface has a radius of curvature of +15.00 cm. Answer the questions in Problem 1.

4. Two thin lenses, located in air, are separated by 25.00 mm. The power of the first lens is −10.00 D and the power of the second lens +1.00 D. A real object, which is 45.00 mm in height, is located 30.00 cm in front of the first lens. (a) How far is the image from the second lens? (b) What is the height of the image? (c) Is the image real or virtual? (d) Is the image erect or inverted?

6

Thick Lenses

In the previous chapter, we learned how to use a surface-by-surface approach to locate images formed by thick lenses. In this chapter, we'll learn how to construct what is referred to as an **equivalent lens** to solve thick lens problems. This approach is particularly helpful when dealing with complex optical systems. We'll also discuss front and back vertex power, two commonly encountered clinical measurements.

DEFINITIONS

To refresh your memory, Figure 6-1A reviews how we can locate an image by taking into account the refraction that occurs at each lens surface. Light rays that emerge from the object, O, are refracted at the front surface and subsequently refracted again by the back lens surface to result in the image, I. An alternative strategy is to construct an equivalent lens. This lens, which doesn't exist physically, has two imaginary principal planes; these are drawn as dotted vertical lines in Figure 6-1B, and labeled H (the primary principal plane) and H' (the secondary principal plane). The principal planes are redrawn in Figure 6-1C without the lens, but with the object and image.

When working with an equivalent lens, all refraction is assumed to occur at the principal planes. Object distance is measured from the primary principal plane to the object, and image distance is measured from the secondary principal plane to the image. Object and image vergences are calculated using the refractive index of the medium in which the lens exists (generally air), not the lens's index of refraction. Later in this chapter we'll solve a problem with this approach, but before doing so, we'll learn how to specify the power of a thick lens.

Figure 6-2 shows a thick glass lens situated in air. Labeled are the primary (H) and secondary (H') principal planes and the primary (F) and secondary (F') focal points. *This thick lens does not have a single focal length—it has several focal lengths.* The

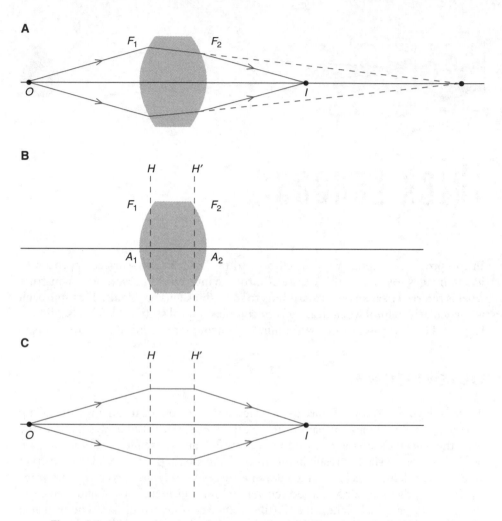

Figure 6-1. A. In a surface-by-surface approach to locating an image formed by a thick lens, the image formed by the first surface serves as an object for the second surface. In this example, the object for the second surface is virtual. **B.** A thick lens showing the location of its primary (*H*) and secondary principal planes (*H'*). The front and back surface apices are labeled A_1 and A_2, respectively. **C.** For an equivalent lens, all refraction is assumed to occur at the principal planes.

focal length can be measured from a principal plane, the anterior surface of the lens, or the posterior surface of the lens. When the focal length is measured from the primary equivalent plane to the primary focal point, it is called the **primary equivalent focal length** (f_e), and when it is measured from the secondary equivalent plane to the secondary focal point, it is called the **secondary equivalent focal length** (f_e'). [Since this lens is surrounded by a single medium (air), the primary and secondary equivalent focal lengths are equal to each other.] The **back vertex**

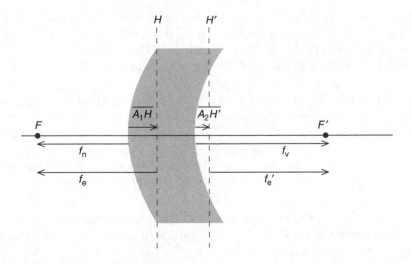

Figure 6-2. Equivalent lens showing the front vertex (f_n), back vertex (f_v), and equivalent focal lengths (f_e and f_e'). Also shown are distances from the front surface apex to the primary principal plane ($\overline{A_1H}$) and back surface apex to the secondary principal plane ($\overline{A_2H'}$).

focal length (f_v) is measured from the back *surface* of the lens to the secondary focal point, and the **front vertex focal length (f_n)** is measured from the front *surface* of the lens to the primary focal point.

For each of these focal lengths, there is a corresponding power, which is simply the reciprocal of the focal length in meters.[1] These three powers—equivalent power (F_e), back vertex power (F_v), and front vertex power (F_n)—are discussed in the following sections.

BACK AND FRONT VERTEX POWER

For most clinical applications, we are interested in the power of a lens with respect to its front or back surface, not its equivalent planes. The power specified with respect to the back surface (which is called the ocular surface in an ophthalmic lens), is called the **back vertex power**, abbreviated F_v. **When using a lensometer to neutralize the distance prescription in a patient's spectacle lenses, we typically measure the back vertex power.** It can be calculated with the following formula:

$$F_v = \frac{F_1}{1 - \left(\dfrac{t}{n}\right) F_1} + F_2$$

---

1. This assumes the lens is situated in air, which has a refractive index of 1.00.

where F_1 is the power of the front surface, F_2 is the power of the second surface, t is the thickness of the lens in meters, and n is the lens's index of refraction.

As is the case for all the thick lens formulae in this chapter, thickness (t) is in meters and the index of refraction (n) is that of the lens.

In clinical practice, the nominal power, F_T (which does not take into account lens thickness), and the back vertex power, F_V, are sometimes very similar to each other. *Take, for example, a polycarbonate lens that has a front surface power of +2.00 DS and a back surface power of +8.00 DS. Assume a central thickness of 2.00 mm. What is the nominal power of this lens? How does this compare to the back vertex power, which is more accurate because it takes thickness into account?*

The nominal power is, of course, +10.00 D, the sum of the two surfaces. This value is an estimate of the lens power that ignores its thickness. To determine the back vertex power, we substitute as follows:

$$F_v = \frac{F_1}{1 - \left(\dfrac{t}{n}\right)F_1} + F_2$$

$$F_v = \frac{+2.00\ \text{D}}{1 - \left(\dfrac{0.002\ \text{m}}{1.586}\right)(+2.00\ \text{D})} + 8.00\ \text{D} = +10.01\ \text{D}$$

In this case, the nominal and back vertex powers are essentially the same. Now, let's look at a lens that has the same nominal power (+10.00 D) but is made with a much more curved front surface ($F_1 = +15.00$ D) and a back surface power of −5.00 D. Substituting into the front vertex power formula, we have

$$F_v = \frac{+15.00\ \text{D}}{1 - \left(\dfrac{0.002\ \text{m}}{1.586}\right)(+15.00\ \text{D})} + (-5.00\ \text{D}) = +10.28\ \text{D}$$

In this case, there is a difference of 0.28 D between the estimate provided by adding the two surfaces together ($F_T = +10.00$ D) and the actual lens power ($F_V = +10.28$ D). This difference could be clinically significant.

By examining the denominator of the back vertex power formula, we can arrive at a general rule that will help us to know when we should worry about the effect of lens thickness. **As the curvature of the front surface and/or thickness of the lens increases, the back vertex power will become increasingly different than the nominal power. For plus lens, the back vertex power will become more positive and for minus lenses, it will become less minus.** High plus lenses, which generally have highly curved front surfaces, are especially likely to have nominal and back vertex powers that are significantly different from each other.

We can also specify lens's power with respect to its front surface (see f_n in Fig. 6-2). Referred to as the **front vertex** or **neutralizing power** and abbreviated F_n, it is given by following formula:

$$F_n = \frac{F_2}{1 - \left(\frac{t}{n}\right) F_2} + F_1$$

In the procedure called hand neutralization, trial lenses of known power are held against the front surface of a lens of unknown power to neutralize the movement seen through the unknown lens as it is moved. When the movement has been neutralized, the power of the trial lens is equal and opposite the unknown lens's front vertex power. Front vertex power may also be used to specify the power of bifocal adds (see Chapter 8 and Fig. 11-9).

Let's take this opportunity to point out a source of confusion that is common when first learning this material. Students sometimes confuse F_1 and F_2 with F_v and F_n. Let's be sure we understand that F_1 and F_2 refer to the powers of the front and back surfaces of the lens, while F_v and F_n give the power of the lens itself (taking into account the lens's two surfaces).

EQUIVALENT LENSES

Equivalent Power

As we discussed earlier in this chapter, the equivalent power of a lens, F_e, specifies the lens's power with respect to its principal planes. It can be calculated using the following formula:

$$F_e = F_1 + F_2 - \left(\frac{t}{n}\right) F_1 F_2$$

Equivalent power can be used in the vergence equation to determine the location of an image (or object) relative to the principal planes.

Locating the Principal Planes

As the shape of a lens changes, the positions of its principal planes change even when the equivalent power of the lens remains constant. This can be seen in Figure 6-3, which shows how the principal planes for plus and negative lenses move as the front surface becomes more convex. Note that when the front surface is very convex, principal planes can be located outside of the lens itself.

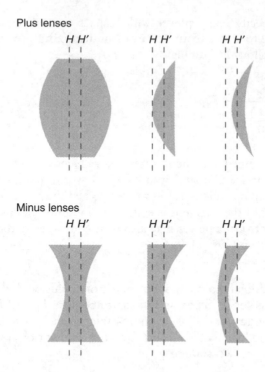

Figure 6-3. The positions of the principal planes are dependent on the curvature of the front surface of the lens relative to the curvature of the back surface. Note that as the front surface becomes steeper, the principal planes move out of the lens.

When a lens is surrounded by air, the locations of the principal planes (with respect to the lens apices, A_1 and A_2) can be determined with the following formulae:

$$\overline{A_1 H} = \frac{\left(\frac{t}{n}\right) F_2}{F_e}$$

and

$$\overline{A_2 H'} = \frac{-\left(\frac{t}{n}\right) F_1}{F_e}$$

where $\overline{A_1 H}$ is the distance from the front surface apex to the primary principal plane and $\overline{A_2 H'}$ is the distance from the back surface apex to the secondary principal plane. These distances are in meters.

Sample Problem

Now that we've learned how to determine the equivalent power of a thick lens and the location of its principal planes, let's try a problem. We'll work on the thick lens problem that we solved previously in Chapter 5. *An object is located 25.00 cm in front of a biconvex crown glass lens that has an front radius of curvature of 10.00 cm and a back radius of curvature of –5.00 cm (Fig. 5-6). The lens has a thickness of 20.00 mm. Using an equivalent lens approach, locate the image with respect to the posterior surface and calculate the magnification produced by the lens. Is the image real or virtual? Is the image erect or inverted?*

In Chapter 5, we solved this problem by taking a surface-by-surface approach. Now, let's see how we can solve it using an equivalent lens strategy.

We previously determined the front (F_1) and back surface (F_2) powers to be +5.20 D and +10.40 D, respectively. First, we determine the equivalent power as follows:

$$F_e = F_1 + F_2 - \left(\frac{t}{n}\right)F_1 F_2$$

$$F_e = 5.20 \text{ D} + 10.40 \text{ D} - \left(\frac{0.02 \text{ m}}{1.52}\right)(5.20 \text{ D})(10.40 \text{ D})$$

$$F_e = +14.89 \text{ D}$$

Next, we locate the primary principal plane as follows:

$$\overline{A_1 H} = \frac{\left(\frac{t}{n}\right)F_2}{F_e}$$

$$\overline{A_1 H} = \frac{\left(\frac{0.02}{1.52}\right)(10.40 \text{ D})}{14.89 \text{ D}}$$

$$\overline{A_1 H} = +0.0092 \text{ m or } +0.92 \text{ cm}$$

Similarly, we can locate the secondary principal plane

$$\overline{A_2 H'} = \frac{-\left(\frac{t}{n}\right)F_1}{F_e}$$

$$\overline{A_2 H'} = \frac{-\left(\frac{0.02}{1.52}\right)(5.20 \text{ D})}{14.89 \text{ D}}$$

$$\overline{A_2 H'} = -0.0046 \text{ m or } -0.46 \text{ cm}$$

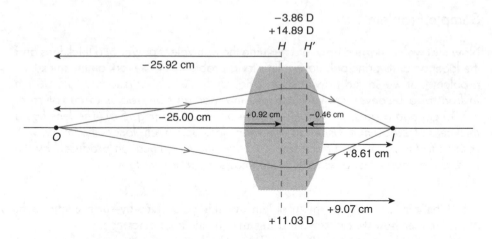

Figure 6-4. When locating the image formed by an equivalent lens, the object distance is measured from the primary principal plane and the image distance from the second-ary principal plane. Object vergence and equivalent lens power are given, respectively, at the top of the equivalent lens and image vergence at the bottom.

Figure 6-4 shows the locations of the equivalent lens's primary and secondary principal planes. The object is located 25.00 cm to the left of the lens. *When we use the vergence equation to solve this problem, should we use an object distance of −25.00 cm?* The answer is "no" because when we create an equivalent lens, object (and image) distances are measured from the principal planes, not the lens surfaces. Thus, the object distance is −25.92 cm (Fig. 6-4). The object vergence is calculated the same as it would be for a thin lens situated in air

$$L = \frac{n}{l}$$

$$L = \frac{(100)(1.00)}{-25.92 \text{ cm}}$$

$$L = -3.86 \text{ D}$$

We can now use the vergence relationship to locate the image

$$L' = L + F_e$$

$$L' = -3.86 \text{ D} + 14.89 \text{ D}$$

$$L' = +11.03 \text{ D}$$

The positive vergence tells us that the image is real. As with a thin lens in air, the image distance is calculated as

$$L' = \frac{n'}{l'}$$

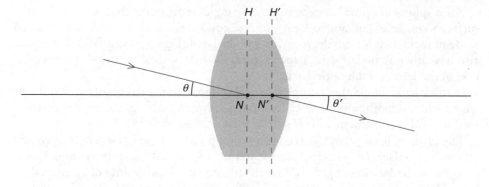

Figure 6-5. A light ray headed toward the primary nodal point emerges from the secondary nodal point at the same angle with respect to the optical axis (i.e., $\theta = \theta'$); therefore, the direction of the ray is unchanged.

$$l' = \frac{(100)(1.00)}{+11.03 \text{ D}}$$

$$l' = +9.07 \text{ cm}$$

This real image is located 9.07 cm to the right of the secondary principal plane or 8.61 cm (9.07 − 0.46 cm = 8.61 cm) to the right of the back surface of the lens. This answer is about the same as what we obtained with a surface-by-surface approach in Chapter 5.

The equivalent lens approach can also be used to calculate the lateral magnification produced by the thick lens. The formula is the same as that for a thin lens[2]:

$$M_L = \frac{L}{L'}$$

$$M_L = \frac{-3.86 \text{ D}}{11.03 \text{ D}}$$

$$M_L = -0.35\times$$

This is what we obtained when treating the lens surfaces independently in Chapter 5. Note that the magnification is negative, confirming that the real image is inverted.

Nodal Points

By definition, when a light ray is directed toward the **primary nodal point** of a lens, N, it emerges from the **secondary nodal point**, N', at the same angle with respect to the optical axis. As can be seen in Figure 6-5, a ray headed toward N leaves N' with its direction unchanged.

---

2. As with a thin lens, the lateral magnification can also be determined using the formula $M_L = \dfrac{l'}{l}$.

For a spherical optical *surface*, there is a single nodal point that is located at the surface's center of curvature. A ray directed toward the center of curvature has an angle of incidence of zero degrees; it is not deviated (Figs. 2-8 and 2-9). A thin lens also has only one nodal point, which is located at its **optical center**—the intersection of the lens and the optical axis.

In thick lenses and other complex optical systems, the nodal points are not coincident with each other. For a thick lens that is surrounded by air (or any other single medium), N is coincident with H and N' is coincident with H'.

The primary focal point (F), secondary focal point (F'), points where the primary (H) and secondary (H') principal planes intersect the optical axis, primary nodal point (N), and secondary nodal point (N') constitute the **cardinal points** of an equivalent lens. The six cardinal points fully describe the equivalent lens and allow the solution of virtually all optical problems involving paraxial light rays. As we will see in subsequent chapters, the cardinal points can be useful for understanding complex optical systems—such as the eye—that are made up of multiple refracting surfaces.

SUMMARY

There are two approaches we can use to locate an image formed by a thick lens. In the surface-by-surface approach, which we discussed in the previous chapter, the image formed by the first lens surface serves as an object for the second surface. Alternatively, as discussed in this chapter, we can construct an equivalent lens, which we can treat like a thin lens. Object and image distances are measured from the principal planes of the equivalent lens.

The power of a thick lens can be quantified with respect to one of the lens's surfaces (back and front vertex powers) or its principal planes (equivalent power). Spectacle lenses are specified by their back vertex power, while bifocal adds are often specified by their front vertex power. Equivalent power is used when locating an image formed by a thick lens.

KEY FORMULAE

Back vertex power:

$$F_v = \frac{F_1}{1 - \left(\frac{t}{n}\right) F_1} + F_2$$

Front vertex (neutralizing) power:

$$F_n = \frac{F_2}{1 - \left(\frac{t}{n}\right) F_2} + F_1$$

Equivalent power:

$$F_e = F_1 + F_2 - \left(\frac{t}{n}\right)F_1 F_2$$

Locations of principal planes:

$$\overline{A_1 H} = \frac{\left(\frac{t}{n}\right)F_2}{F_e}$$

$$\overline{A_2 H'} = \frac{-\left(\frac{t}{n}\right)F_1}{F_e}$$

SELF-ASSESSMENT PROBLEMS

1. A 30.00-mm-thick biconvex crown glass lens has an index of refraction of 1.52. The front surface has a radius of curvature of +5.00 cm and back surface has a radius of −2.50 cm. The lens is surrounded by air. (a) Calculate F_e, F_v, *and* F_n and determine the following distances: $\overline{A_1 H}$, $\overline{A_2 H'}$, f_e, and f_e'. (b) A real object that is 30.00 mm in height is located 25.00 cm in front of the lens. Treating the optical system as an *equivalent lens*, locate the image with respect to A_2 and determine its size. (c) Using a *surface-by-surface approach*, locate the image with respect to A_2 and determine its size.

2. A crown glass lens has a front surface radius of curvature of +25.00 mm and a back surface radius of curvature of +75.00 mm. The lens is 10.00 mm thick and located in air. (a) Calculate F_e, F_v, *and* F_n and calculate the following distances: $\overline{A_1 H}$, $\overline{A_2 H'}$, f_e, and f_e'. (b) A real object that is 1.00 cm in height is located 15.00 cm in front of the lens. Treating the optical system as an *equivalent lens*, locate the image with respect to A_2 and determine its size. (c) Using a *surface-by-surface approach*, locate the image with respect to A_2 and determine its size.

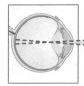

Ametropia

The eye is a sophisticated optical system constituted of multiple refracting surfaces, and to solve certain optical problems it is necessary to consider the optical properties of the eye in all their complexity. For many problems and clinical cases, however, a satisfactory solution can be obtained by using a simplified optical model of the eye, referred to as a **schematic eye**.

There are various schematic eyes. For our purposes, we will work with what is called the **reduced eye**, which is given in Figure 7-1. It consists of a single spherical refracting surface[1] with a radius of curvature of 5.55 mm that separates air from aqueous, which is assumed to have an index of refraction of 1.333. There is a single nodal point located at the center of curvature of the refracting surface. As is the case for all spherical refracting surfaces, the principal planes are coincident with the surface. The distance from the surface to the retina—the **axial length**—is 22.22 mm.

The reduced eye is **emmetropic**, meaning that as illustrated in Figure 7-2, light rays originating at infinity are focused on the retina.[2] Let's look at this in more detail. First, we'll determine the power of the reduced eye. Since we know its radius of curvature and the relevant refractive indices, the surface's refractive power can be calculated as follows:

$$F = \frac{n' - n}{r}$$

$$F = \frac{1.333 - 1.000}{0.00555}$$

$$F = +60.00 \text{ D}$$

---

1. The refracting surface of the reduced eye is located 1.67 mm posterior to the cornea. We ignore this small distance in this book and use the terms "anterior surface of the eye" and "cornea" interchangeably.

2. Both the cornea and relaxed crystalline lens contribute to the reduced eye's refractive power. Accommodation is discussed in the next chapter.

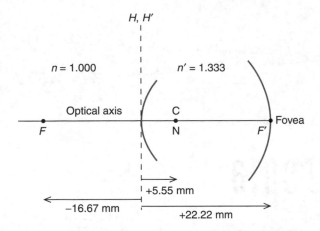

Figure 7-1. The reduced eye consists of a single refracting surface (with a radius of curvature of +5.55 mm) that separates air and aqueous. The principal planes are coincident with the refracting surface, and the nodal point is located at its center of curvature. The primary and secondary focal lengths are −16.67 and +22.22 mm, respectively.

Now we'll calculate the location of the image when this eye views an infinitely distant object. The vergence for such an object is zero. The image vergence can be determined with the ever-so helpful vergence relationship.

$$L' = L + F$$

$$L' = 0.00 \text{ D} + 60.00 \text{ D}$$

$$L' = +60.00 \text{ D}$$

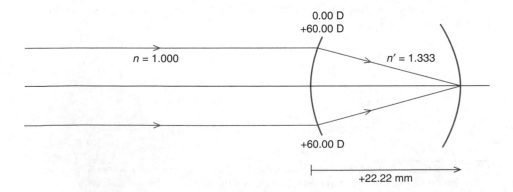

Figure 7-2. An infinitely distant object is imaged on the retina of the reduced eye. The eye has a refractive power of +60.00 D and an axial length of +22.22 mm.

What is the image distance? The key is to realize that the rays forming the image exist in aqueous, the secondary medium. This can be seen in Figure 7-2. The image distance is calculated as

$$L' = \frac{n'}{l'}$$

$$+60.00 \text{ D} = \frac{1.333}{l'}$$

$$l' = +0.02222 \text{ m, or } +22.22 \text{ mm}$$

This calculation confirms what we already know—the distance from the refractive surface to the retina in the reduced eye is 22.22 mm.

To summarize, an infinitely distant object is focused on the retina of the reduced eye. Such an eye is said to be **emmetropic** (or have the condition of emmetropia). Another way of saying this is that in emmetropia, the retina is conjugate with infinity.

In **ametropia**, an infinitely distant image is not focused on the retina. The remainder of this chapter discusses the quantification of two common forms of ametropia—myopia and hyperopia—and their correction.

MYOPIA

In the myopic eye, an infinitely distant object is focused anterior to the retina.[3] Relative to the reduced eye, the eye can be too long (an axial length greater than 22.22 mm), too strong (a refractive power greater than +60.00 D) or a combination thereof.[4] Consider an eye that is too long—it has an axial length of 23.22 mm rather than 22.22 mm. The eye's power is +60.00 D. As can be seen in Figure 7-3A, an infinitely distant object is focused 22.22 mm behind the refracting surface, or 1.00 mm anterior to the retina of this eye.

A large part of our practices as eye doctors is to quantify a patient's myopia so that we can prescribe appropriate corrective lenses. How would we quantify the myopia in the previous paragraph? Answering the following question will help us to do this: *Where must an object be located for it to be imaged on the retina of an eye that has an axial length of 23.22 mm and power of +60.00 D?*

Figure 7-3B guides us through the solution of this problem. First, we determine the vergence required for an image to be focused on the retina. Since the eye has

---

3. A patient who is myopic has the condition of *myopia*.
4. In Chapter 13, we'll learn about axial and refractive myopia. Clinically, these terms are typically used when comparing the refractive states of a patient's two eyes. If, for example, one eye is more myopic than the other and this is due to a difference in axial length between the two eyes, the myopia is labeled as axial. Likewise, if the difference in myopia is due to a difference in corneal power, the myopia is refractive.

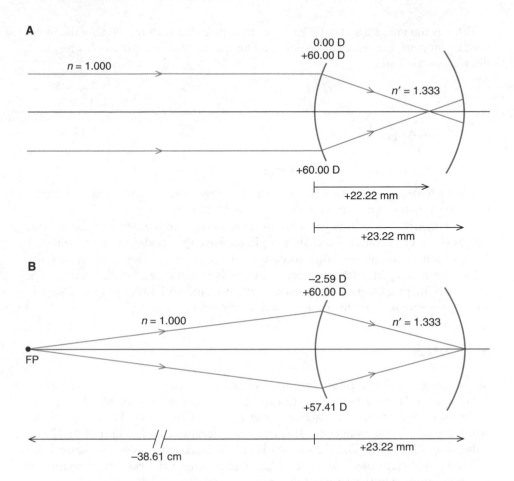

Figure 7-3. A. In myopia, an infinitely distant object is imaged anterior to the retina. **B.** The far point of the eye (FP) is conjugate with the retina, meaning that an object located at the far point is imaged on the retina. Object vergence and eye power are given at the top of the refracting surface and image vergence at the bottom. See text for further details. [Note that object distance (−38.61 cm) is given in centimeters and image distance (+23.22 mm) in millimeters.]

an axial length of 23.22 mm and the rays that form the image exist in aqueous, the image vergence must be[5]

$$L' = \frac{n'}{l'}$$

$$L' = \frac{(1000)(1.333)}{23.22 \text{ mm}}$$

$$L' = +57.41 \text{ D}$$

---

5. We have placed a factor of 1000 in the numerator because we are keeping the axial length in millimeters.

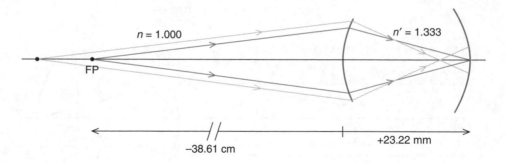

Figure 7-4. An object located farther from the myopic eye than the far point will be imaged in front of the retina.

Next, we use the paraxial relationship to determine the object vergence required to produce this image vergence.

$$L' = L + F$$

$$+ 57.41 \text{ D} = L + 60.00 \text{ D}$$

$$L = -2.59 \text{ D}$$

Object light rays with a vergence of –2.59 D are focused on the retina. **This is referred to as the *far-point vergence*, and the eye is said to be 2.59 D myopic.**

To produce this vergence, the object must be located in front of the anterior surface of the reduced eye. The distance from the surface to the object is[6]

$$L = \frac{n}{l}$$

$$l = \frac{(100)(1.00)}{-2.59 \text{ D}}$$

$$l = -38.61 \text{ cm}$$

As can be seen in Figure 7-3B, an object located 38.61 cm anterior to the reduced eye's front surface—at what is defined as the **far point of the eye (FP)**—is focused on the retina. **That is, the far point is conjugate with the retina.** In myopia, it is always located anterior to the eye's surface. Figure 7-4 shows that an object located farther from the eye than the far point is focused anterior to the retina.

What power contact lens is required to image an infinitely distant object on the retina of this myopic eye?

---

6. Because we have placed a factor of 100 in the numerator, the calculated distance is in centimeters.

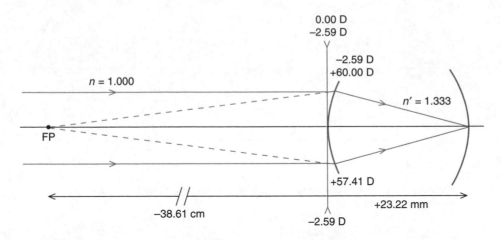

Figure 7-5. A corrective contact lens images an infinitely distant object at its secondary focal point, which is coincident with the eye's far point. Since the far point is conjugate with the retina, a focused image is formed on the retina. Note that the image vergence emerging from the corrective lens (−2.59 D) serves as the object vergence for the myopic eye. (At the top of both the contact lens and eye surface are the object vergence and refractive power, respectively. Image vergence is given below these refracting elements.)

A contact lens,[7] which we'll assume rests on the reduced eye's anterior surface, must have a power of −2.59 D. Figure 7-5 shows that when light rays from an infinitely distant object strike this lens, an image is formed at its secondary focal point, which is coincident with the far point of the eye; this image serves as an object for the eye and is focused on the retina. **Note that the contact lens power (−2.59 D) is equal to the eye's far point vergence.**

In summary, to correct myopia, the secondary focal point of a minus correcting lens must be coincident with the far point of the eye. When this is the case, an infinitely distant object is imaged at the far point. Since the far point is conjugate with the retina, an image is focused on the retina.

Just a slight increase in axial length can cause clinically significant myopia. *What is the axial length of a 1.00 D myopic eye that has a refractive power of +60.00 D?*

An object with a vergence of −1.00 D (the far point vergence) will be focused on the retina. The vergence relationship can be used to determine the axial length as follows:

$$L' = L + F$$

$$L' = -1.00 + 60.00 \text{ D}$$

$$L' = +59.00 \text{ D}$$

---

7. We'll discuss correction with spectacle lenses when we talk about lens effectivity later in this chapter.

The light rays that form the retinal image exist in aqueous. Therefore, the image distance is

$$L' = \frac{n'}{l'}$$

$$+59.00\ D = \frac{1.333}{l'}$$

$$l' = +0.02259\ m,\ or\ +22.59\ mm$$

An increase in the axial length of only 0.37 mm (22.59 − 22.22 mm = 0.37 mm) causes 1.00 D of myopia. This points to the exquisite coordination of growth that is required for eyes to become emmetropic, a process referred to as **emmetropization. A useful rule of thumb is that for every 1/3-mm increase in the eye's axial length, the eye becomes 1.00 D more myopic.** Consequently, an eye that is 1.00 mm too long is approximately 3.00 D myopic.

HYPEROPIA

In hyperopia (sometimes called hypermetropia), an infinitely distant object is focused posterior to the retina. Relative to the reduced eye, the eye can be too short (axial length less than 22.22 mm), too weak (refractive power less than +60.00 D), or a combination of these two factors. Consider an eye that is too short—it has an axial length of 21.22 mm and a power of +60.00 D. As can be seen in Figure 7-6, an infinitely distant object is focused 22.22 mm behind the refracting surface, or 1.00 mm posterior to the retina of this eye.

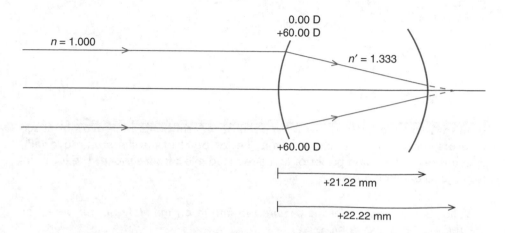

Figure 7-6. In hyperopia, an infinitely distant object is imaged behind the retina.

How do we quantify the hyperopia in the previous paragraph so that corrective lenses can be prescribed? Similar to myopia, answering the following question is helpful: *Where must an object be located if its image is to be focused on the retina of an eye that has an axial length of 21.22 mm and power of +60.00 D?*

Figure 7-7A guides us through the solution of this problem. If the image is to be focused on the retina, the image vergence must be

$$L' = \frac{n'}{l'}$$

$$L' = \frac{(1000)(1.333)}{21.22 \text{ mm}}$$

$$L' = +62.82 \text{ D}$$

To determine the object vergence required to produce this image vergence, we use the vergence relationship.

$$L' = L + F$$

$$+62.82 \text{ D} = L + 60.00 \text{ D}$$

$$L = +2.82 \text{ D}$$

Light rays with +2.82 D of vergence are focused on the retina. **This is referred to as the far-point vergence, and the eye is said to be 2.82 D hyperopic.**

Note that the far-point vergence is positive. What does this mean? It means that the object must be located behind the anterior surface of the reduced eye—it is a *virtual* object (Fig. 7-7A). The light rays that form this virtual object exist in air. Therefore, the distance from the cornea to the virtual object is calculated as

$$L = \frac{n}{l}$$

$$l = \frac{(100)(1.00)}{+2.82 \text{ D}}$$

$$l = +35.46 \text{ cm}$$

Light rays that are headed toward a point 35.46 cm behind the eye's front surface are focused on the retina. This is the far point of the hyperopic eye (FP), which is always located posterior to the reduced eye's front surface. The far point is conjugate with the retina.

What power contact lens is required to image an infinitely distant object on the retina of this hyperopic eye?

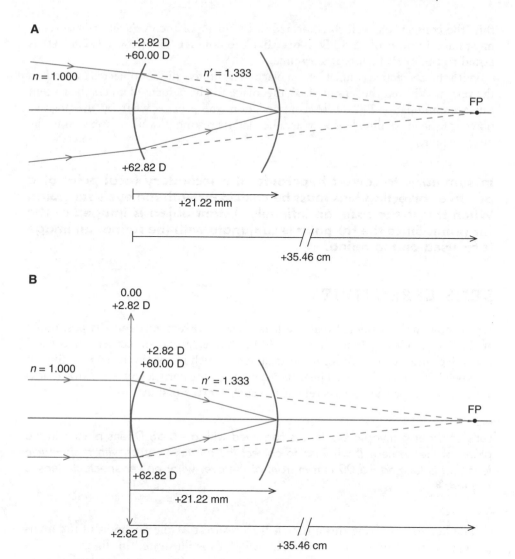

Figure 7-7. A. For light rays to be focused on the retina of this hyperopic eye, they must enter the eye with a vergence of +2.82 D. That is, they must form a virtual object at the far point of the eye, +35.46 cm behind the cornea. **B.** A corrective lens images an infinitely distant object at its secondary focal point, which is coincident with the far point of the eye. Since the far point is conjugate with the retina, a focused image is formed on the retina. The image vergence emerging from the corrective lens (+2.82 D) serves as the object vergence for the hyperopic eye.

The lens must form an image at the far point of the eye; this image serves as an object for the eye and is focused on the retina. Therefore, the secondary focal point of the correcting lens must be coincident with the far point (Fig. 7-7B). To achieve this, the contact lens, which is located in the plane of the eye's anterior surface, must have a power of +2.82 D. **Note that the contact lens power (+2.82 D) is equal to the eye's far point vergence.**

With the corrective contact lens in place, an infinitely distant object is focused on the retina. Without the lens in place, the image will be defocused unless the patient can accommodate +2.82 D. (Accommodation, the process whereby the positive power of the crystalline lens increases beyond its resting power, is discussed in the next chapter.)

In summary, to correct hyperopia, the secondary focal point of a positive correcting lens must be coincident with the eye's far point. When this is the case, an infinitely distant object is imaged at the far point. Since the far point is conjugate with the retina, an image is focused on the retina.

LENS EFFECTIVITY

Up to now, we've assumed that the lens used to correct ametropia is positioned at the eye's anterior surface. This would be the case for a contact lens or corneal refractive surgery, but not for a spectacle lens, which is positioned at a significant distance in front of the eye. The distance between the cornea and the ocular (back) surface of the spectacle lens is referred to as the **vertex distance**.

Let's consider a myopic eye that is corrected with a −6.68 D lens placed in the plane of the cornea. *If we wish to correct the refractive error with a spectacle lens that is located 15.00 mm in front of the eye, what power spectacle lens is required?*

The key to answering this question is to realize that the far point of the myopic eye is at a fixed distance from the eye. This is illustrated in Figure 7-8. To correct the refractive error, the secondary focal point of the correcting lens must be coincident with this far point. In the case at hand, the far point is 14.97 cm anterior to the cornea. If the correcting lens is 15.00 mm anterior to the cornea, its secondary focal length must be −13.47 cm [(−14.97 cm) − (−1.50 cm) = −13.47 cm]. The power of a minus lens with a secondary focal length of −13.47 cm is

$$F = \frac{n'}{f'}$$

$$F = \frac{(100)(1.00)}{-13.47 \text{ cm}}$$

$$F = -7.42 \text{ D}$$

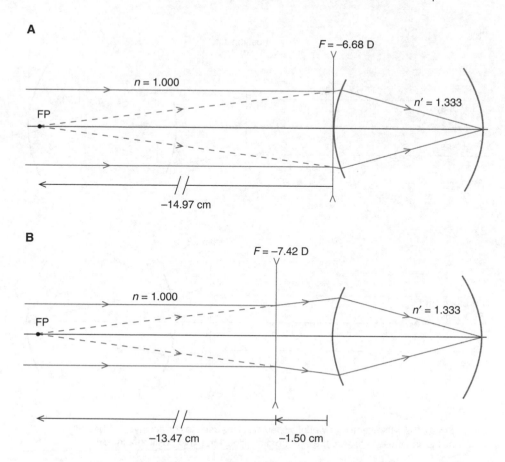

Figure 7-8. This refractive error can be corrected with (**A**) a –6.68 D contact lens or (**B**) a –7.42 D spectacle lens. In both cases, an infinitely distant object is focused at the eye's far point.

This myopic eye can be corrected with either a –6.68 D contact lens or a –7.42 D spectacle lens at a vertex distance of 15.00 mm. Both have the same *effective* power. Note that when we replace a myopic patient's contact lens with a spectacle lens, the power must be increased. Think of it this way: since we are moving the corrective lens closer to the far point, it must now have a shorter focal length.

Understanding lens effectivity is critical to understanding and solving common clinical symptoms. For instance, patients with myopia sometimes report that blurred distant objects become clearer when they push their spectacles very close to their eyes. How can we explain this? Most likely, the corrective lenses are not sufficiently strong. As illustrated in Figure 7-9, by pushing the lenses closer to the eyes, the secondary focal points of the corrective lenses are made coincident with the far points, thereby increasing the lens effectivity.

A

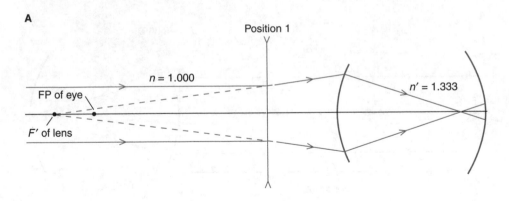

B

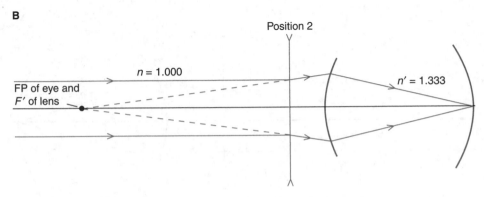

Figure 7-9. The effective power of a spectacle lens used to correct myopia is increased by moving the lens toward the eye [from position 1 in (**A**) to position 2 in (**B**)].

The principles of lens effectivity also apply to hyperopia. *Consider the 2.82 D hyperope who we discussed earlier in the chapter. This hyperopic patient requires a corrective lens of +2.82 D in the plane of the cornea (i.e., a contact lens whose power is +2.82D). What power spectacle lens is required to correct this refractive error? Assume a vertex distance of 15.00 mm.*

The secondary focal point of the corrective lens, whether it is a contact lens or a spectacle lens, must be coincident with the far point of the eye (which is 35.46 cm to the right of the cornea). From Figure 7-10, we see that the secondary focal length of the spectacle lens must be 36.96 cm (35.46 + 1.50 cm = 36.96 cm). The power of this spectacle lens is

$$F = \frac{n'}{f'}$$

$$F = \frac{(100)(1.00)}{36.96 \text{ cm}}$$

$$F = +2.71 \text{ D}$$

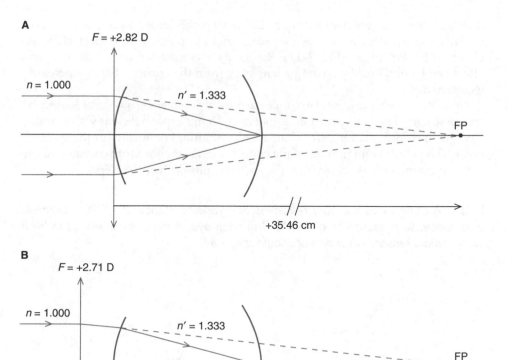

Figure 7-10. This refractive error can be corrected with (**A**) a +2.82 D contact lens or (**B**) a +2.71 D spectacle lens. In both cases, an infinitely distant object is focused at the eye's far point. Although lens effectivity is relatively small with this low power prescription, it can be significant with higher power lenses.

This hyperope can be corrected with either a +2.82 D contact lens or a +2.71 D spectacle lens. The contact lens has a higher power because it must have a shorter focal length if its secondary focal point to be coincident with the eye's far point. In this example, the difference between the power of the contact lens and the spectacle lens is small. For higher powers, however, lens effectivity is an important clinical factor. For instance, a patient who is corrected with a +10.00 D contact lens requires a spectacle lens whose power is +8.70 D.

Hyperopic patients sometimes notice that their distance visual acuity improves when they slide their spectacles down their nose so that they are farther from their eyes. What is happening here? Most likely, the lenses—when worn at the normal distance—are not sufficiently strong. By moving the lenses away from his eyes, the hyperopic patient is moving the secondary focal points of the spectacle lenses closer to his far points (Fig. 7-11). Rather than using a stronger lens, the same effect can be obtained by moving a lens away from the cornea, thereby increasing its effectivity.

Up to now, we've discussed examples that involve replacing a contact lens with a spectacle lens. The same principles apply to replacing a spectacle lens with a contact lens. As a practical matter, refractions are almost always performed at the spectacle plane, about 15.00 mm in front of the cornea. Therefore it is more common to calculate the contact lens power from the spectacle power than vice versa.

Let's look at an example. Your refraction at a vertex distance of 15.00 mm results in a spectacle prescription of –9.00 D in each eye. If the patient wishes to be fit with contact lenses, what power should they be?

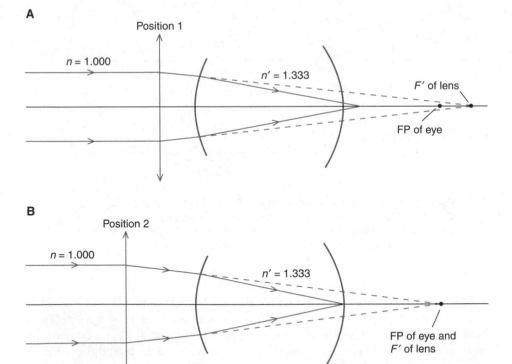

Figure 7-11. The effective power of a plus spectacle lens that is used to correct hyperopia is increased by moving the lens away from the eye [from position 1 in (**A**) to position 2 in (**B**)].

First, without doing any calculations, you should know that the power of the contact lenses will be less than the spectacle lenses. Since the contact lenses are closer to the eyes, they are farther from the far point and consequently have a longer focal length and lower power.[8] To be specific, whereas the secondary focal length for the spectacles is −11.11 cm (e.g., 100/−9.00 D = −11.11 cm), the secondary focal length for the contact lenses is −12.61 cm [e.g., (−11.11 cm) + (−1.5 cm) = −12.61 cm]. A −7.93 D contact lens has this focal length (e.g., 100/−12.61 cm = −7.93 D).

Just to be sure we have these important concepts down, let's do one more example. If we perform a trial-lens refraction at a distance of 12 mm and find +12.00 D, what power contact lens should be prescribed?

Before we do any calculations, we know that the contact lens must have a shorter focal length than the spectacle lens, which means it has more power. Rather than a focal length of 8.33 cm (for the spectacle lens), the contact lens focal length is 1.2 cm shorter, or 7.13 cm. Such a contact lens has a dioptric power of +14.02 D.

Lens effectivity can also be calculated using equations. Although some people prefer to use equations, I think it's better to solve these problems without them. It's all too easy to forget equations, but once you understand the basic concepts of lens effectivity, they should stay with you over the course of your professional career.

CORRECTION OF AMETROPIA WITH LASER AND SURGICAL PROCEDURES

Ametropia is most often corrected with an ophthalmic lens positioned in the spectacle plane or a contact lens in the corneal plane. In recent years, it has become commonplace to compensate (or partially compensate) for refractive errors with surgical and laser procedures.

The first widely utilized surgical procedure was *radial keratotomy* (RK). This procedure was used primarily to compensate for myopia. Radial incisions are made in the cornea, leading to the flattening of this tissue and a resultant decrease in the eye's refractive power (Fig. 7-12).

Photorefractive procedures that utilize excimer laser technology have supplanted radial keratotomy. In *photorefractive keratectomy* (PRK), the corneal epithelium is removed prior to using an excimer laser to sculpt the underlying stroma. With *laser-assisted in situ keratomileusis* (LASIK), a microtome or laser is used to create a corneal flap (Fig. 7-13). The exposed stroma is sculpted with the goal of adjusting

---

8. When we say that one corrective lens is stronger (or more powerful) than another, we are typically referring to the absolute power of the lenses. That is, a −10.00 D lens is said to be stronger than a −5.00 D lens.

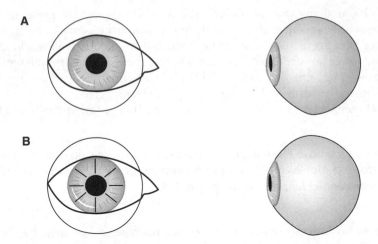

Figure 7-12. **A.** Views of the cornea prior to radial keratotomy. **B.** Following radial keratotomy, the cornea is flattened.

the refractive power of the eye and reducing the amount of ametropia. Once the laser has sculpted the underlying stroma, the corneal cap is repositioned.

Surgical corneal implants can also be used to compensate for ametropia. The implants can typically be removed if they are unsuccessful in providing an acceptable correction.

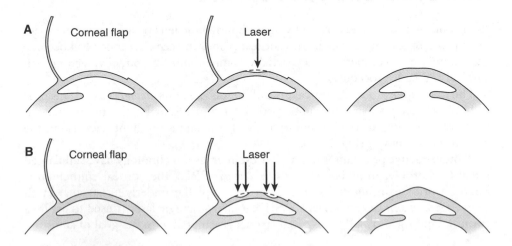

Figure 7-13. **A.** When myopia is corrected with LASIK, the central cornea is flattened. **B.** When hyperopia is corrected with LASIK, the central cornea is steepened. (This diagram is a simplification.)

In these various laser and surgical procedures, the ametropic correction is in the plane of the cornea. The principles of lens effectivity apply to laser and surgical corrections in much the same manner as they apply to the correction of ametropia with contact lenses.

SUMMARY

When an emmetropic eye views a distant object, an image is focused on the retina. This is not the case in ametropia, where there is a mismatch between the eye's refractive power and axial length. In myopia, the image is focused anterior to the retina; in hyperopia, it is focused posterior to the retina.

Both myopia and hyperopia can be corrected with lenses that focus an infinitely distant object at the far point of the eye. When the far point is anterior to the cornea, which is the case in myopia, a minus corrective lens is required. In hyperopia, the far point is posterior to the cornea necessitating a plus lens for its correction.

The power of the lens required to correct ametropia is dependent on its distance from the eye, a phenomenon referred to as lens effectivity. A myopic patient requires less minus power in her contact lens prescription than in her spectacles, whereas a hyperopic patient requires more plus power in her contact lens prescription than in her spectacles.

SELF-ASSESSMENT PROBLEMS

1. A myopic eye is fully corrected with a –6.00 DS spectacle lens. (a) What is the power of the contact lens required to fully correct this eye? (b) Answer the same question for a hyperopic eye that is fully corrected with a +6.00 DS spectacle lens. Assume a vertex distance of 12.0 mm.

2. A patient's left eye is fully corrected with a –7.00 DS contact lens. (a) What is the power of the spectacle lens required to correct this eye? (b) Answer the same question for an eye that is corrected with a +7.00 DS contact lens. Assume a vertex distance of 12.0 mm.

3. A reduced eye has 10.00 D of myopia as measured at its anterior surface. (a) If the myopia is axial, what is the axial length of the eye? (b) If the myopia is refractive, what is the refractive power of the eye?

4. A reduced eye is corrected with a +5.00 DS spectacle lens. If the ametropia is axial, what is the axial length of the eye? Assume a vertex distance of 15.0 mm.

5. The farthest distance at which a patient can see clearly with her right eye is 25.00 cm anterior to her cornea. What is the power of the spectacle lens that will correct her ametropia? Assume a vertex distance of 15.0 mm.

6. A patient was last examined 2 years earlier and is currently wearing a –4.00 DS spectacle lens over his right eye. Today, you determine that his far point is

100.00 cm anterior to the spectacle plane. Assuming a vertex distance of 15.0 mm, what is the power of the contact lens you would prescribe for this patient to correct his ametropia?

7. An object is located 15.00 cm anterior to the cornea of an emmetropic eye. What power spectacle lens is required for the object to be focused on the retina if the vertex distance is 12.0 mm? (Assume the patient cannot accommodate.)

8. An image is located 2.00 mm posterior to the retina of an emmetropic reduced eye of standard axial length (i.e., 22.22 mm). Where is the object located? (Ignore accommodation.)

Accommodation

When an eye is corrected for distance, the retinal image of a near object will be defocused unless the power of the eye increases. The process whereby the refractive power of the eye increases, thereby allowing near objects to be imaged clearly on the retina, is called **accommodation** (Fig. 8-1). When accommodation is relaxed (i.e., when the eye is focused for distance), the anterior surface of the crystalline lens is comparatively flat and the power of the lens is at a minimum. (Even in this relaxed state, the lens contributes about one-third of the dioptric power of the eye. The cornea contributes two-thirds of the relaxed eye's refractive power.) During accommodation, the anterior surface of the crystalline lens becomes more curved, thereby increasing the dioptric power of the lens and allowing near objects to be imaged on the retina.

The physiology and physical processes of accommodation are complex. The young lens apparently has a natural proclivity to be in a rounded state. When the sphincter-like ciliary muscle is relaxed, the lens zonules are pulled outward and exert tension at the equator of the lens. This tension causes the anterior surface of the lens to flatten (Fig. 8-1). When the ciliary muscle constricts during accommodation—much like a sphincter constricting—the tension on the zonules is reduced, thereby allowing the lens to assume its "preferred" rounded shape. In this rounded shape, the radius of curvature of the anterior lens surface is decreased, increasing the dioptric power.

The surface of the lens, referred to as the **lens capsule**, is pliable in the young eye. As we age, the lens capsule is thought to become less pliable, which may explain the progressive decrease in accommodative capacity that occurs over time. Whereas a 10-year-old child may be able to accommodate 12.00 D (i.e., the total refractive power of the eye increases from +60.00 D for distance to +72.00 D for near), a 75-year-old adult has no ability to accommodate. Table 8-1 shows the average maximum accommodative capacity—clinically referred to as the **amplitude of accommodation**—at various ages.

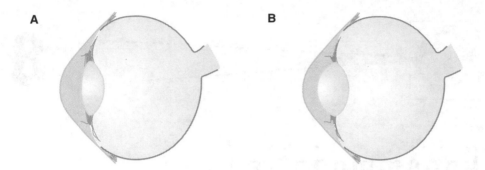

Figure 8-1. A. When distant objects are viewed, the anterior surface of the crystalline lens is at its flattest, thereby minimizing the lens' refractive power. The cornea provides about two-thirds of the distance refractive power of the eye, with the remainder provided by the crystalline lens. **B.** When near objects are viewed, the sphincter-like ciliary muscle constricts; this reduces the tension on the zonules, thereby allowing the anterior surface of the lens to bulge forward, decreasing its radius of curvature. As a result, the dioptric power of the lens is increased. (*Reproduced with permission from Schwartz, SH. Visual Perception: A Clinical Orientation, 4th ed. http://www.accessmedicine.com. Copyright © 2010 McGraw-Hill Education. All rights reserved.*)

When the loss of accommodation due to aging leads to clinical symptoms—such as near blur and asthenopia[1]—the condition is referred to as **presbyopia**. Presbyopia is corrected by adding plus lens power to the patient's distance correction. This additional plus lens power is often in the form of a **bifocal add** (see Fig. 11-9).

Presbyopia does not develop at the same rate in all patients. Exposure to high levels of ultraviolet radiation, as occurs with people living close to the equator, appears to accelerate its development.

TABLE 8-1. AMPLITUDE OF ACCOMMODATION AS A FUNCTION OF AGE

Age (years)	Typical Amplitude of Accommodation (diopters)*
10	12.50
20	9.75
30	7.25
40	4.00
50	2.50
60	1.25
70	0.50
75	0.00

*Extrapolated from the data of Donders (1864) and Duane (1912).

---

1. *Asthenopia* is another term for eyestrain.

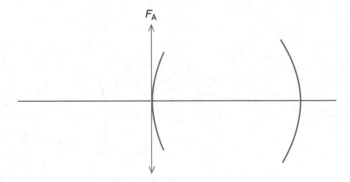

Figure 8-2. A plus lens, F_A, in the plane of front surface of the eye can be used to represent accommodation.

In the model eyes discussed in the previous chapter, the ciliary muscle is assumed to be relaxed and accommodation is zero. In this chapter, we consider various conditions where accommodation comes into play.

VERGENCE RELATIONSHIP FOR ACCOMMODATION

The purpose of accommodation is to image a viewed object at the far point of the eye. When this occurs, the object will, in turn, be imaged on the retina because the far point is conjugate with the retina. As can be seen in Figure 8-2, accommodation is represented as a plus lens, F_A, in the plane of the front surface of the eye (which we'll assume is the corneal plane[2]).

Let's state this in a slightly different way. In order for a near object to be focused on the retina, the vergence leaving the accommodative lens must equal the far-point vergence. We can write this as the vergence relationship for accommodation

$$F_{FP} = L + F_A$$

where F_{FP} is the far-point vergence as measured at the cornea, L is the **near stimulus vergence** (i.e., the vergence that the object produces at the cornea), and F_A is the accommodation, measured in the plane of the cornea, required to focus the object on the retina.

---

2. As discussed in Chapter 7, the anterior surface of the reduced eye is situated 1.67 mm posterior to the cornea. We ignore this small distance in this book.

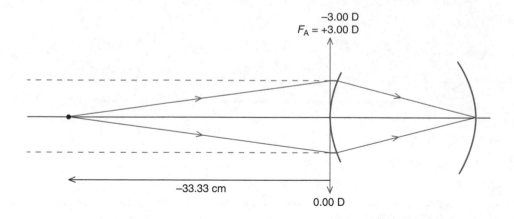

Figure 8-3. An object located 33.33 cm anterior to the cornea results in −3.00 D of vergence (at the cornea). This is the near stimulus vergence. For the object to be imaged on the retina, the emmetropic eye must accommodate 3.00 D.

Let's consider the simplest case, that of an emmetrope. *An object is located 33.33 cm in front of the cornea of an emmetropic eye. How much must the eye accommodate for the object to be imaged on the retina?*

As indicated in Figure 8-3, the object distance is −33.33 cm, making the near stimulus vergence −3.00 D [e.g., (1.00)(100)/−33.33 cm = −3.00 D]. Since the far point of an emmetropic eye is at infinity, the far-point vergence is 0.00 D. Substituting into the vergence relationship for accommodation, we have

$$F_{FP} = L + F_A$$

$$0.00 \text{ D} = -3.00 \text{ D} + F_A$$

$$F_A = +3.00 \text{ D}$$

Note that the accommodation required by an emmetropic eye is equal (and opposite) to the near stimulus vergence. The emmetropic eye must accommodate 3.00 D in order for an object at 33.33 cm to be imaged on the retina.

This calculation may seem unnecessarily cumbersome. After all, it makes intuitive sense that the emmetropic eye must accommodate 3.00 D to image an object at 33.33 cm on the retina. In subsequent examples, however, we will learn that the determination of the required accommodation is not always so straightforward.

ACCOMMODATION IN AMETROPIA

Now that we've determined how much an emmetropic eye must accommodate for an object located at 33.33 cm to be imaged on the retina, let's compare this to a myopic eye. *How much must a patient with 1.00 D of uncorrected myopia,*

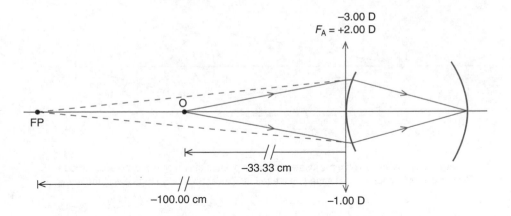

Figure 8-4. For an object located 33.33 cm anterior to the cornea (near stimulus vergence of −3.00 D) to be imaged on the retina, an uncorrected 1.00 D myopic eye must accommodate 2.00 D.

as measured at the surface of the eye, accommodate for an object located at a distance of 33.33 cm to be imaged on the retina?

The object vergence at the plane of the cornea—where accommodation is posited to occur—is −3.00 D. This is the near stimulus vergence. As illustrated in Figure 8-4, following accommodation the vergence must equal the far-point vergence of −1.00 D. From the vergence relationship for accommodation, we have

$$F_{FP} = L + F_A$$
$$-1.00 \text{ D} = -3.00 \text{ D} + F_A$$
$$F_A = +2.00 \text{ D}$$

For an object located 33.33 cm anterior to the eye, the uncorrected myope must accommodate less than the emmetrope. This makes intuitive sense because the myopic eye has an excess of plus power—it is too strong for its axial length.

How does correction of a refractive error affect the amount of accommodation that is required? *If a 1.00 D myopic eye is corrected with a contact lens, how much accommodation is required to see clearly an object located at a distance of 33.00 cm?*

The corrected myopic eye is focused for infinity, meaning that its far point is at infinity. As with an emmetropic eye, the far-point vergence, as measured at the cornea, is zero. The near stimulus vergence is the reciprocal of the distance from

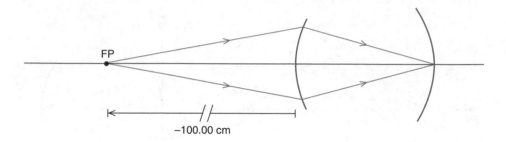

Figure 8-5. When an object is located at the far point of the myopic eye, no accommodation is required for it to be imaged on the retina. The far point is conjugate with the retina.

the eye to the object (in meters). Substituting into the vergence relationship for accommodation, we find

$$F_{FP} = L + F_A$$

$$0.00 \text{ D} = -3.00 \text{ D} + F_A$$

$$F_A = +3.00 \text{ D}$$

As with the emmetropic eye, the required accommodation is 3.00 D. **When an eye is corrected in the corneal plane with a contact lens (or refractive surgery), the required accommodation is equal (and opposite) to the near stimulus vergence.**

We'll look at one more example for this 1.00 myopic eye. *Suppose an object is located at a distance of 100 cm. How much accommodation is now required if the eye is uncorrected?*

Since the object is located at the far point of the eye, as indicated in Figure 8-5, it is by definition imaged on the retina. No accommodation is required. Alternatively, we could use the vergence relationship for accommodation

$$F_{FP} = L + F_A$$

$$-1.00 \text{ D} = -1.00 \text{ D} + F_A$$

$$F_A = +0.00 \text{ D}$$

Next, let's consider uncorrected hyperopia. *To image an object located at a distance of 33.33 cm on the retina, how much must an uncorrected 1.00 D hyperopic eye, as measured in the plane of the cornea, accommodate?*

Figure 8-6 shows that following accommodation, the vergence must equal the far-point vergence of +1.00 D. Using the vergence relationship for accommodation, we have

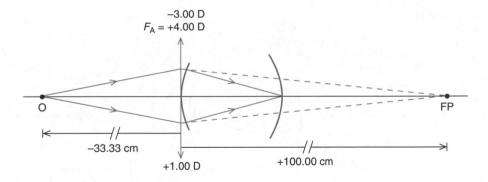

Figure 8-6. To image an object located 33.33 cm anterior to the cornea (near stimulus vergence of −3.00 D) upon the retina, an uncorrected 1.00 D hyperopic eye must accommodate 4.00 D.

$$F_{FP} = L + F_A$$
$$+1.00 \text{ D} = -3.00 \text{ D} + F_A$$
$$F_A = +4.00 \text{ D}$$

For an object located 33.33 cm anterior to the eye, the uncorrected hyperope must accommodate more than the emmetrope. This makes sense because the hyperopic eye has a shortfall of refractive power—it is too weak for its axial length.

How much must the hyperopic eye accommodate when corrected with a contact lens? As with emmetropia, the far-point vergence of a hyperopic eye corrected with a contact lens is zero. Consequently, to image a near object on the retina, the corrected hyperopic eye will need to accommodate the same amount as the emmetropic eye.

These examples show that to image a near object on the retina, the *uncorrected* hyperopic eye must accommodate the most, the emmetropic eye less, and the myopic eye even less. In fact, the uncorrected myopic patient may continue to have acceptable near vision even as she ages and loses the ability to accommodate. For instance, at the age of 75 years, a patient with 3.00 D of *uncorrected* myopia and no accommodative reserve will still be able to see an object at 33.33 cm clearly, whereas the object will appear blurred to emmetropic and uncorrected hyperopic patients of the same age. It is for this reason that aging myopes can sometimes remove their distance spectacles to view near objects.

As he or she ages, the *uncorrected* hyperopic patient may have increasing difficulty not only seeing near objects, but distant objects as well. An uncorrected 3.00 D hyperope, for example, must accommodate 3.00 D to image an infinitely distant object on the retina. A young patient (e.g., 12 years old) will generally be able to accommodate 3.00 D, but doing so may result in asthenopia (i.e., eyestrain) and/or other symptoms such as intermittent blur (Fig. 8-7A). Focusing on near objects will require additional accommodation and may be more difficult and uncomfortable.

A 12-year-old

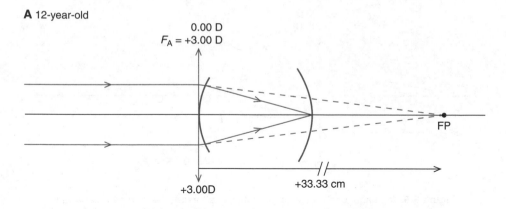

B 70-year-old

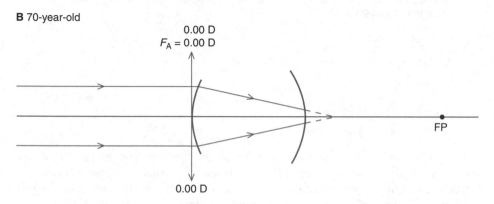

Figure 8-7. A. When viewing a distant object, a 12-year-old uncorrected 3.00 hyperopic child can accommodate the 3.00 D required to focus the image on the retina. The patient may, however, manifest symptoms of asthenopia and/or intermittent blur. **B.** A 75-year-old uncorrected hyperope does not have the ability to accommodate. Therefore the retinal image is out of focus.

As the patient ages and the amplitude of accommodation progressively decreases, the symptoms will become more pronounced, with the uncorrected patient initially not able to see clearly at near and ultimately not able to see clearly at distance (Fig. 8-7B).

NEAR POINT OF ACCOMMODATION

The advantage of uncorrected myopia for viewing near objects can be nicely illustrated by determining how near an object can be to the eye and still be imaged clearly on the retina—the so-called **near point of accommodation (NPA)**.

Consider three 50-year-old patients. Each has an amplitude of accommodation of 2.00 D. One patient has emmetropia, another has 2.00 D of uncorrected myopia, and the third has 2.00 D of uncorrected hyperopia (all measured in the corneal plane). Determine the NPA for each patient.

First consider the emmetropic eye (Fig. 8-8A). The amplitude of accommodation is 2.00 D and the far-point vergence is zero (i.e., the far point is at infinity). From the vergence relationship for accommodation, we have

$$F_{FP} = L + F_A$$

$$0.00 = L + 2.00$$

$$L = -2.00 \text{ D}$$

When the eye is maximally accommodated, objects located as close as 50.00 cm (100/–2.00 D = –50.00 cm) in front of the cornea can be imaged on the retina (i.e., the NPA is 50.00 cm). An object that is closer than 50.00 cm, however, cannot be imaged on the retina because the eye does not have sufficient accommodative power. For instance, for an object located 40.00 cm from this eye to be imaged on the retina, the eye would need to accommodate 2.50 D. Since the eye has only 2.00 D of accommodation, the image is blurred.

Now, let's determine the NPA for the uncorrected 2.00 D myopic eye (Fig. 8-8B). The maximum amount of accommodation is the same as it is for the emmetropic eye (2.00 D), but the far-point vergence is –2.00 D. Therefore,

$$F_{FP} = L + F_A$$

$$-2.00 = L + 2.00$$

$$L = -4.00 \text{ D}$$

For this uncorrected myopic eye, the NPA is 25.00 cm: objects located as close as 25.00 cm anterior to the eye can be imaged on the retina. For the emmetropic eye, an object at 25.00 cm will be out of focus. The uncorrected myopic eye is better able to focus near objects than the emmetropic eye.

Now it's time to look at a 2.00 D uncorrected hyperopic eye that also has an amplitude of accommodation of 2.00 D. Substituting in the vergence relationship for accommodation, we have

$$F_{FP} = L + F_A$$

$$+2.00 = L + 2.00$$

$$L = 0.00 \text{ D}$$

The NPA is at infinity (100/0.00 D = ∞); consequently, when this hyperopic patient is uncorrected, any object closer than optical infinity will be out of focus (Fig. 8-8C). With the same amplitude of accommodation, an emmetrope has an NPA of 50.00 cm and an uncorrected 2.00 D myope has an NPA of 25.00 cm. The uncorrected myope has an advantage when viewing near objects, whereas the

A

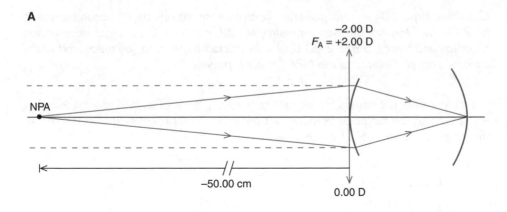

B

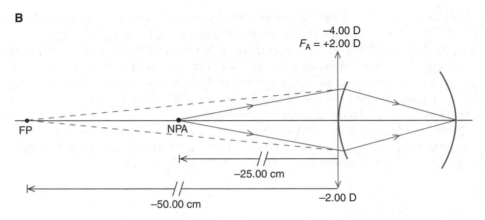

C

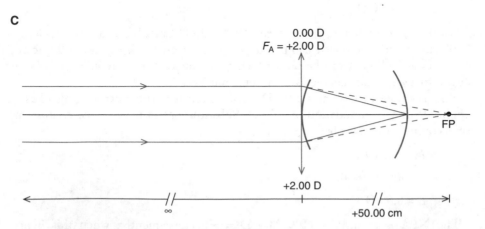

Figure 8-8. A. For an emmetropic eye that has an amplitude of accommodation of 2.00 D, the near point of accommodation (NPA) is 50.00 cm. **B.** For an uncorrected 2.00 D myopic with the same amplitude, the NPA is 25.00 cm. **C.** A 2.00 D uncorrected hyperopic eye with the same amplitude has an NPA at infinity.

uncorrected hyperope suffers a disadvantage. [When corrected with contact lenses, all three patients will have the same NPA (50.00 cm) since each has a corneal far-point vergence of 0.00 D.]

ACCOMMODATION WHEN AMETROPIA IS CORRECTED WITH SPECTACLES

Ametropia can be corrected in the plane of the cornea (with, for example, contact lenses, laser procedures, or orthokeratology) or in the spectacle plane. The amount of accommodation that is required to image a near object on the retina depends on whether the ametropic correction is in the plane of the cornea or in the spectacle plane.

First consider the case of a myopic patient who is fully corrected with a –5.00 D contact lens. How much accommodation is required to image an object located 10.00 cm anterior to the cornea onto the retina?

Recall that when an eye is corrected with a contact lens, the required accommodation is equal (and opposite) to the near stimulus vergence. In this example, the required accommodation is 10.00 D (which is equal to the accommodation required by an emmetropic eye for the same near stimulus vergence).

The patient needs spectacles (vertex distance of 15 mm) to use for those times when she is not wearing her contact lenses. What should be the power of the spectacle lenses? When wearing the spectacles, how much accommodation is required to see clearly an object that is located 10.00 cm anterior to the cornea?

In Chapter 7, we learned how to perform calculations involving lens power effectivity. You should confirm that at the spectacle plane of 15 mm, the required spectacle lens has a power of –5.41 D. (The focal length is 200 – 15 mm = 185 mm.)

As shown in Figure 8-9, the object is located 85.00 mm in front of the –5.41 D spectacle lens. The resulting image vergence is

$$L' = L + F$$

$$L' = \left[\frac{(1000)(1.000)}{-85.00 \text{ mm}}\right] + (-5.41 \text{ D})$$

$$L' = -17.17 \text{ D}$$

The vergence leaving the spectacle lens is –17.17 D, but because the lens is 15 mm anterior to the cornea, this is not the vergence at the eye. To calculate the vergence at the eye, we must first locate the image formed by the spectacle lens.

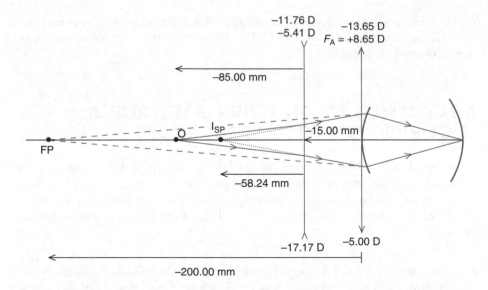

Figure 8-9. Accommodation required when a 5.00 myopic eye (as measured at the front surface of the eye) is corrected with a −5.41 D spectacle lens at a vertex distance of 15.00 mm. An object located 85.00 mm in front of the spectacle lens is imaged 58.24 mm in front of the spectacle lens. This virtual image (I_{SP}) serves as an object for the accommodative lens, F_A. It is 73.24 mm to the left of the accommodative lens, which images it at the far point of the eye (200 mm to the left of the accommodative lens).

This image is virtual and located to the left of the spectacle lens. The image distance is calculated as

$$L' = \frac{n'}{l'}$$

$$l' = \frac{(1000)(1.000)}{-17.17 \text{ D}}$$

$$l' = -58.24 \text{ mm}$$

The virtual image formed by the spectacle lens (labeled I_{SP} in Fig. 8-9) is located 58.24 mm to the left of the spectacle lens and 73.24 mm to the left of the cornea (58.24 mm + 15 mm = 73.24 mm). This image creates the near stimulus vergence. Following accommodation, the vergence must be −5.00 D (the corneal far-point vergence). The required accommodation is given by the vergence relationship for accommodation

$$F_{FP} = L + F_A$$

$$-5.00 \text{ D} = \left[\frac{(1000)(1.000)}{-73.24 \text{ mm}}\right] + F_A$$

$$F_A = +8.65 \text{ D}$$

TABLE 8-2. ACCOMMODATION TO VIEW AN OBJECT AT 10.00 CM

Correction in Corneal Plane	Prescription Worn	Required Accommodation*
−5.00 DS	−5.00 DS contact lens	+10.00 D
−5.00 DS	−5.41 DS spectacle lens	+8.65 D
+5.00 DS	+5.00 DS contact lens	+10.00 D
+5.00 DS	+4.65 DS spectacle lens	+11.42 D

*As measured in the corneal plane.

When properly corrected with spectacles, this myope must accommodate 8.65 D to see an object located at a distance of 10.00 cm from the cornea. The same myope must accommodate 10.00 D when wearing contact lenses (Table 8-2). This has important clinical implications. Consider a 45-year-old patient who wears spectacles and wishes to be fitted with contact lenses or to undergo a laser procedure. More accommodation is required when the correction is moved to the plane of cornea, and this may lead to asthenopia and/or near blur. It is important for the clinician to be aware that the accommodative demand increases when a spectacle-wearing myopic patient is corrected with contact lenses or a laser refractive procedure.[3]

Now, let's consider a patient with hyperopia. *When corrected with contact lenses, how much accommodation is required for a 5.00 D hyperopic patient to see clearly an object located at a distance of 10.00 cm from the cornea?*

As with a myopic eye corrected with contact lenses, or an emmetropic eye, the required accommodation is equal in magnitude to the near stimulus vergence, 10.00 D.

How much accommodation is required when this hyperopic patient wears her spectacles? Assume a vertex distance of 15 mm.

Applying the principles of lens effectivity, you should verify that the spectacle lens must have a power of +4.65 D. (The focal length is 200 + 15 mm = 215 mm). As can be seen in Figure 8-10, the object vergence at the spectacle lens plane is −11.76 D, resulting in an image vergence of −7.11 D. The virtual image (labeled I_{SP} in Fig. 8-10), which serves as the object for the accommodation lens, is located

---

3. To minimize near symptoms, one eye of a bilateral presbyopic myopic patient is sometimes undercorrected (i.e., the eye remains slightly myopic after it has been fitted with a contact lens or following a laser procedure). The undercorrected eye is used to view near objects, and the fellow eye, which is typically fully corrected, is used to view distant objects. This type of correction is referred to as **monovision**.

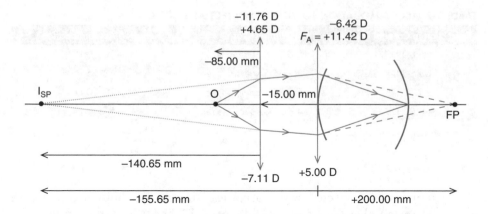

Figure 8-10. Accommodation required when a 5.00 hyperopic eye (as measured at the front surface of the eye) is corrected with a +4.65 D spectacle lens at a vertex distance of 15.00 mm. An object located 85.00 mm in front of the spectacle lens is imaged 140.65 mm in front of the spectacle lens. This virtual image (I_{SP}) serves as an object for the accommodative lens, F_A. It is 155.65 mm to the left of the accommodative lens, which images it at the far point of the eye (200 cm to the right of the front surface of the eye).

140.65 mm to the left of the corrective lens and 155.65 mm to the left of the accommodative plane. To determine the required amount of accommodation, we use the vergence relationship for accommodation as follows:

$$F_{FP} = L + F_A$$

$$+5.00 \text{ D} = \left[\frac{(1000)(1.000)}{-155.65 \text{ mm}}\right] + F_A$$

$$F_A = +11.42 \text{ D}$$

Compare these results with those obtained with a myopic eye. Whereas the myopic eye's accommodation decreases when going from contact lenses to spectacles, the hyperopic eye's accommodation increases. The results of these calculations are summarized in Table 8-2.

How is this information clinically relevant? Suppose that your 47-year-old patient, who is corrected with +6.50 DS contact lenses that provide her with satisfactory distance and near vision, wishes to obtain a pair of spectacles. You correct for lens effectivity (vertex distance of 15 mm) and prescribe +6.00 DS spectacle lens. After receiving her new spectacles, your patient calls to let you know that she is not comfortable reading with them. What's happening here? Because of the patient's age, she may not have sufficient accommodative reserves to provide the increased accommodation necessitated by the change from contact lenses to spectacles.

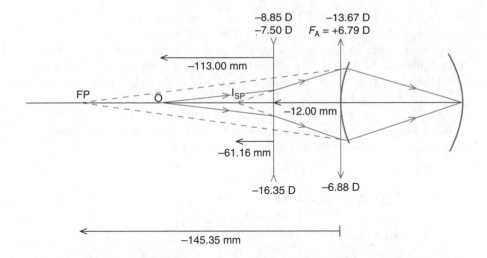

Figure 8-11. Accommodation required when a 7.50 D myopic eye (as measured in the spectacle plane) views an object located 125.00 mm from the eye. The spectacle lens forms a virtual image (I_{SP}) 61.16 mm in front of the lens and 73.16 mm anterior to the eye. This image serves as an object for the accommodative lens, which must image it at the eye's far point (145.35 mm to the left of the eye's surface).

Before we leave this section, let's try a problem where we are given the refractive error as measured in the spectacle, not corneal, plane. *An eye is corrected with a –7.50 D spectacle lens. How much accommodation is required when viewing an object 12.50 cm from the eye while wearing the spectacle lens? Assume a vertex distance of 12.0 mm.*

First, we'll locate the image formed by the spectacle lens. As illustrated in Figure 8-11, the object is located 113.00 mm (125.00 – 12.00 mm = 113.00 mm) to the left of the spectacle lens, giving us

$$L' = L + F$$

$$L' = \left[\frac{(1000)(1.000)}{-113.00 \text{ mm}}\right] + (-7.50 \text{ D})$$

$$L' = -16.35 \text{ D}$$

$$L' = \frac{n'}{l'}$$

$$l' = \frac{(1000)(1.000)}{-16.35 \text{ D}}$$

$$l' = -61.16 \text{ mm}$$

Since this image is located 61.16 mm to the left of the spectacle lens, it is located 73.16 mm (61.16 + 12.00 mm = 73.16 mm) to the left of the cornea.

Next, we must determine the correction required in the plane of the cornea. For a vertex distance of 12.0 mm, a −7.50 D spectacle lens has an effective power of −6.88 D at the cornea. [We've already learned how to do this, but in case you need a quick refresher: the focal length of corrective lens required in the plane of the cornea is (1000/−7.5 D) + (−12 mm) = −145.33 mm; the power is 1000/−145.33 mm = −6.88 D.] This is the far-point vergence as measured at the cornea. Substituting into the vergence relationship for accommodation, we have

$$F_{FP} = L + F_A$$

$$-6.88 \text{ D} = \left[\frac{(1000)(1.000)}{-73.16 \text{ mm}} \right] + F_A$$

$$F_A = +6.79 \text{ D}$$

When wearing a spectacle lens, the eye must accommodate 6.79 D. This is less than the 8.00 D of accommodation that would be required if the eye were corrected with a contact lens.

CORRECTION OF PRESBYOPIA

In developed countries, presbyopia, with its symptoms of near blur and asthenopia, probably prompts more visits to the eye doctor than any other single diagnosis. Fortunately, it's usually straightforward to alleviate presbyopic symptoms by prescribing plus power beyond that required for distance viewing. This can take the form of single-vision lenses for near use or multifocal lenses that allow correction of the patient's distance refractive error when viewing through the upper portion of the lens and correction of presbyopia when looking through the lower portion. The difference between the distance and near powers of a multifocal lens is referred to as the add. If, for example, a 5.00 D myopic patient requires a +2.00 D add, the near portion of the correction has a total power of −3.00 D.

How is the patient's add determined? It is based on the patient's amplitude of accommodation, which is defined as the total amount the patient can accommodate. In general, the goal is to prescribe an add that requires the patient to use one-half of her accommodative amplitude at her habitual reading distance. So, if a 50-year patient has an amplitude of accommodation of 2.50 D, the goal is to allow the patient to use only half of this amplitude (+1.25 D) when reading. By doing so, the patient's range of clear vision at near will be centered *dioptrically* at her reading distance. That is, she can relax her accommodation 1.25 D to see objects further away than her reading distance or accommodate another 1.25 D to see nearer objects.

Near-point testing to determine the patient's add is often performed in the phoropter. The doctor selects a tentative add based on the patient's age and history, and the patient is then instructed to view near-threshold letters located at her near working distance (when looking through her combined distance correction and the tentative add). In probably the most commonly used method, the doctor first adds plus power to the tentative add until the patient reports that the letters are blurred. This occurs when the patient has fully relaxed his accommodation. The maximum amount of plus that the patient accepts is equal to the amount of accommodation used to resolve the letters through the tentative add and is called the **negative relative accommodation (NRA)**.

Next, minus power is added until the letters are blurred. (The patient is still looking through the same tentative add.) The letters become blurred when the patient can no longer accommodate—she has used all of her accommodation. The maximum amount of minus that the patient accepts is the **positive relative accommodation (PRA)**. The total of the NRA and PRA is equal to the patient's amplitude of accommodation (as measured in the spectacle plane).[4] The doctor then adjusts the tentative add so that the NRA and PRA are equal.

Let's consider an example. A 50-year-old myopic patient requires −3.00 D spectacles for distance use. When he reads with his distance glasses, he suffers asthenopia and near blur. Although he can take his glasses off to see near objects, it is inconvenient. The patient does most of his near work at a distance of 40 cm from the spectacle plane. How would the bifocal add be determined? What is the patient's range of clear vision when looking through the add?

We'll use the NRA/PRA method to determine the add. Assume that based on the patient's age and history, the doctor selects a tentative of add of +1.25 D. Through this tentative add (and the distance prescription), the patient is instructed to view near-threshold text at his reading distance of 40.00 cm. Suppose that the NRA is +1.25 D and the PRA is −1.75 D. In this case, the amplitude of accommodation is 3.00 D. To dioptrically center the near reading range at 40 cm, the add would need to be adjusted to +1.00 D. When this is done, the NRA and PRA are expected to be, respectively, +1.50 D and −1.50 D. The patient is in now using one-half of her accommodation to view at 40 cm.

We've used the term "dioptrically centered" without yet fully explaining what is meant by it. In the current example, the patient's near vision is dioptrically centered at −2.50 D, which corresponds to a distance of −40 cm (i.e., 100/−40 cm = 2.50 D). The patient can accommodate an additional 1.50 D or relax his accommodation 1.50 D, making the dioptric range of clear vision from −4.00 D to −1.00 D. While this dioptric range is centered at −2.50 D, it is important to note that it is not linearly centered at −40 cm; the linear range of clear vision is from −25 cm (i.e., 100/−4.00 D = −25 cm) to −100 cm (i.e., 100/−1.00 D = −100 cm).[5]

---

4. In previous examples in this chapter, we've specified accommodation with respect to the corneal plane, but when determining the NRA and PRA, we test the patient in the spectacle plane. A person with emmetropia must accommodate 4.00 D, as measured in the corneal plane, to see an object located at 25.00 cm. The effective power of a +4.00 D lens at a vertex distance of 15.00 mm is about +4.25 D.

5. As we will learn in Chapter 11, depth of field increases the range of clear vision.

SUMMARY

For near objects to be clearly imaged on the retina, the eye's crystalline lens must increase in power, a process referred to as accommodation. Through accommodation, near objects are imaged at the far point of the eye, which is conjugate with the retina.

Since the uncorrected myopic eye is too strong for its length, it requires less accommodation to image near objects on the retina than the uncorrected hyperopic eye, which is too weak for its length. The manner in which ametropia is corrected determines the amount of accommodation that is required. A myopic eye corrected with a spectacle lens accommodates less than when corrected with a contact lens. In comparison, the hyperopic eye must accommodate more when corrected with a spectacle lens compared to a contact lens.

As we age, there is a decrease in the accommodative amplitude. When this produces symptoms such as near blur and asthenopia, the condition is referred to as presbyopia. Presbyopia may be corrected by adding plus power to the distance prescription.

KEY FORMULA

Vergence relationship for accommodation:

$$F_{FP} = L + F_A$$

SELF-ASSESSMENT PROBLEMS[6]

1. An object is located 10.00 cm anterior to the cornea of a 3.50 D myopic eye (as measured at the corneal plane). How much accommodation is required to image the object on the retina if (a) the eye is uncorrected? (b) corrected with a contact lens? and (c) corrected with a spectacle lens? Assume a vertex distance of 15.00 mm.

2. A 5.00 D hyperopic eye (as measured in the corneal plane) views an object that is located 10.00 cm anterior to his cornea. If the eye is wearing a +4.00 DS contact lens, how much accommodation is required to image the object on the retina?

3. An emmetropic presbyopic patient has a range of clear vision from infinity to 20.00 cm from the cornea. What power contact lens would allow the patient to see clearly at 15.00 cm when using only one-half of her total amplitude of accommodation? (Ignore depth of field.)

4. To image an object located 33.00 cm anterior to its cornea onto its retina, an uncorrected 2.00 D hyperopic eye (as measured in the corneal plane) exerts one-half of its accommodative amplitude. What is the eye's amplitude of accommodation? (Ignore depth of field.)

---

6. In solving these problems, assume that accommodation is measured in the corneal plane.

5. A hyperopic eye is corrected with a +6.00 D lens in the spectacle plane. Assuming a vertex distance of 12.00 mm, how much accommodation is required to view an object at a distance of 10.00 cm from the eye?

6. A 5.00 D myopic eye, as measured in the spectacle plane, views an object through a −4.00 D lens held 10 cm in front of the eye. If the object is 15 cm from the eye, how much accommodation is required for the image to be focused on the retina? (Assume that the spectacle plane is at a distance of 1.3 cm.)

7. A 45-year-old patient is corrected in each eye with a −6.00 D spectacle lens. The patient undergoes LASIK, which fully corrects the ametropia. (a) Prior to the surgery, how much accommodation is required to view an object located 20.00 cm from the cornea when the patient is wearing his spectacles? (Assume a vertex distance of 15.0 mm.) (b) Following the surgery, how much accommodation is required to view this same object? (c) What is the clinical significance of this finding?

Cylindrical Lenses and the Correction of Astigmatism

Myopia and hyperopia are spherical refractive errors that can be corrected with spherical lenses. By definition, a spherical lens has the same refractive power in all of its meridians. As can be seen in Figure 9-1A, whether it is measured across the horizontal meridian, the vertical meridian, or anywhere between these two meridians, the dioptric power is the same.

Another common form of ametropia, **astigmatism**, is not a spherical refractive error and cannot be fully corrected with a spherical lens, but it can be corrected with what is referred to as a **cylindrical lens**. A cylindrical lens has maximum dioptric power in one meridian, while the orthogonal (perpendicular) meridian has no dioptric power.

Figure 9-1B shows a glass cylinder fashioned as a cylindrical lens. This cylinder is positioned so that its axis is horizontal. Along the **axis**, the cylinder is flat—the radius of curvature is infinity—and there is no dioptric power. Perpendicular to the axis is the **power meridian** in which the cylinder has its maximum power (+5.00 D).

LENS CROSSES

It can be very useful to represent lens power on a lens cross,[1] such as in Figure 9-2A, which shows a lens cross for a +5.00 D spherical lens. Although only two meridians are shown, all others also have a power of +5.00 D.

When drawing a lens cross for a cylindrical lens, powers in the power meridian and axis are indicated. For the lens in Figure 9-2B, the horizontal meridian (which

---

1. A lens cross is sometimes referred to as an optical cross.

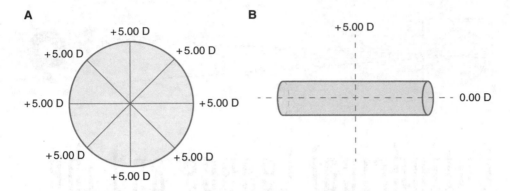

Figure 9-1. A. A spherical lens has the same power in all of its meridians. **B.** This glass cylinder has no power along the horizontal meridian and +5.00 D of power along the vertical meridian.

is the axis of the lens) has a power of zero and is designated by the term **plano** (abbreviated as **pl**). The vertical meridian (the power meridian) is labeled +5.00 D.

Spherical and cylindrical powers are often combined to form what is called a **spherocylindrical** lens. Figure 9-3 illustrates a +2.00 D spherical lens combined with a cylindrical lens that has a maximum power of +5.00 D and a horizontal axis. The resultant spherocylindrical lens has +7.00 D of power in the vertical meridian and +2.00 D of power in the horizontal meridian. This lens has two secondary focal points: +14.29 cm for the vertical meridian and +50.00 cm for the horizontal meridian.[2]

A spherocylindrical lens's meridians of maximum power and minimum power, which are perpendicular to each other, are called the **major**, or **principal**,

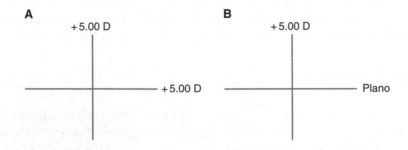

Figure 9-2. A. A lens cross for a +5.00 D spherical lens. **B.** A lens cross for a cylindrical lens shows powers in the power and axis meridians.

---

2. The lens also has two *primary* focal points.

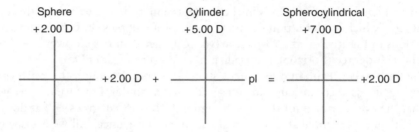

Figure 9-3. A spherocylindrical lens can be conceptualized as a combination of spherical and cylindrical lenses.

meridians. For the lens in Figure 9-3, the meridians whose powers are +7.00 D and +2.00 (i.e., the vertical and horizontal meridians) are the principal meridians.

By convention, lens meridians are specified in degrees measured *counterclockwise* from the 3 o'clock position when facing the patient (Fig. 9-4).[3] Horizontal is always labeled as 180 degrees, not 0 degrees. Using this convention, the power of the

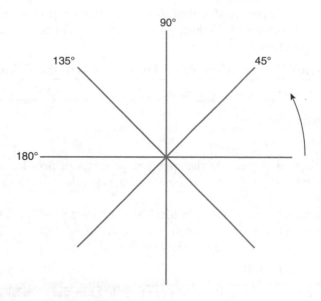

Figure 9-4. Lens meridians (and axes) are specified in degrees as measured counterclockwise from the 3 o'clock position. The horizontal should be referred to as 180 degrees—not 0.00 degrees.

---

3. When the doctor is facing a patient, the 3 o'clock position is on the doctor's right.

cylindrical lens in Figure 9-2B is in the 90 degree meridian. The axis of this cylindrical lens, which by definition has no power, is 180 degrees. For the spherocylindrical lens in Figure 9-3, the 90-degree (vertical) meridian has a power of +7.00 D and the 180-degree (horizontal) meridian has a power of +2.00 D.

The term **axis meridian** often elicits student groans. Although this term can be confusing, it's used commonly and you should understand it. For instance, we could say that the axis meridian for the lens in Figure 9-2B is 180 degrees. What does this mean? It's not as complicated as it might seem at first glance. All we are saying is that the cylinder axis is in the 180-degree meridian (i.e., there is no power along the 180 meridian).

LENS FORMULAE/PRESCRIPTIONS

When writing a prescription (formula) for a correcting (ophthalmic) lens, it is important to avoid any confusion or ambiguity. For a spherical prescription, this can be done by designating the lens power as diopters sphere, which is abbreviated as *DS*. Sometimes the abbreviations *S* or *Sph*, which stand for sphere, are used. Using these conventions, the spherical lens in Figure 9-1 may be labeled as +5.00 DS, +5.00 S, or +5.00 Sph.

The formula for a cylindrical lens gives (1) the spherical power (which is zero), (2) the cylindrical power, and (3) the axis of the cylinder. For the cylindrical lens in Figure 9-2, these values are:

Spherical Power	Cylindrical Power	Axis of the Cylinder
pl	+5.00	180

The lens formula is written as

pl +5.00 × 180

This formula tells us that (1) the spherical power is plano (i.e., zero), (2) the cylindrical power is +5.00 D, and (3) the axis of the cylinder (i.e., the axis meridian) is 180 degrees.

Now, let's return to the spherocylindrical lens in Figure 9-3. Think of this lens as the combination of a spherical lens that has a power of +2.00 DS and a cylindrical lens whose power is pl +5.00 × 180. The lens formula is

+2.00 +5.00 × 180

This spherocylindrical lens has a power of +7.00 D in the vertical meridian and +2.00 D in the horizontal meridian. Since the cylindrical power is positive, this is referred to as the **plus-cylinder form** of the lens prescription. The major meridians are at 90 and 180 degrees.

In Figure 9-5, we have redrawn the lens cross. On the top of the figure, we have broken down the lens into a +2.00 sphere and pl +5.00 × 180 cylinder (just as we did in Fig. 9-3). On the bottom, we show that there is another way to conceptualize

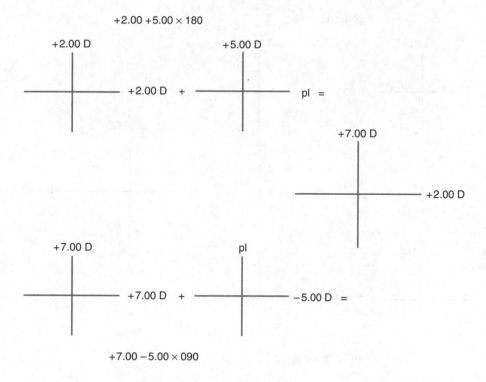

Figure 9-5. The spherocylindrical lens on the right can be conceptualized as a combination of the two lenses on the top (plus-cylinder form) or the two on the bottom (minus-cylinder form).

this lens. The lens can be considered as a combination of lenses whose powers are +7.00 DS and pl −5.00 × 090. When conceptualized this way the lens formula is

$$+7.00 -5.00 \times 090$$

This is the **minus-cylinder form** of the prescription (because the cylinder power is minus).

It is important to keep in mind that the plus- and minus-cylinder forms of the prescription represent the same lens—namely, the spherocylindrical lens in Figure 9-5, which has a power of +7.00 D in the vertical meridian and +2.00 D in the horizontal meridian. **Plus-cylinder and minus-cylinder prescription forms are simply different ways of designating the same lens**. Figure 9-6 provides another example. Traditionally, optometrists tend to write lens prescriptions in minus-cylinder form, while ophthalmologists tend to write lens prescriptions in plus-cylinder form.

Students and practitioners alike often confuse the written form of a prescription with the shape of the lens. With respect to shape, one of the surfaces of a sphero-cylindrical lens is toric, meaning that it has two curves that are at right angles to

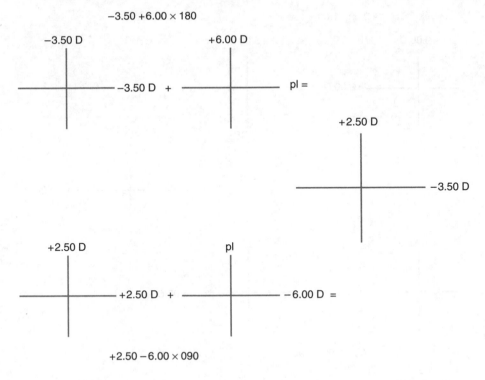

Figure 9-6. The plus-cylinder (top) and minus-cylinder forms of the spherocylindrical lens (on the right).

each other. Another way of saying this is that a spherocylindrical lens can be ground with the cylinder on either the front or the back surface. The former is called a front toric lens, while the latter is a back toric lenses. Almost all modern lenses are back toric designs. It is sometimes *mistakenly* assumed that a plus cylinder prescription is synonymous with a front toric design and a minus cylinder prescription is synonymous with a back toric design. This is not the case!

It's relatively straightforward to transpose a plus-cylinder prescription into minus-cylinder form and vice versa. The rule is as follows:

- Keeping the signs, add the sphere and cylindrical powers to arrive at the new sphere value.
- Reverse the cylinder sign to arrive at the new cylinder power.
- Change the axis by 90 degrees to arrive at the new axis. (Remember that the axis is never greater than 180 degrees.)

You should confirm that these rules apply to the examples in Figures 9-5 and 9-6.

IMAGE FORMATION: POINT SOURCES

Image formation by spherocylindrical lenses can be confusing. With some persistence, however, you will be able to master this material. The concepts associated with image formation by spherocylindrical lenses have myriad clinical applications, and it is worth the effort to understand them.

A spherocylindrical lens does not have the same power in all meridians. For instance, the lens in Figure 9-7 has a power of +5.00 D in the vertical meridian and a power of +3.00 D in the horizontal meridian. A point source (the object) located at infinity is not imaged by this lens in a single plane. The image that is formed by the vertical meridian is focused in one plane and the image focused by the horizontal meridian is located in another plane. (In contrast, a spherical lens forms an image in one plane.)

For the purposes of our discussion, we assume that the light rays emitted by a point source diverge either vertically or horizontally.[4] First, consider the

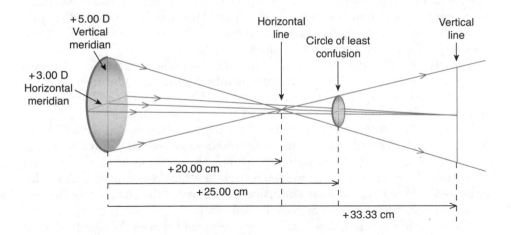

Figure 9-7. A spherocylindrical lens (which has a power of +5.00 D in the vertical meridian and +3.00 D in the horizontal meridian) focuses an infinitely distant point source in two image planes. Centered dioptrically between these two planes is the circle of least confusion.

---

4. Hold your hands together so that the fingers and palm of one hand are touching the fingers and palm of the other. Rotate your hands so that your palms are horizontal. Next, keep your wrists together while separating your hands. Think of your fingers as vertically diverging light rays. To mimic horizontally diverging light rays, again hold your hands together so that the fingers and palm of one hand are touching the fingers and palm of the other, but rotate your palms so that they are vertical. When your palms are now separated (but your wrists are together), you can think of your fingers as horizontally diverging light rays.

image formed by the vertical meridian, which is the stronger meridian of the lens in Figure 9-7. The vertical meridian focuses those rays that diverge vertically from the object. These rays, which are said to have vertical divergence, are focused by the vertical meridian at a plane that is +20.00 cm from the lens. If you place a screen at this plane, however, there is not a point, but a thin horizontal line.

The upper and lower edges of the horizontal image are sharply focused because they are formed by the in-focus vertical meridian. If the lens were spherical, we would have a point image, but because the horizontal meridian has a different power, the image is smeared in a horizontal dimension (and has blurred left and right edges). Think of it this way: the horizontal dimension of the line occurs because the horizontally diverging object rays are focused by the horizontal meridian at +33.33 cm, not at 20.00 cm. At 20.00 cm, these rays have not yet been focused and are smeared horizontally to create the horizontal dimension of the line.

Now, consider the image formed by the weaker horizontal meridian. This meridian focuses rays that have horizontal divergence—rays that diverge from the object in the horizontal dimension. These horizontally diverging rays are focused by the horizontal meridian at a plane that is +33.33 cm from the lens. At this plane, however, there is not a point, but a vertical line. This is because the vertically diverging object rays are focused by the vertical meridian at +20.00 cm; beyond +20.00 cm, these rays diverge, forming a vertical smear at +33.33 cm.

The left and right edges of the vertical line are in sharp focus at 33.33 cm because they are formed by the in-focus horizontal meridian of the lens. The image is, however, smeared in the vertical dimension (and has blurred upper and lower edges) because the vertical meridian is in focus at 20.00 cm, not 33.33 cm.

If we place a screen directly behind the lens and move it away from the lens, we will see that a horizontal line is found at +20.00 cm and a vertical line at +33.33 cm. The interval that is bracketed by these two images is referred to as the **interval of Sturm**. Within this interval, we find a circle at +25.00 cm from the lens. This circle—called the **circle of least confusion**—is located at the plane where the vertical and horizontal meridians are equally defocused.

The circle of least confusion is *not* linearly centered between the planes of focus of the two principal meridians, but *centered dioptrically*. For the point source located infinitely far from the lens in Figure 9-7, the *dioptric* location of the circle of least confusion—the dioptric midpoint between the horizontal and vertical image planes—is calculated as follows:

$$+3.00 \text{ D} + \frac{5.00 \text{ D} - 3.00 \text{ D}}{2} = +4.00 \text{ D}$$

Therefore, the *linear* location is

$$\frac{(100)(1.00)}{+4.00 \text{ D}} = +25.00 \text{ cm}$$

The circle of least confusion is located 25.00 cm to the right of the lens.

IMAGE FORMATION: EXTENDED SOURCES

An extended source, such as a cross, is formed by an infinite number of point sources. In Figure 9-8, we show the images formed by major meridians of a +3.00 +2.00 × 180 lens (the same lens as in Figure 9-7) when a cross is located at infinity.

First, consider the horizontal line of the object. The points that constitute this line emit light rays with vertical and horizontal divergence. Those rays with vertical divergence are focused by the vertical meridian to form a horizontal line at +20.00 cm. The upper and lower edges of this line are sharply focused by the vertical meridian. In comparison, the left and right edges are blurred. Horizontally diverging rays emitted by the horizontal line, which are focused at +33.33 cm, form these fuzzy edges.

The vertical line of the object is also made up of points that emit vertically and horizontally diverging rays. Those rays with horizontal divergence are focused by the horizontal meridian at +33.33 cm to form a vertical line with sharply focused left and right edges. In comparison, the upper and lower borders of this line are blurred. The vertical line's vertically diverging rays, which are focused by the vertical meridian at 20.00 cm, form these blurred upper and lower edges.

Where is the circle of least confusion for this extended object? As is the case for a point source, the circle is dioptrically centered between the focused images of the two principal meridians (i.e., the point where the *defocus* of the vertical meridian is equal to the *defocus* of the horizontal meridian). For the example in Figure 9-8, this corresponds to a linear distance of 25.00 cm.

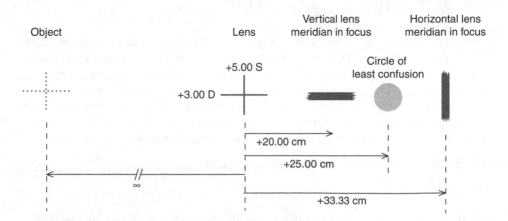

Figure 9-8. A spherocylindrical lens focuses an extended object in two planes. See the text for further details.

Let's summarize a few key points on image formation by spherocylindrical lenses. Assume that the major meridians of the lens are at 90 and 180 degrees and that both have positive power.

- You can think of a point source (i.e., point object) as emitting light rays that diverge vertically and horizontally. Vertically diverging object rays are focused by the vertical meridian of the lens and horizontally diverging object rays are focused by the horizontal meridian.
- For a point source, a horizontal line is formed where the vertical meridian is in focus. The upper and lower edges of the line are in sharp focus because they are formed by the in-focus vertical meridian, while the smeared horizontal extent of the line is due the out-of-focus horizontal meridian.
- For a point source, a vertical line is formed where the horizontal meridian is in focus. The left and right edges of the line are sharply focused by the in-focus horizontal meridian, while the smeared vertical extent of the line is due to the out-of-focus vertical meridian.
- The vertically diverging rays emitted by a horizontal line (object) are focused by the vertical meridian as a horizontal line.
- The horizontally diverging rays emitted by a vertical line are focused by the horizontal meridian as a vertical line.

This material can be difficult to conceptualize, so don't fret if you are finding it confusing. Take a break—maybe sleep on it—and then reread the sections on image formation for point and extended sources. It will click!

POWER IN AN OBLIQUE MERIDIAN OF A CYLINDRICAL LENS

Consider the pl −5.00 × 030 lens in Figure 9-9. The power in the axis meridian (30 degrees) is zero, and the power in the 120-degree meridian (the power meridian) is −5.00 D. What about the other meridians of the lens? Can we determine the power at, say, 180 degrees? The answer is "yes," we can calculate a power for this meridian, but it may not be all that meaningful of a value. Let's first do the calculation and then I'll tell you the problem with it. The formula to determine the power in the oblique meridian of a cylindrical lens—sometimes called the **sine-squared formula**—is as follows:

$$F_\theta = (F_{cyl})\sin^2\theta$$

where F_θ is the power in the oblique meridian, F_{cyl} is the power in the power meridian, and θ is the angle between the oblique meridian and the cylinder axis.

In the current example, the oblique meridian is 180 degrees. We are asked to determine the power in this meridian. The power in the power meridian

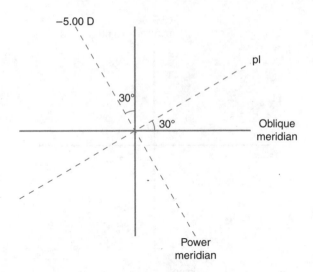

Figure 9-9. Lens cross used to determine power in the 180 degree (horizontal) meridian of a pl − 5.00 × 030 lens.

is −5.00 D and the angle between the oblique meridian (180 degrees) and the cylinder axis (30 degrees) is 30 degrees. Substituting into the sine-squared formula, we have

$$F_\theta = (-5.00 \text{ D})\sin^2(30)$$

$$F_\theta = -1.25 \text{ D}$$

According to our calculations, the power in the 180-degree meridian is −1.25 D.

The problem with specifying the power in an oblique meridian is that there is no focal point for the 180 meridian. There is a focal point for the power meridian (at −20 cm), but not for the 180-degree meridian. Nonetheless, the power value obtained with the sine-squared formula may sometimes be useful when making calculations that deal with lens thickness and the prism in decentered cylindrical lenses. For more details see Brooks and Borish (2007).

Let's look at a spherocylindrical lens. What's the power in the vertical meridian of a +2.00 − 3.00 × 160 lens?

To solve this problem, we need to treat the spherical (+2.00 DS) and cylindrical components (pl − 3.00 × 160) of the lens separately. While the sphere has the same power (+2.00 D) in all meridians, including the vertical meridian, this is not the case for the cylinder. Figure 9-10 shows the lens cross we use to determine the power in the cylinder's vertical meridian. Since the oblique meridian (90 degrees)

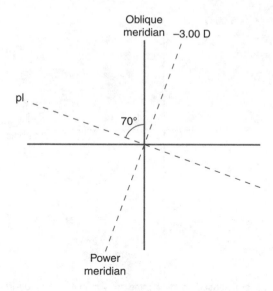

Figure 9-10. Lens cross used to determine power in the vertical meridian of a pl −3.00 × 160 lens.

and axis meridian (160 degrees) make an angle 70 degrees, this value is substituted into the sine-squared formula as follows:

$$F_\theta = (F_{cyl})\sin^2\theta$$

$$F_\theta = (-3.00 \text{ D})\sin^2(70)$$

$$F_\theta = -2.65 \text{ D}$$

Combining −2.65 D with the +2.00 D sphere component gives a power of −0.65 D in the vertical meridian.

ASTIGMATISM: DEFINITIONS AND CLASSIFICATIONS

The power of an *astigmatic eye* is spherocylindrical.[5] In **regular astigmatism**, the two major meridians of the eye are perpendicular to each other. This form of astigmatism, which is by far the more common form, can be corrected with spherocylindrical spectacle lenses. **Irregular astigmatism** is generally secondary to

---

5. The Greek term *stigma* refers to a point or small mark. Astigmatism is a refractive error that results in an image that is not a point.

trauma, surgery, or a disease process. The major meridians are not perpendicular to each other, and the eye cannot be fully corrected with a spherocylindrical spectacle lens.

When an astigmatic eye views an infinitely distant point source, an image is formed by each of the eye's two principal meridians, just as in Figure 9-7. As illustrated in Figure 9-11, regular astigmatism is classified according to the locations of the images with respect to the retina (with accommodation relaxed). The tilted image line is intended to depict the horizontal line formed by the vertical meridian,

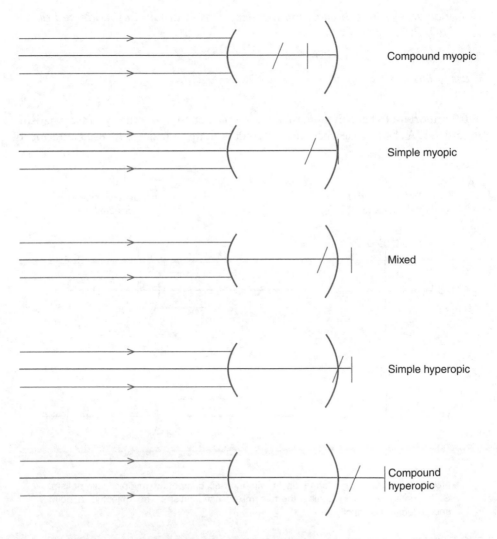

Compound myopic

Simple myopic

Mixed

Simple hyperopic

Compound hyperopic

Figure 9-11. Image formation in the various forms of ocular astigmatism when the object is a point source located at infinity.

while the vertical image line is formed by the horizontal meridian. This same convention is used for subsequent figures in this chapter.

In addition to classifying astigmatism based on image location, it is common to classify it according to the meridian of the eye that has the most converging refracting power. If the vertical meridian *of the eye*[6] is strongest, we call the astigmatism **with-the-rule**. **Against-the-rule** astigmatism is present when the horizontal meridian *of the eye* is strongest. When the strongest meridian *of the eye* is neither vertical nor horizontal but falls somewhere between the two (e.g., 135 ± 15 degrees or 45 ± 15 degrees), we have **oblique astigmatism**.

Consider an eye that requires the following lens to obtain best corrected acuity (e.g., 20/20):

$$-5.00 - 2.00 \times 180$$

Classify this eye's astigmatism.

It's important to keep in mind that this lens is used to *correct* the eye's astigmatism. Figure 9-12A shows that when uncorrected, both meridians are focused anterior to

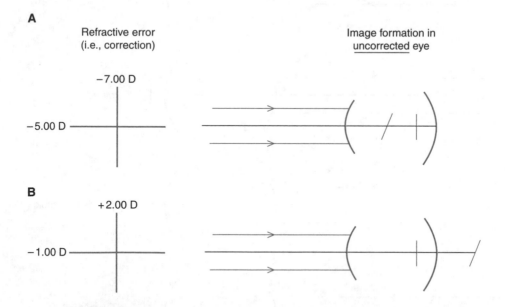

Figure 9-12. A. Image formation in with-the-rule compound myopic astigmatism. **B.** Image formation in against-the-rule mixed astigmatism. The object is a point source located at infinity.

---

6. The phrase "of the eye" is italicized to emphasize that we are referring to the power of the eye, not the correction.

the retina, making the astigmatism compound myopic. The vertical meridian of the eye, which is focused closest to the reduced eye's front surface, requires a correction of −7.00 D and the horizontal meridian requires −5.00 D. Since the eye's vertical meridian has the most converging power (requiring more minus power to correct it), the patient has with-the-rule compound myopic astigmatism.

Let's take another example. Classify the astigmatism when the following corrective lens is required:

$$+2.00 - 3.00 \times 090$$

As can be seen in Figure 9-12B, the correction for the vertical meridian is +2.00 D and for the horizontal meridian it is −1.00 D. This is a case of mixed astigmatism because one meridian (the horizontal meridian) is focused anterior to the retina and the other (the vertical meridian) posterior to the retina. Since the eye's horizontal meridian has the greater converging power, the eye has against-the-rule mixed astigmatism.

It is not uncommon for young human infants to have 0.75 to 2.00 D of astigmatism (Howland et al., 1978). The nature of the astigmatism is apparently related to race, with Chinese infants tending to have with-the-rule astigmatism and Caucasian infants tending to have against-the-rule (Thorn et al., 1987). This astigmatism generally decreases by school age (Gwiazda et al., 1984).

In the fifth decade of life and beyond, the astigmatism is apt to become more against-the-rule. This is apparently due to aging of the crystalline lens.

JACKSON CROSSED-CYLINDER TEST

The Jackson crossed-cylinder (JCC) test is the most commonly used subjective clinical procedure to determine the amount of a patient's astigmatism. The power in one of the principal meridians of a crossed cylinder is equal and opposite to the power in the other principal meridian. In the example in Figure 9-13A, one meridian has a power of +0.25 D and the other meridian has a power of −0.25 D. The crossed cylinder is mounted in front of the patient's eye such that it can be quickly flipped between the position where the vertical meridian has plus power and the position where it has minus power.

How can a crossed cylinder be used to determine the amount of astigmatism? Figure 9-13B shows the position of the retinal images formed when an emmetropic eye views a distant object through a crossed cylinder. The circle of least confusion is located on the retina. When the crossed cylinder is flipped, the sequence of the line images reverses but the amount of astigmatism remains the same (i.e., 0.50 D) and the circle of least confusion remains on the retina. Consequently, the patient will report that the image is more-or-less equally blurred for both positions of the crossed cylinder.

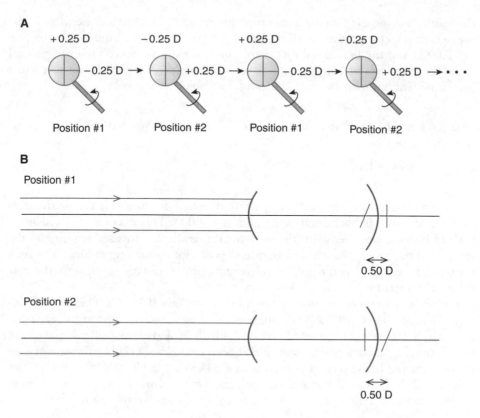

Figure 9-13. A. A crossed-cylinder lens can be flipped quickly between position 1 where the vertical meridian has positive power and position 2 where the vertical meridian has negative power. To flip the crossed cylinder, the stem is twisted between the thumb and forefinger. **B.** Image formation in an emmetropic eye when looking through a crossed-cylinder lens in position 1 (top) and position 2 (bottom). Note that the sequence of the (line) images reverses when the crossed cylinder is flipped.

Now consider the astigmatic eye in Figure 9-14A, which has a power of +62.00 D in the vertical meridian and +58.00 D in the horizontal meridian (with-the-rule mixed astigmatism). When a crossed-cylinder lens is placed in front of the eye so that its positive meridian is oriented vertically (Fig. 9-14B, position 1), the amount of astigmatism is 4.50 D (i.e., 62.25 − 57.75 D = 4.50 D). When the crossed cylinder is flipped so that its vertical meridian now has negative power (Fig. 9-14, position 2), the amount of astigmatism is 3.50 D (i.e., 61.75 − 58.25 D = 3.50 D). Given a choice, the patient will say that position 2 is clearer than position 1 because the amount of astigmatism is less in position 2. The doctor can then add minus power to the vertical meridian (i.e., minus cylinder with an *axis* of 180 degrees) and repeat the crossed-cylinder test until the patient reports that the image is equally blurred in positions 1 and 2, as is the case in Figure 9-14C (at

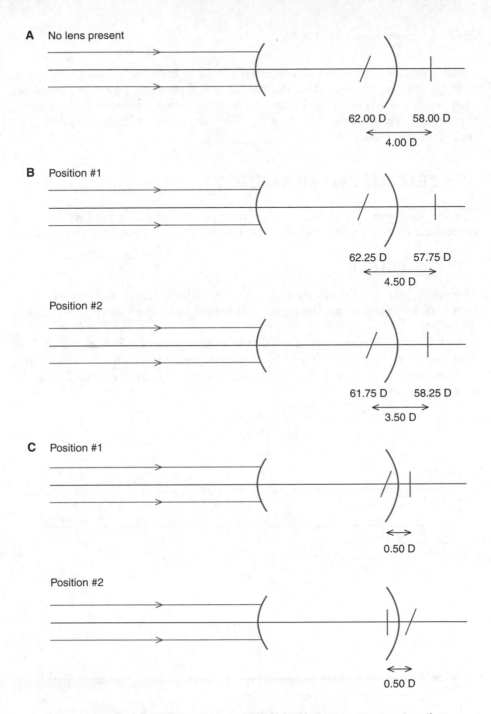

Figure 9-14. A. Image formation in uncorrected with-the-rule mixed astigmatism. **B.** Image formation when this eye views through a crossed-cylinder lens positioned so that the vertical meridian is positive (position 1) and negative (position 2). **C.** After correction of the astigmatism (and any spherical refractive error), the amount of image blur is the same whether the crossed-cylinder lens is in position 1 or 2. Note that the sequence of the (line) images reverses when the crossed cylinder is flipped.

which point the astigmatism is corrected). If the examiner adds too much minus power to the vertical meridian, the patient will report that position 1 is clearer than position 2. (As discussed in the next section, during crossed-cylinder testing, the doctor adds plus spherical power to keep the circle of least confusion positioned on the retina.)

SPHERICAL EQUIVALENCY

The eye in Figure 9-15A has simple hyperopic with-the-rule astigmatism. The vertical meridian has a power of 60.00 D and is focused on the retina. The prescription is

pl + 5.00 × 090

Suppose that you do not have access to cylindrical lenses and can prescribe only a spherical lens to correct this eye. What would be the best spherical lens to prescribe?

To minimize the amount of distortion that the patient experiences, the circle of least confusion should generally be located on the retina. This can be accomplished by prescribing a **spherical equivalent** lens whose power is determined with the following relationship:

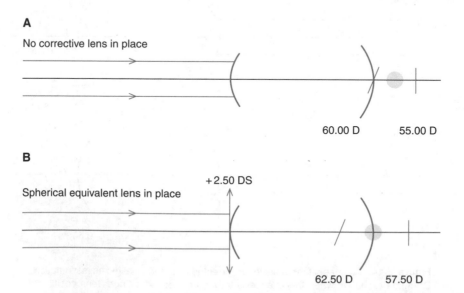

Figure 9-15. When a spherical equivalent lens centers the interval of Sturm dioptically (not linearly) on the retina, the circle of least confusion falls upon the retina. In this figure, the spherical equivalent is +2.50 D.

$$\text{spherical equivalent} = \text{spherical correction} + \frac{\text{cylindrical correction}}{2}$$

For the current example, the spherical equivalent power is determined as follows:

$$\text{spherical equivalent} = 0.00\ D + \frac{5.00\ D}{2}$$

$$\text{spherical equivalent} = +2.50\ D$$

As can be seen in Figure 9-15B, the +2.50 DS lens causes the interval of Sturm to be *dioptrically* centered on the retina, which means that the circle of least confusion is located in the plane of the retina.

For the JCC test to produce accurate results, the circle of least confusion must remain on the retina. For each −0.50 of cylindrical power that is added during the testing procedure, the spherical equivalent power changes by −0.25 DS. That is, if the circle of least confusion initially falls on the retina, the addition of −0.50 D of cylinder will cause the circle to fall −0.25 DS behind the retina. To keep the circle of least confusion on the retina during the JCC test, the examiner can increase the spherical power by +0.25 DS each time he or she increases the cylinder power by −0.50 D.

WHAT DOES A PERSON WITH ASTIGMATISM SEE?

A patient with uncorrected myopia or uncompensated hyperopia experiences uniform blur—the image is equally blurred in all orientations: up and down, left and right, and every orientation in between. For example, when an uncorrected myope views a distant point source, he or she perceives a blurred circle (Fig. 9-16A).

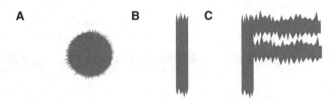

Figure 9-16. **A.** Appearance of a point source to a patient with uncorrected myopia. **B.** Appearance of a point source to a patient with uncorrected with-the-rule simple myopic astigmatism. **C.** Appearance of the optotype **F** to a patient with uncorrected with-the-rule simple myopic astigmatism.

What does a patient with the following uncorrected astigmatic correction perceive when viewing a distant point source?

pl −2.00 × 180

This patient has simple with-the-rule myopic astigmatism. The horizontal meridian of the eye requires no correction. This meridian focuses the point source's horizontally diverging rays onto the retina. Now consider the stronger vertical meridian. This meridian focuses the vertically diverging rays in front of the retina. These rays subsequently diverge vertically and fall upon the retina to form a smeared vertical line. The patient reports seeing a vertical line with sharp lateral edges and fuzzy vertical edges (Fig. 9-16B).

Suppose we ask this patient to read a visual acuity chart. *Are there any optotypes that the patient will find particularly difficult to resolve?*

Consider the **F** optotype. To correctly identify this optotype (which is an extended object), it is necessary to resolve the gap between the two horizontal line segments. The vertically diverging light rays emanating from the horizontal lines are focused by the vertical meridian *in front* of the retina. The rays then diverge vertically to form vertically smeared horizontal lines on the retina. As illustrated in Figure 9-16C, this makes the gap difficult to see; consequently, patients with myopic with-the-rule astigmatism often mistakenly identify an **F** as a **P**.

This astigmatic patient will have less difficulty identifying the vertical line in the **F**. The horizontal meridian of the eye focuses the vertical line on the retina. Its lateral edges will be sharply focused, but its vertical edges will be smeared because they are formed by the out-of-focus vertical meridian.

SUMMARY

Image formation by a converging spherocylindrical lens can be understood by visualizing a point source as producing light rays that have vertical and horizontal divergence. Rays with vertical divergence are focused by the vertical lens meridian as a horizontal line, while rays with horizontal vergence are focused as a vertical line by the horizontal lens meridian. For an extended source, such as a cross, the vertical lens meridian focuses the horizontal line and the horizontal lens meridian focuses the vertical line.

An astigmatic eye has two focal points separated by the interval of Sturm. Dioptrically centered between these two points is the circle of least confusion. The Jackson crossed cylinder test is commonly used to determine the amount of ocular astigmatism.

KEY FORMULAE

Power in an oblique meridian (sine-squared formula):

$F_\theta = (F_{cyl})\sin^2\theta$

Spherical equivalent:

$$\text{spherical equivalent} = \text{spherical correction} + \frac{\text{cylindrical correction}}{2}$$

REFERENCES

Brooks, CW, Borish IM. *System for Ophthalmic Dispensing*, 3rd ed. St. Louis: Butterworth-Heinemann, 2007.

Gwiazda J, Scheiman M, Mohindra I, Held R. Astigmatism in infants: changes in axis and amount from birth to six years. *Invest Ophthalmol Vis Sci.* 1984;25:88.

Howland HC, Atkinson J, Braddick O, French J. Infant astigmatism measured by photorefraction. *Science.* 1978;202:331–333.

Thorn F, Held R, Fang L. Orthogonal astigmatic axis in Chinese and Caucasian infants. *Invest Ophthalmol Vis Sci.* 1987;28:191.

SELF-ASSESSMENT PROBLEMS

1. A lens has the following formula: −1.00 − 1.00 × 090. (a) Draw a lens cross. (b) Write the prescription in plus-cylinder form.

2. A point source is located 50.00 cm in front of the following lens: +4.00 +2.00 × 180. (a) Which meridian is focused closest to the lens? (b) Is the line that is focused closest to the lens horizontal or vertical? (c) How far is this image located from the lens? (d) Answer questions *b* and *c* for the image that is located furthest from the lens (i.e., the image formed by the other meridian of the lens). (e) Calculate the linear extent of the interval of Sturm. (f) Locate the circle of least confusion.

3. A point source is located 25.00 cm in front of the following lens: +5.00 +2.00 × 090. Answer all the questions asked for Problem 2.

4. A cross is located 40.00 cm in front of the following lens: +6.00 − 1.00 × 090. (a) At what distance is the horizontal line imaged? (b) At what distance is the vertical line imaged? (c) What is the linear extent of the interval of Sturm? (d) Locate the circle of least confusion.

5. A cross is situated 40.00 cm in front of the following lens: +6.00 − 2.00 × 180. Answer all the questions asked for Problem 4.

6. Consider the following lens crosses:

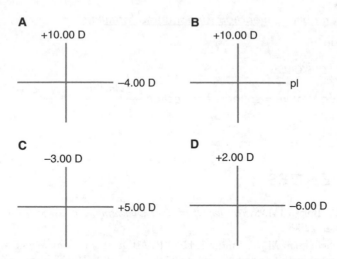

Write the lens prescriptions in both minus-cylinder and plus-cylinder forms.

7. A patient's refractive error is corrected with the following lens: +4.00 − 3.00 × 090. (a) Is the patient's astigmatism with-the-rule or against-the-rule? What form of astigmatism does the patient have (see Fig. 9-11)? (b) Answer the same questions for a prescription of −1.00 − 2.00 × 180. (c) Answer the same questions for a prescription of −3.00 + 4.00 × 090.

8. A patient with uncorrected compound myopic astigmatism compares a grating consisting of horizontal bars to a grating consisting of vertical bars. The gratings are located 20 feet from the patient. He reports that both gratings appear blurry, with the vertical bars appearing clearer than the horizontal bars. Is the patient more likely to have with-the-rule or against-the-rule myopic astigmatism? Explain your answer.

9. What is the power in the (a) vertical meridian of a (a) +5.00 − 3.00 × 030 lens? (b) horizontal meridian of a +4.50 + 2.75 × 110 lens?

10. A patient's prescription is −4.00 − 1.50 × 170. What power spherical lens do you expect would provide this patient with the best visual acuity?

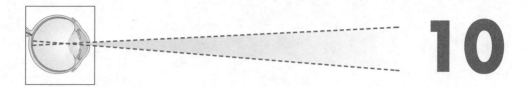

Prisms

Prisms are useful clinical tools that refract light, changing the direction of incident light rays. Since their surfaces are flat, prisms do not affect the vergence of light. Another way of saying this is that prisms have no dioptric power—they do not affect light vergence and do not have focal points.

Figure 10-1 shows the refraction that occurs at the two surfaces of a prism. Refraction at each surface is predictable from Snell's law. For this prism (and all ophthalmic prisms), **light rays are deviated toward the base of the prism**. When an observer views an object through the prism, he or she sees an image of the object. **The image is displaced toward the apex of the prism.** Images formed by prisms are virtual.

Those readers who have used a lensometer to neutralize prism know that the lensometer target is displaced toward the prism base, not the apex as you'd expect from our discussion so far. What's happening here? A Keplerian telescope, which produces an inverted image (Chapter 12), is incorporated into the lensometer design, resulting in the target being displaced toward the prism base.

THICK AND THIN PRISMS

The refractive properties of a prism are dependent on its index of refraction and apical angle, α. As the refractive index or apical angle increases, the angle of deviation, d, also increases. The apical angle and angle of deviation are labeled in Figure 10-1.

Based on the size of their apical angle, prisms may be divided into thick and thin prisms, with thin prisms having an apical angle less than 10 degrees. For thick prisms, the angle of deviation is dependent on the angle that light rays strike the prism (i.e., the angle of incidence). This can be seen in Figure 10-2, which shows the prism deviation angle for a thick prism as a function of the angle of incidence. Note that the prism has a minimum angle of deviation given by the trough in the curve.

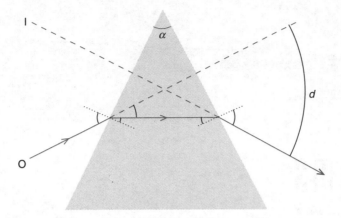

Figure 10-1. A light ray originating from an object, O, is refracted by a prism so that it appears to come from a virtual image, I. The angle that the ray emerging from the prism is deviated from its original course is the angle of deviation, *d.* The prism's apical angle is labeled α.

Figure 10-2 also shows the behavior of a thin prism. Although the angle of deviation for the thin prism is dependent on the angle of incidence, it is less so than for the thick prism, and there is a fairly broad range of incident angles over which it remains relatively stable. That is, the extensive trough for the thin prism shows that the minimum angle of deviation holds true for a wide range of incident angles. For a thin prism in air, the relationship between the minimum angle of deviation, the apical angle, and index of refraction is as follows:

$$d_{min} = \alpha(n - 1)$$

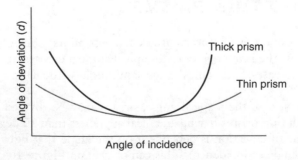

Figure 10-2. This schematic representation shows the angle of deviation for a thick and thin prism as a function of the angle of incidence. As discussed in the text, the angle of incidence is less important for thin prisms.

where d_{min} is the minimum angle of deviation in degrees, α is the apical angle, and n is the prism's index of refraction.

It's important to note that this formula gives the minimum angle of deviation in degrees. Clinical prisms are almost always quantified in prism diopters—our next topic—not degrees.

PRISM DIOPTERS

Figure 10-3A shows a light ray, which after refraction by a prism falls upon a screen that is at a distance of 1.00 m. The light ray is deviated 1.00 cm from its original destination. **A prism that deviates a light ray 1.00 cm at a distance of 1.00 m is said to have a power of 1 *prism diopter*** (abbreviated pd or denoted by the symbol Δ). If the ray is deviated 5.00 cm at a distance of 1.00 m, the power of the prism is 5^Δ. Likewise, a prism that deviates a ray of light 8.00 cm at a distance of 400.00 cm has a power of 2^Δ. More formally, we can determine the power of a prism in prism diopters with the following formula, where the distances are defined in Figure 10-3B:

$$P = (100)\left(\frac{x}{y}\right)$$

where P is the prism power in diopters, x is the distance that the light ray is deviated, and y is the distance at which the deviation is measured.

Since $\tan(d) = x/y$, it follows that

$$P = (100)\tan(d)$$

where d is the angle of deviation in degrees.

Let's look at an example. *What is the power of a prism, in prism diopters, that deviates a light ray 6.00 cm at a distance of 500.00 cm?* Substituting, we have

$$P = (100)\left(\frac{x}{y}\right)$$

$$P = (100)\left(\frac{6 \text{ cm}}{500 \text{ cm}}\right)$$

$$P = 1.2^\Delta$$

PRISMATIC EFFECTS OF LENSES

Not only does a spherical lens have dioptric power, meaning that it changes the vergence of incident light rays, it also has prismatic power because it changes the direction of the incident rays. Consider Figure 10-4, which shows lenses that are

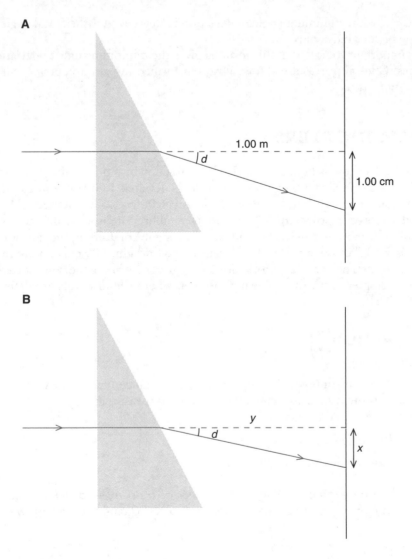

Figure 10-3. A. A prism that deviates a light ray 1.00 cm at a distance of 1.00 m has a power of 1 prism diopter. **B.** Distances pertinent to defining a prism diopter. See the text for further details.

dissected into segments. The central segments have no prismatic power because their surfaces are approximately parallel to each other. Adjacent segments do not have parallel surfaces, giving them prismatic power. Compare these to the prism segments furthest from the lens center. Here, the sides of the segments form larger angles with each other, giving them more prism power than those closer to the center.

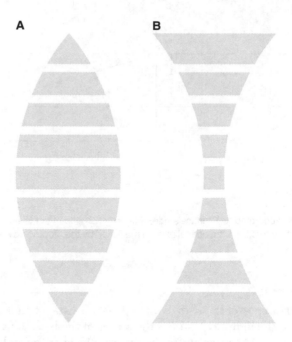

Figure 10-4. Lenses can be conceptualized as a series of prisms whose prismatic power increases from the center of the lens to its edge.

To summarize, when looking along the optical axis of a lens, there is no prism power, but when viewing through more peripheral regions of the lens, there is. Prismatic power increases as the distance from the optical axis increases. This has important clinical implications in management of conditions that require the prescription of prisms.

Figure 10-5 shows how the prismatic power of a lens can be quantified. A light ray, originating from infinity, strikes a lens at a distance c from its optical axis. After refraction, this ray intersects the optical axis at the secondary focal point of the lens, F'. Let's assume the distances are in centimeters. From the definition of a prism diopter, we have

$$P = (100)\left(\frac{c}{f'}\right)$$

Since the distances are in centimeters, we know that

$$f' = \frac{100}{F}$$

Substituting, we have

$$P = (c)(F)$$

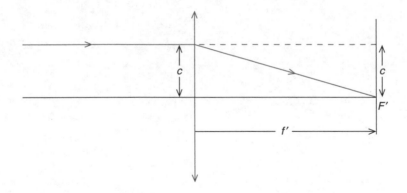

Figure 10-5. According to Prentice's rule, a lens's prismatic effect is equal to the distance in centimeters from the optical axis (*c*) multiplied by the dioptric power of the lens.

where *P* is the prism power in prism diopters,[1] *c* is the distance **in centimeters** from the optical axis to the light ray, and *F* is the power of the lens. This handy relationship, which allows us to calculate the prismatic power of an ophthalmic lens, is referred to as **Prentice's rule**.

Figure 10-6 illustrates two important manifestations of Prentice's rule. First, as the distance from the optical axis (*c*) increases, the prismatic power increases. Second, as the power of the lens increases (*F*), the prismatic power increases.

Let's look at some examples. *A +6.00 D ophthalmic lens is decentered so that its optical center is 3.0 mm nasal to a patient's pupil. What is the prismatic effect at the point where the patient is looking through the lens?*

Figure 10-7A schematically illustrates this from the perspective of looking down onto the patient's head. Applying Prentice's rule, we have

$$P = (c)(F)$$

$$P = (0.3 \text{ cm})(6.00 \text{ D})$$

$$P = 1.8^{\Delta}$$

Since the base of the prism is facing nasally, the prismatic power is designated as 1.8^{Δ} *base in.* If a +6.00 DS the lens were decentered so that its optical center was 3.00 mm temporal to a patient's pupil, as in Figure 10-7B, the prismatic power would now be 1.8^{Δ} *base out* because the prism base is temporal.

---

1. The symbol "Δ" is sometimes used instead of "*P*."

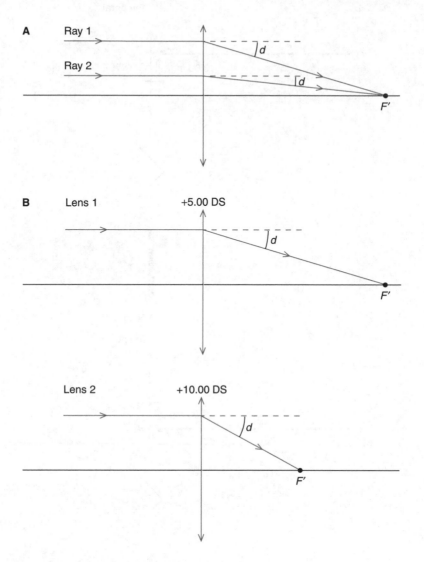

Figure 10-6. A. The prismatic power of a lens increases as the distance from the optical axis increases (i.e., ray 1 is more deviated than ray 2). **B.** A lens's prismatic power increases as the dioptric power of the lens increases.

A spectacle lens may be decentered vertically as well as horizontally. *When a −7.00 DS lens is decentered 3 mm nasally and 2 mm inferiorly with respect to the patient's pupil, how much prism is induced?*

Figure 10-8 shows this how this would look when facing the patient. The dashed lines represent the lens cross. The patient is looking through a point 3 mm temporal

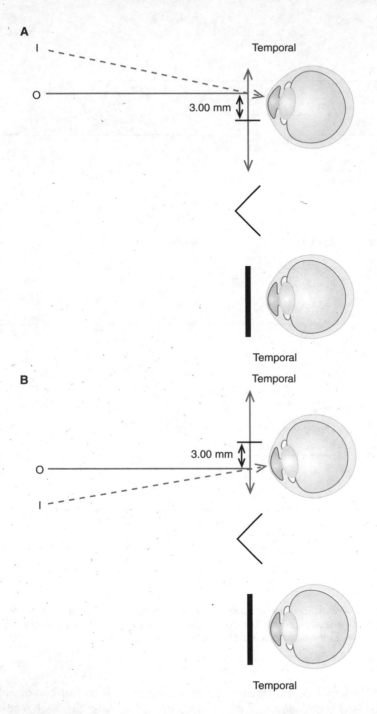

Figure 10-7. A. Prentice's rule can be used to calculate the amount of base-in prism induced when a patient looks through a point that is 3.00 mm temporal to the optical axis (short horizontal line) of a +6.00 DS lens. You are looking-down upon the patient's head. The left eye is occluded. **B.** Likewise, Prentice's rule can be used to calculate the amount of base-out prism induced when a patient looks through a point that is 3.00 mm nasal to the optical axis (short horizontal line) of a +6.00 DS lens.

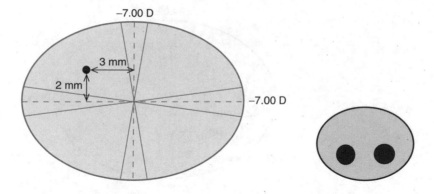

Figure 10-8. When a patient looks through a –7.00 DS right lens at a point 3 mm temporal and 2 mm superior to the optical center, she experiences 2.1 pd base out and 1.4 pd base up. The black dot within the lens represents the patient's pupil.

and 2 mm superior to the lens's optical center. Applying Prentice's rule to the horizontal decentration gives us

$$P = (c)(F)$$
$$P = (0.3 \text{ cm})(7.00 \text{ D})$$
$$P = 2.1^\Delta$$

Is the prism base in or base out? As can be seen in Figure 10-8, which schematically illustrates the prismatic components of the lens, the prism is base out.

The vertical prismatic effect is determined in a similar manner. Substituting into Prentice's rule, we have

$$P = (c)(F)$$
$$P = (0.2 \text{ cm})(7.00 \text{ D})$$
$$P = 1.4^\Delta$$

As can be seen in Figure 10-8, the induced prism is base up.

A decentered cylindrical lens may also induce prism. *A patient views through a pl + 4.00 × 180 lens that has been decentered 3.5 mm temporal and 2.5 mm superior to the pupil. How much prism does she experience?*

Figure 10-9 illustrates this case. Let's first consider the horizontal decentration. To use Prentice's rule, we need to know the dioptric power of the lens's horizontal meridian. Since this is the axis meridian, there is no lens power! As a result, there is no horizontal prism power.

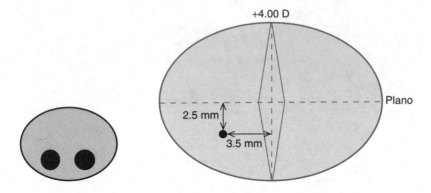

Figure 10-9. When a patient looks through a pl + 4.00 × 180 left lens at a point 3.5 mm nasal and 2.5 mm inferior to the optical center, she experiences 1.0 pd base up. Since the lens has no power in its horizontal meridian, it does not induce horizontal prism. The black dot within the lens represents the patient's pupil.

For the vertical meridian, the decentration is 2.5 mm, giving us a prismatic power of

$$P = (c)(F)$$

$$P = (0.25 \text{ cm})(4.00 \text{ D})$$

$$P = 1.0^{\Delta}$$

As can be seen in Figure 10-9, the prism is base up.

Things become more complicated when we need to determine the prismatic effect caused by decentration of a cylindrical or spherocylindrical lens that has an oblique axis. Brooks and Borish (2007) provides a nice treatment of this material.

CLINICAL APPLICATIONS

Prisms have important clinical applications because of their ability to displace an image in a direction that benefits visual function and/or comfort. The most common applications are in disorders of binocular vision, such as strabismus or heterophoria. Consider a patient with exophoria, a tendency for the eyes to turn outward. Figure 10-10 shows how prisms may be used to treat this patient. Prescription of base-in prisms allows the patient to view a distant object while her eyes are turned in an outward position. This may provide relief for asthenopic and other symptoms.

Prism is commonly incorporated in spectacle prescriptions by decentering the optical center of a lens relative to the patient's pupil. What do we mean by this? When a patient's pupils are aligned with the optical centers of their lenses, the patient does not experience prism power. If, however, the lens optical centers

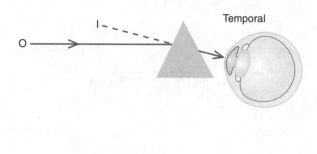

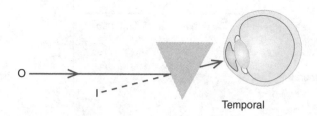

Figure 10-10. When viewing a distant object (O), this patient's eyes have a tendency to turn outward (i.e., the patient has exophoria). The base-in prisms form images (I) temporal to the object, thereby allowing the patient's eyes to turn outward while viewing the object. (You are looking down upon the patient's head.)

are not aligned with the pupils, the patient may experience prism. By intentionally decentering a lens so that its optical center does not coincide with the patient's pupil, we can create therapeutic prism. The amount of prism is given by Prentice's rule.

*Let's look at an example. A patient with exophoria is fully corrected with −4.00 DS lenses in the spectacle plane. The patient requires a prescription of 2.0Δ base-in prism to alleviate symptoms of asthenopia. The distance between her pupils, commonly called the **interpupillary distance (abbreviated as IPD)**, is 60.0 mm. How can we use decentration to incorporate the prism correction into the −4.00 D lenses?*

It is common clinical practice to divide equally the prismatic correction between the two eyes. Where must the patient look through a −4.00 DS lens to obtain 1.0Δ base-in? Prentice's rule is very helpful in cases like this.

$$P = (c)(F)$$

$$1^\Delta = (c)(4.00 \text{ D})$$

$$c = 0.25 \text{ cm} \quad \text{or} \quad 2.5 \text{ mm}$$

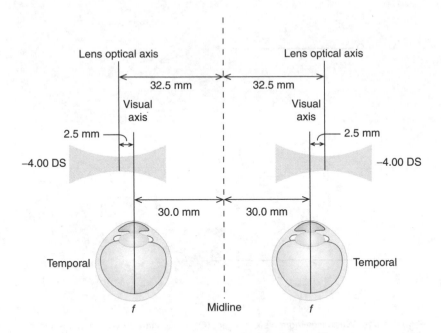

Figure 10-11. A total of 2.0$^\Delta$ base-in prism will be included in a spectacle prescription of −4.00 DS OU if each eye looks through a point 2.5 mm nasal to the optical axis. The visual axis intersects the fovea, *f*. (You are looking down upon the patient's head.)

If the lens is decentered 2.5 mm temporal to the patient's pupil, she experiences 1.0$^\Delta$ base-in. To obtain a total prismatic effect of 2.0$^\Delta$, the optical center of each lens must be decentered 2.5 mm temporally. As can be seen in Figure 10-11, this will occur if the optical centers of the two lenses are separated by a distance of 65 mm rather than the patient's IPD of 60 mm.

Prisms can be used to assist patients who manifest visual field defects. Because they are thin, light, and easily changed, **Fresnel prisms** are often used for this purpose. They come in a thin (on the order of 1 mm thick) flexible plastic sheet that can be cut to a customized size and applied to the patient's lenses. If the initial choice of prism power needs to be changed, the Fresnel prism can be removed easily and replaced by a prism of a more appropriate power. Figure 10-12 shows that the prismatic power is due to a series of small prism apexes contained in the sheet.

Consider a patient with right homonymous hemianopia.[2] Objects to the right of his fixation point are not visible unless he turns his eyes/head to the right. To see things far to the right, he would need to turn his eyes/head far in that direction. By prescribing a prism with its base pointed to the patient's right, objects located in the blind area are imaged to the left allowing the patient to see them with less movement of his eyes/head. As can be seen in Figure 10-13, Fresnel prisms can be

---

2. A patient with this condition is blind in the right visual fields of both eyes.

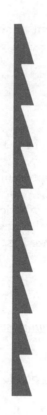

Figure 10-12. A Fresnel prism.

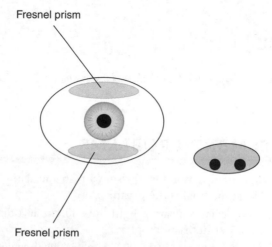

Figure 10-13. Fresnel prisms, positioned above and/or below the patient's line of sight, can be prescribed for visual field loss.

placed above and/or below the patient's line of sight so that the patient can look through prism as needed.

SUMMARY

For clinical applications, prism power is specified in prism diopters. By definition, a prism that deviates a ray of light 1 cm at a distance of 100 cm it is said to have a power of 1 prism diopter.

Spectacle lenses can have both dioptric and prism power. The prism power of a lens increases as the distance from the optical center increases. Prentice's rule can be used to calculate the prism power experienced by a patient when she is looking through a point other than the optical center of the lens. Prism power can be created in a patient's spectacles by decentering the lenses so that the optical centers do not coincide with the patient's pupils.

KEY FORMULAE

Minimum angle of deviation for a thin prism:

$$d_{min} = \alpha(n - 1)$$

Calculation of prism power in prism diopters:

$$P = (100)\left(\frac{x}{y}\right)$$

Prentice's rule:

$$P = (c)(F)$$

REFERENCE

Brooks CW, Borish IM. *System for Ophthalmic Dispensing*, 3rd. St. Louis: Butterworth-Heinemann, 2007.

SELF-ASSESSMENT PROBLEMS

1. The minimum angle of deviation for a prism with an apical angle of 8.00 degrees is 4.69 degrees. What material is the prism?

2. A crown glass prism deviates a ray of light by 4.00 cm at a distance of 5.00 m. What is the prism power in prism diopters?

3. A crown glass prism has a power of 15.00^Δ. At what distance will the prism deviate a light ray by 2.00 cm?

4. What is the prismatic power at a distance of 5.00 mm from the optical center of a +8.00 D plastic lens?

5. A crown glass lens has a power of –6.00 D. At what distance from the optical center is the prism power 2.00$^\Delta$?

6. How much prism is experienced when a +3.00 – 2.50 × 180 lens is decentered 4.00 mm nasally with respect to the pupil?

7. When a +2.00 – 4.00 × 090 lens is decentered 5.00 mm temporally and 3.00 mm superiorly with respect to the pupil, how much prism is experienced?

8. An object is located 13.00 cm in front of a thin 5.00$^\Delta$ polycarbonate prism. What is the vergence of the rays that emerge from the prism?

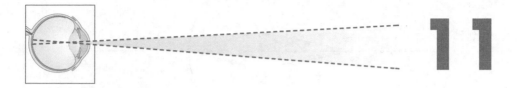

Depth of Field

An object that is conjugate with the retina is by definition focused on the retina. If the object is a point, then the image is a point. Figure 11-1A shows a myopic eye that has no ability to accommodate (i.e., the eye of a patient with **absolute presbyopia**). Point Y is imaged onto the retina at Y'. For an object that is farther from the eye—say at X—the image is focused anterior to the retina at X'. This object produces a blurred image on the retina that is called a **blur circle**. A similar effect occurs for an object at Z: the image is focused at Z' and a blur circle is formed on the retina. Figure 11-1B shows how these blur circles may appear to the observer.

The size of the blur circle depends on both the amount of defocus and the diameter of the pupil. As illustrated in Figure 11-2, as the focused image moves closer to the retina, the diameter of the blur circle decreases. Reducing the size of the pupil blocks peripheral rays, also reducing the size of the blur circle (Fig. 11-3).

BLUR CIRCLES, VISUAL ACUITY, AND PINHOLES

Visual acuity is measured by asking a patient to read optotypes, such as the letter **E**, presented on an eye chart. Optotypes are extended sources, meaning that they are composed of an infinite number of point sources. Figure 11-4A shows how the optotype **E** can thus be conceptualized.

Consider a patient with 1.00 D of uncorrected myopia who observes the optotype **E** on a visual acuity chart that is located 20 ft away (optical infinity). Since the eye is not focused for this distance, each of the point sources forms a blur circle on the retina—similar to what is depicted in Figure 11-4B—and the **E** appears blurry to the patient. Suppose we ask the myopic patient to view the eye chart through a small aperture (approximately 1 mm in diameter) referred to as a **pinhole**, which is smaller than her pupil.[1] As can be seen in Figure11-4C, this causes the diameters

---

1. When a patient looks through an aperture that has a diameter less than her pupil's, the aperture is sometimes referred to as an artificial pupil.

A

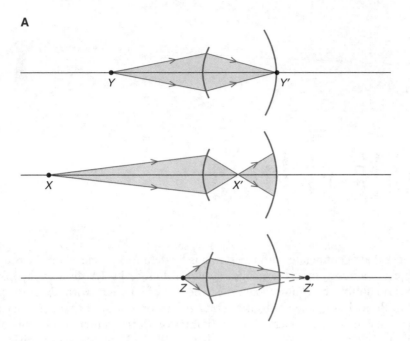

B
Retinal blur circle when the object is located at:

Figure 11-1. **A.** Point source *Y* is imaged on the retina, while point sources *X* and *Z* are out of focus and form blur circles on the retina. **B.** Appearance of a point source that is in focus (*Y*) and point sources that are out of focus (*X* and *Z*). Note that the object that is most out of focus (*X*) produces the largest blur circle.

of the blur circles that constitute the **E** to become smaller, making this and other optotypes on the acuity chart easier to resolve.

An isolated pinhole (or a cluster of pinholes) is an important clinical tool. Common pinhole configurations used in clinic are illustrated in Figure 11-5. When a patient's acuity is reduced due to optical blur, as in the case of ametropia, viewing though a pinhole will typically improve the visual acuity. Consider the patient who has a distance visual acuity of 20/40, but improves to 20/20 when viewing through a pinhole. In such a case, it is highly likely that the reduced visual acuity is due to a refractive error. If the pinhole does not improve visual acuity, we must suspect another etiology (such as disease or amblyopia).

As we age, our pupil becomes smaller. In elderly people, the pupil can be rather small—a condition referred to as **senile miosis**. There are some advantages to this

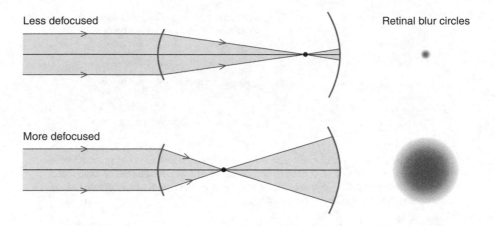

Figure 11-2. As the amount of defocus increases, the diameter of the retinal blur circle also increases.

condition. In uncorrected (or undercorrected) ametropia and presbyopia, the small pupil may improve visual acuity through the so-called pinhole effect.

While the smaller pupil may reduce the diameter of the blur circles, it also reduces the amount of light that reaches the retina. A reduction in retinal illumination may cause a reduction in visual acuity (for physiological, not optical reasons) that offsets

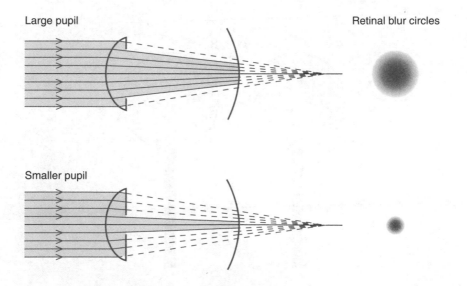

Figure 11-3. Decreasing the pupil diameter reduces the retinal blur circle diameter. The smaller pupil blocks peripheral light rays from reaching the retina, thereby decreasing the size of the blur circle.

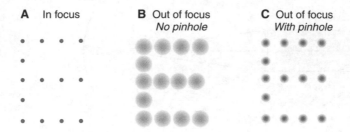

Figure 11-4. **A.** An optotype (or any extended object) is made up of point sources. **B.** If the point sources that constitute the optotype are defocused, the optotype itself appears defocused. **C.** A pinhole decreases the diameters of the blur circles, thereby increasing the resolvability of the optotype.

optical improvements due to the pinhole effect. Bright lighting conditions may help compensate for the reduction in retinal illumination caused by senile miosis.

DIFFRACTION CAUSED BY APERTURES

A small pupil can also limit visual acuity due to **diffraction**, a phenomenon that occurs when light passes by an opaque object such as the pupil. Under these circumstances, light does not behave as the laws of geometrical optics predict; rather, light seems to "bend" around corners. The left side of Figure 11-6A illustrates

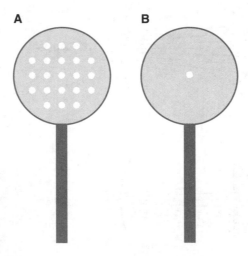

Figure 11-5. In the clinic, it is generally more efficient to use a cluster of pinholes (as in **A**) rather than have the patient search for a single pinhole (illustrated in **B**).

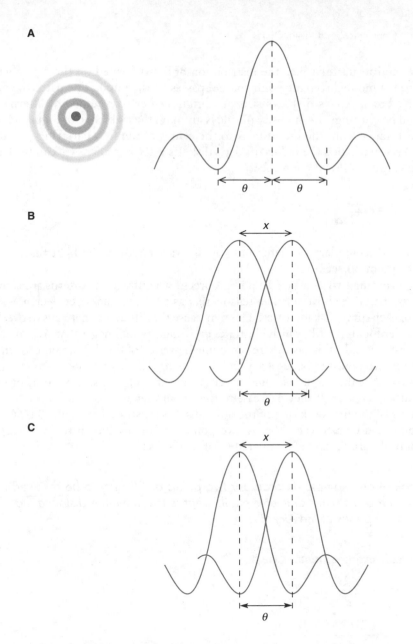

Figure 11-6. A. The diagram on the left shows the diffraction pattern formed on the retina when viewing through a small diameter aperture. To its right is an intensity profile of the diffraction pattern. Peaks represent bright areas and troughs represent dark areas. The distance from the center of the light peak to the first trough (dark ring) is often referred to as the radius of Airy's disk and is designated as θ. **B.** Two objects cannot be resolved unless the peaks of the two Airy's disks are separated by at least the radius of Airy's disk (i.e., the peak of one disk falls on the trough of the other disk). In this diagram, where the retinal images are separated by the distance x, the radii of the Airy's disks are too large to allow resolution. **C.** For a larger pupil size, the radii of the Airy's disks are smaller. Here, the peak of one disk falls on the first trough of the other disk; therefore, resolution is not limited by diffraction.

the **diffraction pattern** (i.e., the distribution of light) formed on the retina when light from a monochromatic point source[2] passes by the pupil. The pattern, which is referred to as **Airy's disk**, consists of a bright center surrounded by alternating dark and bright rings. Its intensity profile is given on the right side of Figure 11-6A.

The distance from the bright peak to the center of the first dark ring (the dark trough) is often called the radius of Airy's disk. Its value in radians (θ) can be determined with the following formula:

$$\theta = 1.22\frac{\lambda}{d}$$

where d is the pupillary diameter and λ is the wavelength of the light that constitutes the point object.

When viewing two side-by-side point sources, two diffraction patterns are formed on the retina. The above formula tells us that as the pupil diameter decreases, the radius of each Airy's disk increases. This may cause the diffraction patterns to overlap.

Consider Figure 11-6B, which illustrates two retinal point images that are separated by the distance x. In this case, there is too much overlap of the diffraction patterns to permit the two points to be resolved, and the patient will see only one point.

Suppose that the pupil becomes larger. When this happens, the radius of each Airy's disk decreases. If they decrease to the extent that an Airy's disk peak falls on the center of the first dark ring of the other disk, as illustrated in Figure 11-6C, the two points can be resolved. That is, two points can be resolved if their diffraction pattern peaks are separated by the radius of Airy's disk.

Let's look at an example. *In order for two points of 555 nm to be resolved by a person with a 5.00-mm-diameter pupil, what is the minimum distance that must separate the peaks of the Airy disks?*

After converting to meters, we have

$$\theta = 1.22\frac{\lambda}{d}$$

$$\theta = \frac{1.22(5.55 \times 10^{-7}\text{ m})}{5 \times 10^{-3}\text{ m}}$$

$$\theta = 1.354 \times 10^{-4}\text{ radians}$$

Converting to minutes of arc (abbreviated as *arcmin*) we have

$$(1.354 \times 10^{-4}\text{ radians})\left(\frac{180\text{ degrees}}{\pi\text{ radians}}\right)\left(\frac{60\text{ arcmin}}{1\text{ degree}}\right) = 0.47\text{ arcmin}$$

---

2. A monochromatic source emits light of a single wavelength.

For a 5.00-mm-diameter pupil, the peaks of the Airy's disks must be separated by at least 0.47 minutes of arc. If we repeat this calculation for a 2.00-mm-diameter pupil, we find that the Airy's disks must be separated by at least 1.16 minutes of arc. As the pupil becomes smaller, the diffraction patterns become larger; consequently the patterns (and point sources) must be farther separated from each other in order to be resolved.[3]

DEPTH OF FIELD AND DEPTH OF FOCUS

Due to what is called **depth of field**, an object, such as the optotype **E**, does not need to be focused on the retina for us to resolve its details. As long as the retinal blur circles are not too large, it can be resolved. (If the blur circles are too large, they will overlap each other, preventing resolution.)

Take a look at Figure 11-7, which shows an eye with 3.00 D of uncorrected myopia that is refractive in origin. Let's assume the eye manifests absolute presbyopia, meaning that it has no ability to accommodate. From Chapter 8, we know that an object located at a distance of 33.00 cm is conjugate with the retina. This eye's depth of field, however, permits objects as far away as 40.00 cm or as close as 28.57 cm to be resolved.

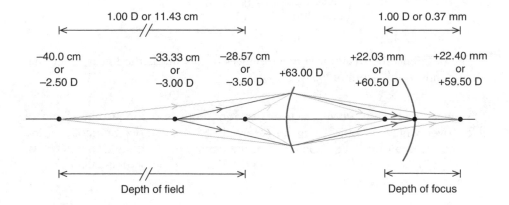

Figure 11-7. The depth of field is conjugate to the depth of focus. Although the depth of field and depth of focus are dioptrically equal (1.00 D), they are not linearly equal (11.43 cm vs. 0.37 mm). (The 3.00 D myopic eye in this figure is uncorrected and unable to accommodate.)

---

3. The packing density of retinal photoreceptors limits our ability to resolve detail less than about 0.50 minarc. In the case of a 5.00-mm-diameter pupil, resolution is not likely to be limited by diffraction but by the density of the photoreceptors and optical aberrations (Chapter 15). As the pupil diameter decreases to about 2.00 to 3.00 mm, diffraction becomes the limiting factor.

By convention, depth of field is given in diopters. In the current example (Figure 11-7), the dioptric equivalent of 40.00 cm is 2.50 D (i.e., 100/40.00 cm = 2.50 D) and the dioptric equivalent of 28.57 cm is 3.50 D (i.e., 100/28.57 cm = 3.50 D cm), making the depth of field equal to 1.00 D. This corresponds to a linear range of 11.43 cm. The depth of field is always dioptrically centered at a point conjugate with the retina, which in this case is 3.00 D (equivalent to 33.33 cm). Another way of saying this is that the depth of focus is ±0.50 D centered at 3.00 D.

Figure 11-7 also shows there is a range centered on the retina—the **depth of focus**—that is conjugate with the depth of field. Like the depth of field, the depth of focus is 1.00 D, but this corresponds to a linear range of only 0.37 mm. You must be wondering, "How did we arrive at this"? Here's how. Keeping in mind what we learned in Chapter 7 and that this myopic eye has a power of +63.00 D, we can locate the image produced when the object distance is 40.00 cm as follows:

$$L' = L + F$$

$$\frac{(1000)(1.333)}{l'} = \left(\frac{-1000}{400.0 \text{ mm}}\right) + 63.00 \text{ D}$$

$$l' = +22.03 \text{ mm}$$

For an object distance of 28.57 cm, we have

$$L' = L + F$$

$$\frac{(1000)(1.333)}{l'} = \left(\frac{-1000}{285.7 \text{ mm}}\right) + 63.00 \text{ D}$$

$$l' = 22.40 \text{ mm}$$

The difference between these two distances (0.37 mm) is the linear range that corresponds to the depth of focus.

Let's summarize what we've discussed so far. There is a range—the depth of field—over which an object can be resolved. It is centered dioptrically at the distance the eye is focused. Conjugate to the depth of field is the depth of focus, which is dioptrically centered on the retina. When in dioptric units, the depth of field is equal to the depth of focus.

The extent of the depth of field (and depth of focus) depends primarily on the pupil diameter. A small pupil decreases the size of the blur circles and thereby increases the depth of field. (If the pupil becomes too small, diffraction and reduced retinal illumination may limit visual resolution, but we'll ignore these factors for now.)

Let's look at an example. *An emmetropic patient with absolute presbyopia wears a near correction of +2.50 D. His total depth of focus is 0.50 D. What is his linear range of near vision when he wears his presbyopic correction? What would be his linear range of clear vision if he wore a near correction of +1.00 D?*

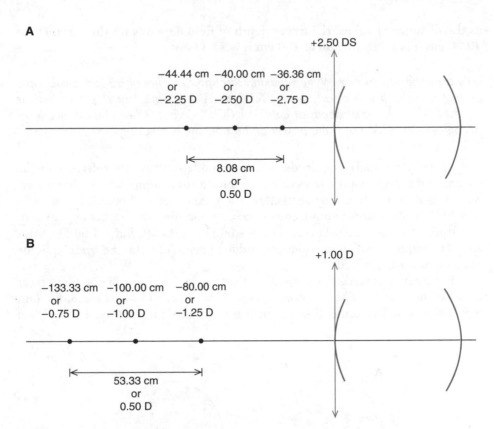

Figure 11-8. Range of clear vision for an emmetropic patient with absolute presbyopia when looking through (**A**) a +2.50 DS near correction and (**B**) a +1.00 DS near correction. Although the depth of field is dioptrically the same at both distances (0.50 D), it is not linearly the same (8.08 vs. 53.33 cm).

Figure 11-8A shows the patient looking through the +2.50 D correction. A point that is 40.00 cm from the eye is conjugate with the retina. What is the patient's depth of field? Recall that the depth of field (in diopters) is equal to the depth of focus (in diopters). This 0.50 D depth of field is centered at the dioptric distance of 2.50 D. Therefore the dioptric boundaries of clear near vision are 2.50 ± 0.25 D, or 2.75 and 2.25 D. In linear units, the patient sees clearly from 36.36 to 44.44 cm when looking through the +2.50 D lens. Although this patient has no ability to accommodate, he is still able to resolve objects over a range of about 8.08 cm due to his depth of field.

Now, let us determine this patient's range of clear vision when wearing a +1.00 D lens. As indicated in Figure 11-8B, a point at 100.00 cm anterior to the cornea is conjugate with the retina. The depth of field, which is still 0.50 D, is centered dioptrically at 1.00 D: its dioptric boundaries are 1.25 and 0.75 D. These correspond to linear boundaries of 80.00 and 133.33 cm, for a range of 53.33 cm. **It is important to note that although the dioptric depth of field does not change**

as the distance changes, the linear depth of field depends on the distance: at 40.00 cm it is 8.08 cm, and at 100 cm it is 53.33 cm.

Let's do another problem. When looking through her bifocal add, a presbyopic patient is able to see clearly from 25.00 to 100.00 cm. Her depth of field is ±0.50 D (i.e., the total depth of field is 1.00 D). What is her true amplitude of accommodation? What is the power of the add she is wearing?

By **true (or actual) amplitude of accommodation**, we are referring to the change in the eye's dioptric power that is solely due to accommodation. In the current example, the patient's range of clear vision, expressed in diopters, is from 4.00 to 1.00 D. The **apparent amplitude of accommodation**, which takes into account the depth of field, is 3.00 D (i.e., 4.00 − 1.00 D = 3.00 D). Since 1.00 D of this apparent amplitude of accommodation is due to depth of field, the *true* amplitude of accommodation is 2.00 D.

For a distance-corrected presbyopic patient to resolve near objects, plus power must be added to the distance prescription. As we learned in Chapter 8, the plus power that is added to the distance correction is called an *add* (Fig. 11-9). When

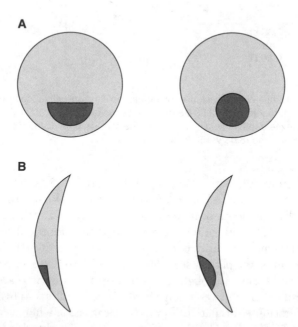

Figure 11-9. A. Flat-top and round bifocal adds. Not shown is a variable-focus lens, often called a progressive lens. In such a lens, the plus power gradually increases going from the center of the lens toward its bottom. **B.** Cross sections of flat-top and round bifocal lenses. The adds in these glass bifocals have a higher index of refraction than the distance carrier lenses.

looking through the add in the current example, the nearest clear distance (i.e., the near point of accommodation) is 25.00 cm in linear units or 4.00 D in dioptric units. Of this 4.00 D, 2.00 D is due to accommodation and 0.50 D to the depth of field. The add provides the remaining power. Hence, the add has a power of 4.00 – 2.00 – 0.50 D = 1.50 D. You'll need to study Figure 11-10A to put this all together.

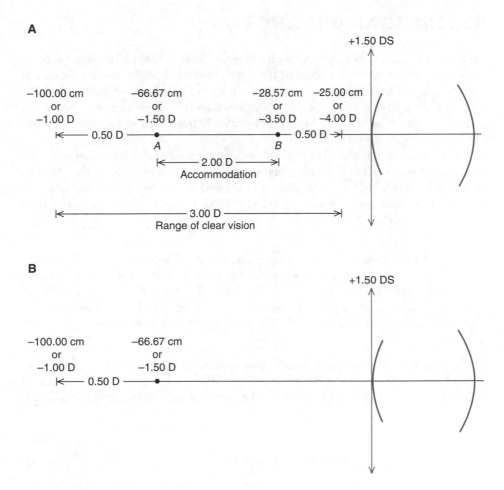

Figure 11-10. A. A presbyopic patient, fully corrected for distance and viewing through her add, has a range of clear vision that extends from –25.00 (or –4.00 D) to –100.00 cm (–1.00 D). If the patient did not have a 1.00 D depth of field, her range of clear vision would be from A (–1.50 D or –66.67 cm) to B (–3.50 D or –28.57 cm); therefore, the true amplitude of accommodation (as measured at the spectacle plane) is 2.00 D. Because the patient's NPA is 25.00 cm, she must be wearing a 1.50 add (i.e., 0.50 + 2.00 + 1.50 D = 4.00 D). **B.** Since the farthest distance the patient can see is –100.00 cm and the depth of field is 1.00 D (i.e., ±0.50 D), the patient must be wearing a +1.50 DS add. See the text for details.

Figure 11-10B shows another approach to determine the add power. When looking through the add, the farthest distance that can be seen clearly is 100 cm. The add focuses the eye at a distance closer than 100 cm, but because of the depth of field, which is ±0.50 D, the patient can see out to 100.00 cm. If the add is 1.50 D, the farthest distance that can be clearly seen is 1.00 D in dioptric units or 100.00 cm in linear units.

HYPERFOCAL DISTANCE

Consider a young emmetropic eye with a depth of field of 1.00 D. If this eye accommodates an amount equal to half of the depth of field, 0.50 D, objects located at infinity can still be resolved because they are within the depth of field. As can be seen in Figure 11-11, when the eye accommodates 0.50 D so that it is focused at 200.00 cm, the range of clear vision is dioptrically from 0.00 D to 1.00 D, or linearly from infinity to 100 cm.

The nearest distance at which the eye can be focused and still resolve infinitely distant objects is referred to its **hyperfocal distance**. The hyperfocal distance can be found by taking half the total depth of field and converting it to linear units. In the current example, the depth of field is 1.00 D, making half the depth of field 0.50 D. This corresponds to a linear distance of 200.00 cm.

It's time for an example. *When taking pilocarpine (a medication that shrinks the pupil, thereby increasing the depth of field) to treat glaucoma, a myopic patient's uncorrected distance visual acuity is 20/20 and her depth of field is 2.00 D. When the patient discontinues the pilocarpine and her pupil returns to its normal size, what is the maximum amount of myopia we expect to find?*

We are asked to determine the maximum amount of uncorrected myopia that is consistent with a distance visual acuity of 20/20 and a hyperfocal distance of 100.00 cm. From Figure 11-12, we see that when an eye is focused at 100.00 cm

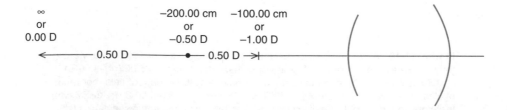

Figure 11-11. Since the depth of field is 1.00 D, the hyperfocal distance is –200.00 cm (i.e., 100/–0.50 D = –200.00 cm). When the eye is focused at a distance of –200.00 cm, objects at infinity can be resolved.

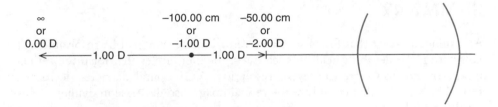

Figure 11-12. When taking pilocarpine, which gives the patient a 2.00 D depth of field, the patient can have up to 1.00 D of uncorrected myopia and still have 20/20 acuity. See the text for details.

(1.00 D), the depth of field extends to infinity, making 20/20 vision possible. Hence, the patient can have up to 1.00 D of myopia and still have an uncorrected distance visual acuity of 20/20. (If the patient discontinues pilocarpine and the pupil returns to its normal size, the depth of focus will be less than ±1.00 D and the distance uncorrected acuity will, therefore, be less than 20/20.)

Let's try one more problem. *An emmetropic patient with absolute presbyopia has a hyperfocal distance of 200.00 cm. What is the range of clear vision in linear units when the patient wears +2.50 DS reading glasses?*

The patient's hyperfocal distance is 200.00 cm in linear units or 0.50 D in dioptric units, making the depth of field 1.00 D. When wearing the +2.50 DS reading glasses, the depth of field is centered at 2.50 D (40.00 cm). As can be seen in Figure 11-13, the depth of field extends from 2.00 to 3.00 D, or from 50.00 to 33.33 cm.

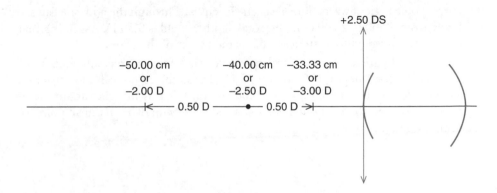

Figure 11-13. Since the hyperfocal distance is –200.00 cm, the depth of field is 1.00 D. When this emmetropic patient with absolute presbyopia wears +2.50 DS reading glasses, the range of clear vision is from –50.00 cm (–2.00 D) to –33.33 cm (–3.00 D).

SUMMARY

An extended object that forms a blurred retinal image may still be resolvable if it falls within the depth of field. In such cases, the blur circles that form the retinal image are not too large to prevent resolution. As the pupil diameter decreases, retinal blur circles that constitute the retinal image also decrease in diameter; this results in both a greater depth of field and depth of focus (the retinal equivalent of depth of field). A small pupil, however, can cause diffraction, which may reduce resolution.

KEY FORMULA

Radius of Airy's disk:

$$\theta = 1.22\frac{\lambda}{d}$$

SELF-ASSESSMENT PROBLEMS

1. A 3.00 D myopic patient who is fully corrected with contact lenses has a hyperfocal distance of 200.00 cm. His near point of accommodation is 10.00 cm. What is his true amplitude of accommodation?

2. A fully corrected 2.00 D hyperopic patient has a total depth of field of 1.00 D. Through her spectacle add, her range of clear vision is from 100.00 to 25.00 cm. What is her range of clear vision through the distance portion of the spectacles?

3. Without any correction, a 1.00 D myopic presbyopic patient has a near point of 20.00 cm. His total depth of field is 1.50 D. What is the furthest distance he can see clearly?

4. A presbyopic patient wears bifocal spectacle lenses. Through the add, she can see clearly from 50.00 to 20.00 cm. Her total depth of field is 0.50 D. Assuming that she is fully corrected for distance, what is the power of the add?

5. A presbyopic patient wears bifocal spectacles that fully correct his 4.00 D of myopia. His total depth of field is 0.75 D. Through his bifocal add, he has a range of clear vision from 40.00 to 20.00 cm. (a) What is his true amplitude of accommodation? (b) Without his spectacles, what would be his near point of accommodation?

12

Magnification and Low Vision Devices

Because of disease, developmental abnormalities or trauma, certain patients do not obtain satisfactory vision even when their ametropia is fully corrected. These patients are said to have **low vision**. A patient with age-related macular degeneration, for instance, may have best corrected acuity[1] of 20/100. This suboptimal visual acuity may limit the patient's ability to participate in various daily activities that others take for granted, such as reading the newspaper and correspondence.

As the population ages, the prevalence of low vision will increase. To obtain satisfactory vision, these patients may use magnifying devices such as plus lenses, electronic magnifiers, or telescopes. In this chapter, we introduce the optics of these important clinical tools with an emphasis on devices used for near vision. This chapter is not intended to be a comprehensive discussion of low-vision devices.

Students and residents often find magnification confusing. This may stem from the various forms of magnification that can be specified. For example, in this book we refer to lateral, relative distance, size, angular, effective, and spectacle magnification. It's important to keep these terms straight. Table 12-1 summarizes the application of these terms in low vision and clinical practice. While these terms might not make much sense at this point, you may find it helpful to refer back to this table as you read through the next sections.

---

1. Best corrected acuity refers to the visual acuity obtained when the patient's ametropia is fully corrected.

TABLE 12-1. **VARIOUS FORMS OF MAGNIFICATION**

Magnification	Clinical Condition Most Relevant to	This Term is Used When
Lateral (transverse or linear)	Low vision	The object is within the focal length of a plus lens, thereby creating a virtual image.
Size	Low vision	The object is made physically larger.
Relative distance	Low vision	The object is moved physically closer to the eye.
Angular	Low vision	The angle an object makes at the eye is increased.
Effective and conventional	Low vision	A manufacturer labels plus lenses to allow consumers to compare their magnifications. Clinicians convert this value to a dioptric value.
Spectacle	Aniseikonia	A patient has anisometropia, and the correcting spectacle lenses create images of different angular sizes for the two eyes. See Chapter 13.

ANGULAR MAGNIFICATION PRODUCED BY PLUS LENSES

Consider a patient who needs to read the small print on the label of a prescription that she received from her pharmacist. If the print is too small for her to resolve when held at her normal reading distance, what are her options? As can be seen in Figure 12-1, if the print were made four times larger, it would subtend an angle that is four times larger at the eye.[2] Another way of saying this is that the angular magnification would be increased by four. This would make it easier for the patient to read the print, but it isn't a practical solution since a medicine bottle is relatively small and the label can't be so large that it won't fit on the bottle.

Another option would be for the patient to hold the label closer to her eye. If she were to hold the bottle one-fourth as far from her eyes, as illustrated in Figure 12-2, the angular magnification would be 4×. This form of magnification is sometimes called **relative distance magnification** and would work as long as the patient has sufficient accommodation to focus at the required distance.

Specifying Print Size

Before going any further, we need to take a slight detour and talk about the specification of print size. Near print size is often expressed in **M-units**. By definition, the detail of 1 M print subtends an angle of 1 min of arc at a viewing distance of 1 m. Overall, the print subtends 5 min of arc at this same viewing distance. Likewise, the detail of 2 M print subtends 2 min of arc at 1 m.

---

2. This is sometimes referred to as size magnification.

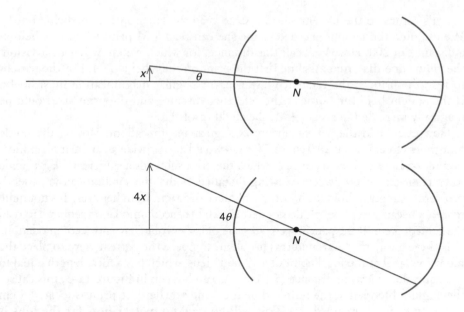

Figure 12-1. Increasing the object size by a factor of 4 increases the angular magnification by a factor of 4. (This diagram shows rays traveling through the eye's nodal point, *N*, because rays headed toward this point do not change direction after refraction.)

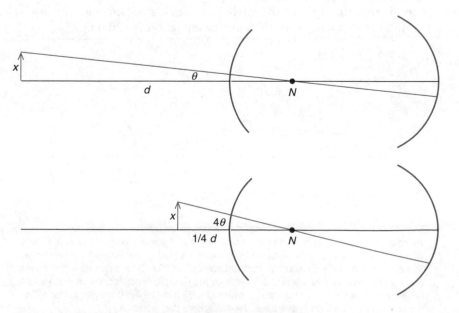

Figure 12-2. Moving an object four times closer to the eye increases the magnification by a factor of 4. This is referred to as relative distance magnification.

Let's return to the patient who needs to read the label on her medicine bottle. We examine the patient and determine she can read 4 M print when it is held at a distance of 20.0 cm. We'll call this distance, for which we know her near vision, the **reference distance**. Assume that the print on the label is 1 M. For the patient to read the print at the reference distance, the angular magnification must be 4×. If the patient held the bottle at the reference distance and the print size could be magically increased in size to 4 M, she could resolve it.

How else could the patient obtain 4× angular magnification? Moving the bottle four times closer—from 20.0 cm to 5.0 cm—would also provide an angular magnification of 4×. Let's call the distance at which the print subtends a sufficiently large angle to be resolved the **equivalent viewing distance**. Is this the solution to the patient's problem—simply to hold the bottle at a distance of 5.0 cm from her eyes? It's not quite that easy because most people do not have the 20 D of accommodation required to read the print at 5 cm. If the patient were 70 years old, she would have no accommodation.

Is there a way to get around this problem? Suppose the patient were to place the medicine label at the focal point of a +20.0 D lens, which has a focal length equal to the equivalent viewing distance (5.0 cm). As can be seen in Figure 12-3, this causes the angle subtended at the retina to be the same as when the print is located 5 cm from the patient's unaided eye. **This will be true no matter how far the lens is located from the patient's eyes as long as the print is at the focal point of the lens.** Be sure to note that the light rays emerging from the lens are parallel. This means that when the patient uses her distance vision correction to look through the magnifying lens, the print will be focused on her retina.

The term **equivalent viewing power**[3] is used to specify the power of a plus lens whose focal length is equal to the equivalent viewing distance. For an equivalent viewing distance of 5 cm, the equivalent viewing power is +20.0 D.

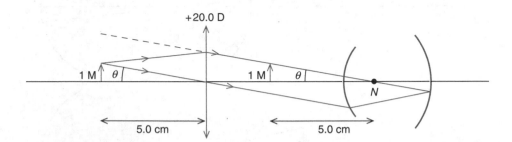

Figure 12-3. An object subtends the same angle at the eye whether it is at the focal point of a plus lens or at a distance from the eye equal to the lens's focal length. In this example, an object placed at the focal point of a +20.0 D lens results in the same angle at the eye as if positioned 5.0 cm from the eye. (To be exact, the object should be 5.0 cm from the eye's nodal point, which is 5.55 mm behind the eye's surface. For the calculations we'll do in this book, we can ignore this distance.)

---

3. Be sure not to confuse equivalent viewing power with equivalent power (F_e).

Let's summarize what we've discussed so far. To read the medicine label, the patient requires angular magnification of 4×. One possibility is to use relative distance magnification by moving the label four times closer, from the reference distance of 20 to 5 cm (the equivalent viewing distance). This is not a practical solution, however, because the patient can't accommodate the 20 D required to view an object located at a reading distance of 5 cm. We can overcome this problem by placing the reading material at the focal point of a lens with a focal length equal to the equivalent viewing distance (5 cm). This lens power has a power of +20 D, which is called the equivalent viewing power. Since the rays emerging from the magnifying glass are parallel, the patient does not need to accommodate if she looks through the magnifying lens with her distance prescription. Furthermore, as long as the object is at the lens's focal point, the angular magnification does not change as the distance from the lens to eye changes.

We've said that angular magnification is the same as long as the reading material remains at the focal point of the magnifying lens. In fact, as the distance between the plus lens and eye increases (with the object remaining at the focal point of the lens), it may *appear* that the image seen through the lens is becoming larger. This illusion occurs because the angle subtended by reading material *not* seen through the magnifying lens becomes smaller as the distance from the eye to the material increases. Consequently, the image seen through the lens *appears* to be growing larger relative to the shrinking background material to which it is being compared. If you were to measure the retinal image size of the material viewed through the lens, however, you would find that it remains constant as the lens moves farther from the eye. There will be no change in the patient's ability to resolve detail in the image seen through the lens.

USE OF PLUS LENSES FOR LOW VISION

The most commonly utilized near magnification devices are plus lenses. These can be mounted in handheld magnifiers, spectacles (high-plus single vision lenses or high-plus bifocal adds), loupes mounted to and positioned in front of the patient's spectacles or stand magnifiers.

Consider a 25-year-old patient who is having difficulty reading personal correspondence. The smallest print this patient can read at 40.0 cm is 2 M. The patient wishes to read print that is half as large—1 M print. What advice should we give to this patient?

The patient requires an angular magnification of 2×. This can be obtained when the patient holds the printed material at one-half the reference distance. Since the reference distance is 40.0 cm, the patient will be able to read his correspondence when it is held 20.0 cm from his eyes. (When 1 M print is at a distance of 20.0 cm, it subtends the same angle as does 2 M print held at a distance of 40.00 cm.)

Suppose this patient's vision deteriorates so that in 2 years the smallest print that can be read at 40.0 cm is 5 M. How can we help this patient?

Because of this deterioration, the patient now requires angular magnification of 5× to resolve 1 M print. He could hold the correspondence five times closer to his eyes—at a distance of 8.0 cm (i.e., 40.0 cm/5 = 8.0 cm). This is the equivalent viewing distance. The patient, however, is not likely to be comfortable holding reading material so close to his eyes. Moreover, the accommodative demand is 12.5 D (i.e., 100/8.0 cm = 12.5 D); it is difficult to sustain this amount of accommodation for very long, even for young patients.

How can a plus lens be used to obtain this same angular magnification? As we've learned, the patient can use a plus lens whose focal length is equal to the equivalent viewing distance. In this case, where the equivalent viewing distance is 8.0 cm, the power of the plus lens—the equivalent viewing power—is +12.5 D. As long as the reading material is held at the focal point of the lens, the print will subtend the same angle at the eye regardless of the distance from the eye to the plus lens.[4]

Let's look at another example. A 70-year-old patient with fully corrected myopia has age-related macular degeneration and can barely see 5 M print at a distance of 40.0 cm when looking through his bifocal add. If our goal is to allow the patient to read 2 M print, what power handheld magnifying lens should we prescribe? How far should the lens be held from the reading material? How far should the lens be held from the patient's eye? Should the patient look through the magnifying lens with his distance correction or bifocal add?

At first glance, this may appear to be a rather confusing problem. If we keep our wits about us and approach it one step at a time, it's not that complicated. The patient can read 5 M print when it is located at the reference distance of 40.0 cm. In order for the patient to read 2 M print, an angular magnification of 2.5× is required (i.e., 5 M/2 M = 2.5×). The equivalent viewing distance is 2.5× closer than the reference distance, which makes it 16.0 cm (i.e., 40 cm/2.5 = 16.0 cm). Therefore, the plus lens must have a power of +6.25 D (i.e., 100/16.0 cm = 6.25 D). (The equivalent viewing power is +6.25 D.)

As long as the print is at the focal point of the plus lens, the patient can hold the lens at whatever distance from the eye he finds most comfortable. The angle subtended at the eye and the ability to see detail remains the same, even though the field of view becomes smaller as the lens is positioned farther from the eye. Since the light rays that emerge from the plus lens are parallel to each other, they

---

4. A slight variation on this approach is to use the formula $M_\theta =$ **(reference distance)**(F), where M_θ is the desired angular magnification and F is the power of the plus lens that will provide this magnification when the reading material is held at the focal point of the lens. The *reference distance* is in meters. In the current example, M_θ is 5× and the *reference distance* is 0.4 m. Solving for F gives a power of +12.5 D.

will be focused onto the retina if the patient looks through the plus lens with the distance portion of his spectacles.

Here's another example. *A patient is able to read 6 M print at a reading distance of 40.0 cm when looking through her bifocal. She goes to the drugstore and purchases a +10.0 D magnifying glass that she holds 10.0 cm from the page. What is the smallest print she can resolve when looking through the magnifying glass?*

When print is held at the focal point of a +10.0 D lens, it subtends the same angle as if held 10.0 cm from the eye. This angle is 4× larger than when the print is at the reference distance of 40.0 cm (i.e., 40.0 cm/10.0 cm = 4×). Therefore the patient can read print that is 4× smaller—she can read 1.5 M print (i.e., 6 M/4 = 1.5 M). Since the material is held at the focal point of the plus lens, the rays that emerge from this lens are parallel to each other; therefore, the patient should look through the magnifier with her distance prescription.

Let's try one more problem. *A patient with age-related macular degeneration has best-corrected distance visual acuity of 20/400. What power magnifying lens is required for the patient to read 2 M print?*

Based on a distance visual acuity of 20/400, we know that the patient's minimum angle of resolution (MAR) is 20 min of arc.[5] Since the detail of 2 M print subtends 2 min of arc at 1.0 m (or 100.0 cm), it will subtend 20 min of arc when it is 10 times closer. This gives us an equivalent viewing distance of 10.0 cm (i.e., 100.0 cm/10 = 10.0 cm). Therefore, the magnifying lens must have a power of +10.0 D (i.e., 100/10.0 cm = 10.0 D).[6]

When prescribing a magnifying lens for presbyopic patients, we usually start off with the assumption that the patient will hold the reading material at the focal point of the lens while looking through his distance correction. What happens if the patient holds the material closer than the focal length? From Chapter 4, we know that a magnified virtual image will be formed on the same side of the lens as the object. For this image to be focused on the retina, the patient must look through his bifocal add. When the distance between the magnifying lens

---

5. The minimum angle of resolution (MAR) is the angle (subtended at the eye) of the smallest detail the patient can resolve. It is the reciprocal of the Snellen visual acuity. For further details see Schwartz (2010).

6. Kestenbaum's rule, which is used commonly in low vision practice, predicts that a plus lens power equal to the reciprocal of the Snellen fraction will allow a patient to read 1 M print (Kestenbaum and Sturnan, 1956). For a distance visual acuity of 20/400, this rule predicts a power of +20.00 D (i.e., 400/20 = 20) to read 1 M print. Therefore, to read 2 M print, the power would be +10.00 D. In clinical practice, Kestenbaum's rule may underestimate the lens power that is needed.

and bifocal add is less than the focal length of the magnifying lens, the patient experiences greater angular magnification (than when the material is held at the focal point of the lens while looking through the distance correction). In the next section, we take a slightly different approach to this issue.

Magnifying Lens and Bifocal Add in Combination

Will a patient obtain more magnification when looking through a handheld magnifying lens with her distance prescription (keeping the object at the primary focal point of the magnifying lens) or with her bifocal add (keeping the object at the primary focal point of the add–magnifier combination)? As we will see from the following examples, it depends on how far the magnifier is held from the add. Consider a patient who wears bifocals that have a 2.50 D add. A +10.00 D handheld magnifying lens (i.e., F_e = +10.00 D) is prescribed to assist the patient with reading.

Suppose the patient holds the magnifying lens 10.0 cm from her add (i.e., the separation between the magnifier and add is equal to the focal length of the magnifier). What is the equivalent power of this magnifier–add combination? To answer this question, we treat the magnifier–add combination as a thick lens. Using the thick lens formula from Chapter 6, we have

$$F_e = F_1 + F_2 - \left(\frac{t}{n}\right)F_1 F_2$$

$$F_e = +2.50 \text{ D} + 10.00 \text{ D} - \left(\frac{0.1 \text{ m}}{1.00}\right)(+2.50 \text{ D})(+10.00 \text{ D})$$

$$F_e = +10.00 \text{ D}$$

When the magnifier is held one focal length from the add, the magnifier–add combination has the same equivalent power as the magnifier itself. Consequently, the same angular magnification is obtained whether the patient looks through the magnifier with her add or distance prescription.

Now suppose the patient holds a magnifying lens less than 10.0 cm from her add, say at 5.0 cm from her add. What is the power of the system?

$$F_e = F_1 + F_2 - \left(\frac{t}{n}\right)F_1 F_2$$

$$F_e = +2.50 \text{ D} + 10.00 \text{ D} - \left(\frac{0.05 \text{ m}}{1.00}\right)(+2.50 \text{ D})(+10.00 \text{ D})$$

$$F_e = +11.25 \text{ D}$$

When the distance between the magnifier and add is less than the focal length of the magnifier, the equivalent power of the magnifier–add combination is greater than that of the magnifier. Consequently, the angular magnification is greater when the patient looks through the magnifying lens with her add than when she looks through it with her distance prescription. (This assumes that the reading material is held at the anterior focal point of the magnifier–add combination, which is less than 10.0 cm from the magnifying lens.[7] Recall from the previous section that when an object is within the focal length of the magnifying lens, a magnified virtual image is created. For this image to be focused on the retina, it must be at the primary focal point at the bifocal add.)

Lastly, what is the equivalent power when the magnifying lens is held farther than 10.0 cm from the add, say at 15.0 cm?

$$F_e = F_1 + F_2 - \left(\frac{t}{n}\right)F_1 F_2$$

$$F_e = +2.50\ D + 10.00\ D - \left(\frac{0.15\ m}{1.00}\right)(+2.50\ D)(+10.00\ D)$$

$$F_e = +8.75\ D$$

If the distance between the magnifier and add is greater than the focal length of the magnifier, the magnifier–add combination has less power than the magnifier. The patient is better off using her distance correction to look through the magnifying lens. This important finding is counterintuitive to both the clinician and the patient.

Let's summarize this section. How can a patient who wears bifocals maximize magnification when using a magnifying lens? She can do so if she looks through the magnifying lens with her add *while holding the magnifying lens closer to the add than its (the magnifying lens's) focal length*. However, if the magnifying lens is held farther from the add than its focal length, the patient experiences less magnification; she is better off looking through the magnifier with the distance prescription. To ensure that the low-vision patient is obtaining the proper magnification, it is important to instruct her on the use of the magnifier and then for the patient to demonstrate that she can use the magnifier properly.

Fixed-Focus Stand Magnifiers

As illustrated in Figure 12-4, a plus lens can be mounted in a stand that rests on reading material. Because it does not need to be held by the patient, a **stand magnifier** may be suitable for a patient with poor motor control (e.g., hand tremors).

The separation between the lens and reading material is usually less than the focal length of the lens. Consequently, an enlarged virtual image is formed. Since this virtual image is not located at infinity, the patient must look through a plus lens

---

7. When the reading material is held at the anterior focal point of the magnifier–add combination, the light rays that emerge from this combination are parallel. They are incident on the distance prescription (which is behind the add) and focused onto the retina.

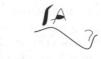

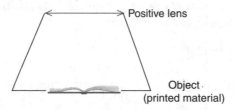

Figure 12-4. Stand magnifiers are designed so that the reading material is at a fixed distance from a plus lens. This distance is often less than the focal length of the lens.

or accommodate to see it clearly. Locating this virtual image allows us to determine where the patient should position her eye and what the accommodative demand will be.

Let's consider an example. *A patient can read 4 M print when it is held 40.00 cm from his spectacles. You prescribe a stand magnifier that contains a +20.00 D lens. The lens is at a fixed distance of 4.00 cm from the reading material. How close must the patient's eye be to the plus lens for him to read 1 M print?*

The first step is to determine the equivalent viewing distance. Since the patient can currently read 4 M print (at the reference distance of 40.00 cm) and wishes to read 1 M print, the required angular magnification is 4×. The equivalent viewing distance, which is four times nearer than the reference distance, is 10.00 cm.

Next, we need to locate the virtual image produced by the stand magnifier and determine its lateral magnification. In Figure 12-5, we have redrawn the stand magnifier so that it is sitting on its side. A stand magnifier is, of course, not typically so positioned, but drawing it this way allows us to use our linear sign conventions. Since the object is located within the focal length of the lens, a virtual image is formed. The image vergence is

$$L' = L + F$$

$$L' = \left[\frac{(100)(1.00)}{-4.00 \text{ cm}}\right] + 20.00 \text{ D}$$

$$L' = -25.00 \text{ D} + 20.00 \text{ D}$$

$$L' = -5.00 \text{ D}$$

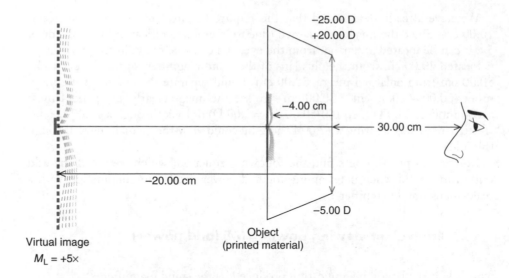

−25.00 D
+20.00 D

−4.00 cm

30.00 cm

−20.00 cm

−5.00 D

Virtual image
$M_L = +5\times$

Object
(printed material)

Figure 12-5. The patient usually looks down into a stand magnifier, but we have drawn the stand magnifier on its side so that we can use our linear sign convention. As is often the case, the distance from the plus lens of the stand magnifier to the reading material is less than the focal length, resulting in an enlarged virtual image. Here, the lateral magnification of the image is 5×. Since the equivalent viewing distance is 10.0 cm, the laterally magnified image can be up to 5× this distance from the eye—50.0 cm—and still be resolved. See the text for further details.

Knowing the image vergence, we can calculate the image location as follows:

$$L' = \frac{n'}{l'}$$

$$-5.00 \text{ D} = \frac{(100)(1.00)}{l'}$$

$$l' = -20.00 \text{ cm}$$

This virtual image is located −20.00 cm from the lens (Fig. 12-5). The lateral magnification is[8]

$$M_L = \frac{L}{L'}$$

$$M_L = \frac{-25.00 \text{ D}}{-5.00 \text{ D}}$$

$$M_L = +5\times$$

---

8. Lateral magnification is discussed in Chapters 2 to 6.

We have already determined that the required equivalent viewing distance is 10.00 cm. Since the image is enlarged (due to lateral magnification) by a factor of 5×, it can be located 5× farther from the eye, at a distance of 50.00 cm. The image is located 20.00 cm from the plus lens of the stand magnifier, so for the eye to be 50.00 cm from enlarged image, 30.00 cm should separate the eye from the magnifier (50.00 − 20.00 cm = 30.00 cm). To see the image clearly, the patient must accommodate 2.00 D (i.e., 100/50.00 cm = 2.00 D) or look through a +2.00 D lens. If the patient was wearing a +2.00 D add, he could view the virtual image through this add.

Low vision practitioners find the following equation, which we'll call the **add equation**, useful when determining the add power needed in conjunction with a fixed-focus stand magnifier[9]:

Equivalent viewing power = (M) (add power)

where *M* is the lateral magnification produced by the stand magnifier.

In the current example, the equivalent viewing distance is 10.00 cm, which means that the equivalent viewing power is +10.00 D. Substituting, we have

Equivalent viewing power = (*M*) (add power)

+10.00 D = (5) (add power)

add power = +2.00 D

Suppose the patient's vision deteriorates to the point where he can read no better than 5 M print at a distance of 40 cm, but he still wishes to read 1 M print. What power bifocal add is required? How far should his eye be from the stand magnifier lens when looking through the add?

The patient requires angular magnification of 5×, making the equivalent viewing distance 8.00 cm (i.e., 40.00 cm/5 = 8.00 cm). This corresponds to an equivalent viewing power of +12.50 D (i.e., 100/8.00 cm = 12.50 D). Substituting, we have

Equivalent viewing power = (*M*) (add power)

+12.50 D = (5) (add power)

add power = +2.50 D

The required add power is 2.50 D. The patient should be taught to position his eye about 20 cm from the lens [i.e., (100/2.50 D) − 20.00 cm = 20.00 cm].[10]

---

9. As we'll learn later in this chapter, the add equation is also useful for determining (1) the add power needed when using an electronic magnifier and (2) lens cap power needed for a telemicroscope.

10. In actual practice, clinicians do not tailor bifocal adds to suit the stand magnifier's image distance. Rather, they often prescribe a stand magnifier whose image is viewable with the patient's current add.

TABLE 12-2. ADVANTAGES AND DISADVANTAGES OF VARIOUS MOUNTINGS OF PLUS LENS AS USED IN LOW VISION

How Mounted	Advantages	Disadvantages
Handheld magnifying lens	Flexibility in viewing distance	1. One hand must be used to hold the device. This can be especially problematic if the patient has poor motor control, as frequently occurs with elderly patients. 2. Lens must be held very close to reading material. 3. Field of view becomes smaller as the lens is held farther from the eye.
Spectacle mounted plus lenses (single vision or bifocal adds)	1. Patient has use of both hands. 2. Wide field of view. 3. For powers less than about +6.00 D, binocular vision may be possible.	1. Head must be held very close to reading material. 2. It may be difficult to illuminate reading material (since the patient's head blocks light).
Loupe	1. Somewhat greater working distance than plus lenses mounted as spectacles. 2. May be removed when not needed.	1. Head must still be held close to reading material. 2. Handling of device may pose a challenge for certain patients.
Stand magnifier	Patient does not need to hold the device. Poor patient motor control is generally not an issue.	1. Eye position is critical. 2. Limited field of view. 3. Patient must accommodate or view through bifocal add.
Lens cap on telescope	Greater working distance	1. Limited field of view. 2. Steady head position required.

In our discussion of plus lenses for low vision, we've concentrated on handheld and fixed-focus stand magnifiers. As mentioned earlier in the chapter, plus lenses can also be mounted in spectacle frames (high-plus single vision lenses or high-plus bifocal adds) or as a loupe that is positioned in front of and attached to the spectacle frame. We'll learn later in the chapter that plus lenses can also be used in conjunction with telescopes for near viewing. Table 12-2 summarizes the advantages and disadvantages of these various configurations.

Effective Magnification

If you go to a pharmacy and look at handheld magnifying glasses, you'll see that they are often specified in terms of magnification. One might be labeled as 2.5×, for instance, while another is 5×. This is the magnification assuming a reference, or standard, distance of 25.0 cm. By assuming this standard reference distance of 25.0 cm, the manufacturer intends to make it possible for a customer to compare the magnification produced by various lenses. When calculated this way, magnification

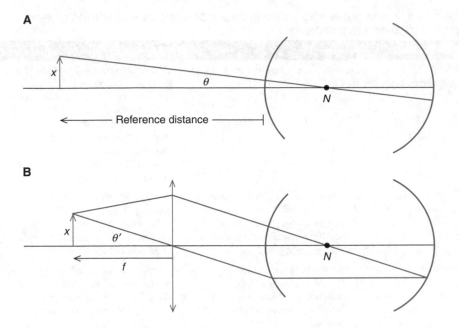

Figure 12-6. A. When specifying effective magnification, manufacturers of magnifying glasses usually assume a reference distance of 25 cm. **B.** The formula for effective magnification assumes the object is held at the focal point of the plus lens.

is sometimes referred to as M_{25} or *effective magnification*. While labeling magnifiers in this way may be of some benefit to people shopping for hand magnifiers, it is of limited utility to practitioners.

Let's derive the formula for effective magnification. Figure 12-6A shows that an object located at the reference distance subtends the angle θ at the eye. Compare this with Figure 12-6B, which shows that an object located at the focal point of a plus lens forms the angle θ' at the eye. The angular magnification, M_{25}, produced by the plus lens is defined as

$$M_{25} = \frac{\theta'}{\theta}$$

where $\theta' =$ object size/focal length of plus lens and $\theta =$ object size/reference distance. Substituting, we have

$$M_{25} = \frac{\text{reference distance}}{\text{focal length}}$$

But since the reference distance is 0.25 m and $F = 1/f$, we can rewrite the equation as

$$M_{25} = \frac{F}{4}$$

This equation may be familiar to you. It's sometimes given in undergraduate physics textbooks for the calculation of magnification produced by magnifying lenses. This formula assumes that the object will be in the focal plane of the lens, creating an image at infinity.

It's not uncommon for a patient to arrive at an eye appointment with a store-bought, handheld magnifying glass that she uses to read at near. Let's look at an example. *A patient purchased a magnifying glass labeled 2.5×. If she can read 4 M print at a distance of 40.0 cm without the magnifier, what size print do you expect her to be able to read with the magnifying lens?*

Once we have determined the power of the magnifying lens, we can solve this problem with the same strategy we have used for other problems on near magnification. The power of the lens is determined as follows:

$$M_{25} = \frac{F}{4}$$

$$2.5 = \frac{F}{4}$$

$$F = +10.0 \text{ D}$$

When reading material is held at the focal point of this +10.0 D lens, it produces the same angle at the eye as if held at 10.0 cm. By being able to decrease her reading distance from 40.0 to 10.0 cm, the patient experiences an angular magnification of 4×. Therefore, she will be able to resolve 1 M print when it's held at the focal point of the magnifier.

Magnification ratings can be tricky. Rather than using effective magnification, certain manufacturers may label lenses by their so-called conventional magnification ($M = 1 + F/4$). Moreover, magnification ratings attached to stand magnifiers are usually based solely on the power of the lens, even though the separation between the lens and the page can have a major effect on final magnification.

ELECTRONIC MAGNIFIERS FOR NEAR

Handheld electronic devices and closed-circuit televisions (CCTVs) are increasingly prescribed for patients with low vision. These devices magnify the original object, creating an enlarged electronic image on a screen. They typically have a variable zoom feature that allows the patient to adjust the magnification, thereby allowing her to remain at a comfortable distance from the device's screen. Patients may also benefit from the capacity of the display screen to reverse the contrast of the print (so that there is white print on a black background rather than black print on a white background) or add color contrast.

Your 70-year-old patient can read 6 M print at a distance of 40.00 cm through her 2.50 add. She would like to read 1 M print using an electronic handheld magnifier that she will rest on her reading material. What is the minimum magnification that must be provided by an electronic magnifier when she uses her bifocal addition?

The patient requires angular magnification of 6×. Since the reading material will remain at 40.0 cm, the magnifier must be set at 6.0×. She will be able to clearly see the material by looking through her bifocal add.

Another approach to this problem is to calculate the equivalent viewing power and then use the add equation to determine required electronic magnification. The equivalent viewing distance is 6.67 cm (i.e., 40.00 cm/6 = 6.67 cm), making the equivalent viewing power +15.00 D (i.e., 100/6.67 cm = +15.00 D). Knowing that the patient's add is +2.50, we can substitute into the add equation as follows:

Equivalent viewing power = (*M*) (add power)

+15.00 D = (*M*) (+2.50 D)

M = 6.0×

Using this approach, we again find that the electronic magnifier must be set at 6.0×.

TELESCOPES

A low-vision patient's distance vision can often be improved by using a telescope. Generally, a telescope is focused for infinity, but—as we will soon learn—telescopes can be adapted for near-vision use.

When an emmetrope or corrected ametrope uses a telescope to view an infinitely distant object, the light rays that enter the telescope have zero vergence, as do the light rays that exit the telescope. Since such a telescope does not have focal points, it is referred to as an **afocal** optical system.

Galilean Telescopes

The design of a Galilean telescope[11] is given in Figure 12-7A. For an infinitely distant object, a converging **objective** lens forms an image at its secondary focal plane, which is coincident with the primary focal plane of the **eyepiece**,[12] a negative lens. Parallel rays emerge from the telescope's eyepiece. Since both the object and the image are at infinity (the bundle of rays entering the telescope are parallel as are the rays emerging from the telescope), lateral magnification is not appropriate; instead, the angular magnification is specified.

---

11. Galilean telescopes are sometimes called **Dutch** telescopes.
12. The eyepiece is also referred to as the **ocular lens**.

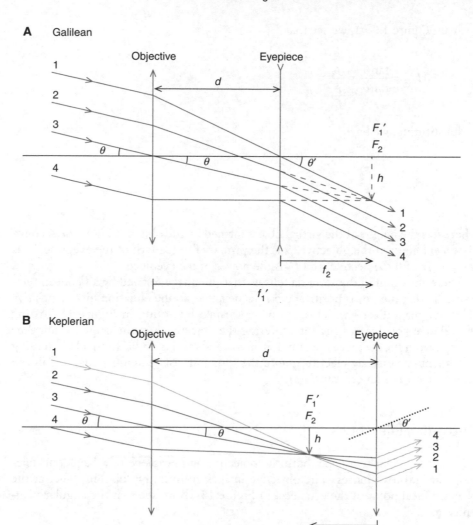

Figure 12-7. A. A Galilean telescope, which consists of a positive objective lens and a stronger minus eyepiece, produces positive angular magnification. **B.** A Keplerian telescope, which consists of a positive objective and a stronger positive eyepiece, produces negative angular magnification unless it is adapted with an inverting element (such as a prism). The tube length of a telescope, *d*, is the distance between the objective and eyepiece.

From Figure 12-7A, we see that

$$M_{ang} = \frac{\tan\theta'}{\tan\theta} = \frac{\dfrac{b}{f_2}}{\dfrac{b}{f_1'}} = \frac{f_1'}{f_2}$$

Substituting, we have

$$\boldsymbol{M_{ang} = -\frac{F_2}{F_1}}$$

where b is the height of the virtual object formed by the objective, f_1' is the secondary focal length of the objective, f_2 is the primary focal length of the eyepiece, F_1 is the power of the objective, and F_2 is the power of the eyepiece.

The minus sign in the formula tells us that the image formed by a Galilean telescope is erect (i.e., F_1 is positive and F_2 is negative, so the equation gives a positive value for magnification). This can be confirmed by noting in Figure 12-7A that the relative positions of the rays entering the objective are unchanged when they emerge from the eyepiece (i.e., ray 1 is on top and ray 4 is on bottom). (When using this formula, you may elect to ignore the sign and just remember that a Galilean telescope creates an erect image.)

Keplerian Telescopes

Unlike a Galilean telescope, both the objective and eyepiece of a Keplerian telescope are positive lenses. The objective images an infinitely distant object at the primary focal point of the eyepiece. In Figure 12-7B we see that the angular magnification is

$$M_{ang} = \frac{\tan\theta'}{\tan\theta} = \frac{\dfrac{b}{f_2}}{\dfrac{b}{f_1'}} = \frac{f_1'}{f_2}$$

Substituting, we have

$$M_{ang} = -\frac{F_2}{F_1}$$

This is the same formula as for a Galilean telescope.

Since both the objective and eyepiece are plus lenses, the magnification is negative, meaning that the image is inverted. Figure 12-7B reveals that the rays emerging from the eyepiece of a Keplerian telescope are in reverse order of the rays that enter the objective (i.e., entering the objective, ray 1 is on top, but it exits the eyepiece on bottom). (When using this formula, you can keep the minus sign in it or just remember that an uncompensated Keplerian telescope creates an inverted image.)

The Keplerian telescope in Figure 12-7B is referred to as **an astronomical telescope**.[13] Such a telescope would be inappropriate for clinical applications due to the inverted image. With the incorporation of prisms or mirrors, however, an astronomical telescope can be converted into a **terrestrial telescope** that produces an erect image. An advantage of Keplerian over Galilean telescopes is that they may provide the patient with a wider field of view, thereby allowing the patient to see a greater expanse of the visual world (for a given amount of magnification).

An Alternative Formula to Determine a Telescope's Angular Magnification

The distance between the lenses of a telescope—**the tube length**—can be used in combination with the power of the objective to calculate a telescope's angular magnification. From Figure 12-7 we can see that tube length, which we'll call d, is calculated as follows[14]:

$$d = f_1' - f_2 = \frac{1}{F_1} + \frac{1}{F_2}$$

By substituting into the formula for angular magnification that we derived previously and rearranging, we have:

$$M_{ang} = \frac{1}{1 - dF_1}$$

Later in this chapter, we'll see how this formula can be useful for understanding magnification when a telescope is used to correct for ametropia.

A Convenient Clinical Method to Determine a Telescope's Angular Magnification

The amount of light that enters an optical system is limited by the size of its **entrance pupil**. Light exits the system through its **exit pupil**. For most telescopes, the entrance pupil is the objective lens. The exit pupil is the image of the objective lens as seen from the eyepiece side of the telescope. A telescope's exit pupil is also called a **Ramsden circle**. Entrance and exit pupils are discussed in more detail in Appendix A.

---

13. Galilean telescopes may also be used in astronomy.
14. Keep in mind that for the negative eyepiece in a Galilean telescope f_2 has a positive value, while for the plus eyepiece of a Keplerian telescope f_2 has a minus value.

A   Galilean

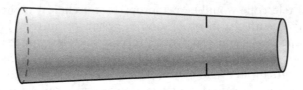

B   Keplerian

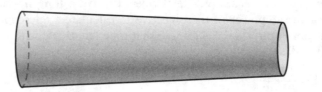

Figure 12-8. A telescope's exit pupil is the image of the objective lens as seen from the eyepiece side of the telescope. **A.** For a Galilean telescope, the exit pupil can be seen floating within the tube; it is a virtual image. **B.** For a Keplerian telescope, the exit pupil can be seen floating in space, outside of the tube; it is a real image.

For a Galilean telescope, the exit pupil is virtual and located within the telescope, while for a Keplerian system, it is real and located outside of the telescope (Figs. 12-8 and A-1 and A-2 in Appendix A). When the eyepiece end of the telescope is viewed from about 40 cm, the Galilean exit pupil is seen as a small circle within the telescope, while the Keplerian exit pupil is seen as a small circle floating in space outside the telescope.

The diameters of the entrance and exit pupils can be used to determine the magnification produced by a telescope. The formula is as follows:

$$M_{ang} = \frac{\text{entrance pupil diameter}}{\text{exit pupil diameter}}$$

This formula is useful to the clinician because it provides a quick and straightforward method to determine (or confirm) angular magnification. Table 12-3 summarizes the characteristics of Galilean and Keplerian systems.

TABLE 12-3. COMPARISON OF GALILEAN AND KEPLERIAN TELESCOPES

Characteristic	Galilean	Keplerian
Objective	Positive	Positive
Eyepiece	Negative	Positive
Image orientation	Erect	Inverted or erect*
Location of exit pupil	Within tube	Outside of tube
Field of view	Less	Greater
Tube length	Shorter	Longer
Shape	Straight	May be bent*
Weight	Generally lighter	Generally heavier

*Image-erecting systems (e.g., prisms or mirrors) are included in Keplerian systems to create the terrestrial systems that are used for clinical purposes. This may result in a bent tube.

Telescope Use in Ametropia

When using a telescope for distance viewing, a person with spherical ametropia has basically two choices. She can wear her distance prescription or she can adjust the tube length so that the vergence emerging from the telescope is equal to her far-point vergence. When wearing her distance prescription, the angular magnification is equal to that of the telescope. If, for instance, a patient with 10.00 D of myopia wears her spectacles when looking through a Galilean telescope that consists of a +10.00 DS objective and −50.00 DS eyepiece, she experiences an angular magnification of +5×.

Suppose the patient prefers to look through the telescope without her spectacles and to adjust the tube length instead. What would be the tube length? What magnification would she experience?

The easiest way to answer this question is to divide the eyepiece into two components: one that corrects the patient's ametropia and the remainder that contributes to the telescope magnification. Since the patient has 10.00 D of myopia, −10.00 D of the eyepiece's power is used to correct this ametropia and the remaining −40.00 D contributes to the telescope.

$$M_{ang} = -\frac{F_2}{F_1}$$

$$M_{ang} = -\frac{(-40.00 \text{ D})}{(10.00 \text{ D})} = +4.0\times$$

We can also solve this problem using the alternative formula for telescope magnification. Since the tube length must be shortened from 8.00 cm (i.e.,

$100/10.00\,\mathrm{D} + 100/{-}50.00\,\mathrm{D} = 8.00\ \mathrm{cm}$) to $7.50\ \mathrm{cm}$ (i.e., $100/10.00\,\mathrm{D} + 100/{-}40.00\,\mathrm{D} = 7.50\ \mathrm{cm}$), we have

$$M_{ang} = \frac{1}{1 - dF_1}$$

$$M_{ang} = \frac{1}{1 - (.0750\ \mathrm{m})(+10.00\ \mathrm{D})} = +4.0\times$$

As you can see, less magnification is provided when the myopic patient compensates for her myopia by shortening a Galilean telescope's tube length.

Now, let's consider a Keplerian telescope. *A patient with 10.00 D of myopia looks through a terrestrial telescope that has an objective of +10.00 D and an ocular of +50.00 D. What is the magnification when the patient wears her −10.00 D spectacles? What would be the tube length and magnification if she were to adjust the tube length to correct for her myopia?*

When viewing through her spectacle correction, the magnification is +5×. If she adjusts the tube length to correct her 10.00 D of myopia, we can conceptualize the eyepiece as a combination of a −10.00 D lens to correct the ametropia and a +60.00 D lens that contributes to the telescope. Our basic angular magnification formula for a telescope gives an angular magnification of +6.0×. (The magnification is positive since the image is erect in a terrestrial telescope.)

The magnification can also be determined using the alternative formula for magnification. As with the Galilean telescope, the tube length must be shortened, this time from 12.00 cm ($100/10.00\,\mathrm{D} + 100/50.00\,\mathrm{D} = 12.00\ \mathrm{cm}$) to 11.67 cm ($100/10.00\,\mathrm{D} + 100/60.00\,\mathrm{D} = 11.67\ \mathrm{cm}$). Substituting, we have

$$M_{ang} = \frac{1}{1 - dF_1}$$

$$M_{ang} = \frac{1}{1 - (.1167\ \mathrm{m})(+10.00\ \mathrm{D})} = -6.0\times$$

Since we are told that this Keplerian telescope has an erecting mechanism, the magnification is actually +6.0×. As you can see, more magnification is provided when the myopic patient compensates for her myopia by shortening a Keplerian telescope's tube length.[15]

In comparison to a myopic patient, a hyperopic patient must lengthen the tube to correct for her ametropia. For a Galilean telescope, this causes increased magnification, while for a Keplerian telescope it results in decreased magnification. Telescope use in ametropia is summarized in Table 12-4.

---

15. Certain low vision telescopes cannot be shortened to correct for myopia because when focused for infinity, they are already at their shortest length.

TABLE 12-4. AMETROPIA, TUBE LENGTH, AND MAGNIFICATION

	Myopia		Hyperopia	
	Galilean	Keplerian	Galilean	Keplerian
Tube length	Must shorten	Must shorten	Must lengthen	Must lengthen
Magnification	Decreased	Increased	Increased	Decreased

Telemicroscopes

Suppose a telescope that is focused for infinity is used to view an object that is at, say, 25.00 cm from the telescope. This situation is illustrated in Figure 12-9, which shows a patient viewing an object with a Galilean telescope that has a +10.00 D objective and a −30.00 D eyepiece. Without the telescope, the object has a vergence of less than −4.00 D at the eye; with the telescope, the vergence is about −20.00 D. The telescope amplifies the object vergence, and this amplification makes it impractical to use a telescope that is focused for infinity to view near objects (because too much accommodation is required to focus the image on the retina).

Lens caps.

A telescope can be adapted for near use by placing a plus lens over the objective and positioning the object at the primary focal point of this lens. The plus lens images the object at infinity; therefore, the rays that enter the telescope have zero vergence. A plus lens used in this manner is called a **lens cap**, and a telescope that is fitted with a lens cap is sometimes called a **telemicroscope**.

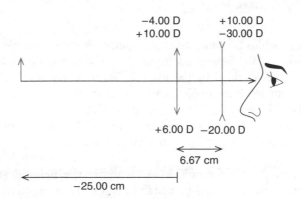

Figure 12-9. When a Galilean telescope (that is focused for distance) is used to view a near object, the vergence is amplified. Without the telescope the vergence at the eye would be less than −4.00 D, but with the telescope it is about −20.00 D. The separation of the objective and eyepiece—the tube length of the telescope—is 6.67 cm.

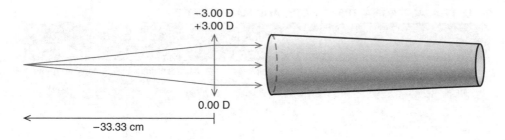

Figure 12-10. A lens cap is placed over the objective to create a telemicroscope. The working distance in this example is 33.33 cm.

Figure 12-10 shows a telemicroscope with a +3.00 D lens cap that would be used to view an object at a distance of 33.33 cm. The telemicroscope is sometimes mounted in a spectacle frame so that the patient has use of his hands. **While telemicroscopes provide patients with a greater working distance than plus lens magnifiers, their field of view is more limited.**

A fully corrected myopic patient with age-related macular degeneration can barely see 5 M print at a distance of 40.0 cm when looking through his bifocal add. He would like to read 1 M print and can do so with his +12.5 D magnifying glass, but must hold the material too close to the lens to allow him to make notes. If we wish to fit this patient with a +2.5× Galilean telescope, what power lens cap should we prescribe? How far should the reading material be held from the telemicroscope? How does this working distance compare with that obtained using the magnifying glass?

The telescope provides 2.5× magnification. Since the patient needs a total of 5.0× magnification (5 M/1 M = 5×), an additional 2.0× magnification (5.0/2.5 = 2.0×) is required. This can be obtained by halving the distance from 40 to 20 cm. For the light rays entering the telescope objective to be parallel, the lens cap must be +5.00 D (100/20 cm = 5 D). The working distance of 20 cm with this telemicroscope is greater than the 8 cm (100/12.5 D) required when using a +12.5 D magnifying glass (and would be more suitable for allowing the patient to make notes).[16]

Another approach to determine the lens cap power is to treat it as an add and use the add equation. This formula works whether the magnification is lateral (as with the virtual image formed by a stand magnifier) or angular, as is the case with telescopes. For the current problem, the equivalent viewing distance is 8.00 cm

16. In clinical practice, the patient's working distance and corresponding lens cap power are often determined first, and the magnification of the telescope is based upon these.

(i.e., 40.00 cm/5 = 8.00 cm), which means that the equivalent viewing power is +12.50 D (i.e., 100/8.00 cm + +12.50 D). Substituting, we have

Equivalent viewing power = (*M*) (add power)

+12.50 D = (2.5) (add power)

add power = +5.00 D

The required lens cap is +5.00 D.

Adjusting tube length.
Lens caps are used because vergence amplification makes it difficult (or impossible) to use a distance-focused telescope to view a near object. Is it possible to focus on near objects with a telescope that does not have a lens cap? Yes, if the tube length is increased sufficiently when viewing near objects, parallel light rays can be made to emerge from the eyepiece. This is the case for both Galilean and Keplerian telescopes.

How does this work? We can conceptualize the objective as consisting of two lenses: one that acts as a lens cap and the other that contributes to the telescope magnification. Think of a Galilean telescope that has a +20.00 D objective and −50.00 D eyepiece. The angular magnification is 2.5×, and the tube length when focused for infinity is 3.00 cm. If the patient wishes to focus at a distance 20.00 cm from the telescope, we consider the +20.00 D lens to consist of a +5.00 D lens cap (i.e., 100/20.00 cm = 5.00 D) and +15.00 D objective that contributes to angular magnification. The angular magnification of the newly created afocal telescope is +3.33× [i.e., −(−50.00 D/(+15.00 D) = 3.33×]. The tube length is 4.67 cm (i.e., 6.67 − 2.00 cm = 4.67 cm).

The same principles apply to a Keplerian telescope. Suppose a patient wishes to use a terrestrial telescope (+20.00 D objective and +50.00 D eyepiece; angular magnification of +2.5×) to view an object located 20.00 cm from the telescope. The tube length when focused for infinity is 7.00 cm. Again, we can think of the +20.00 D lens as consisting of a +5.00 lens cap and a +15.00 D objective lens that contributes to angular magnification. The magnification of the newly created afocal telescope is +3.33×, and the tube length is 8.67 cm (i.e., 6.67 + 2.00 cm = 8.67 cm).

Based on these calculations, which would provide more angular magnification when viewing an object at 20 cm: (1) a lens cap of +5.00 D or (2) increasing the tube length? Using a +5.00 D lens cap with a 2.5× telescope is equivalent to holding the reading material at 8.00 cm (i.e., 20.00 cm/2.5 = 8.00 cm). In comparison, increasing the tube length is equivalent to holding the reading material at 6.01 cm (i.e., 20.00 cm/3.33 = 6.01 cm). Increasing the tube length provides greater angular magnification. (Note that we obtain the same result for Galilean and terrestrial systems.)

SUMMARY

As the population ages, more patients will require the use of magnification devices to carry out daily life functions. This chapter has concentrated on the optics of near magnification. Equivalent viewing distance—the distance at which the reading material subtends the MAR—is a helpful concept for prescribing near devices. Many patients who require near magnification can be helped with a plus lens whose focal length is equal to the equivalent viewing distance. The magnification provided by stand and electronic magnifiers and telemicroscopes is based on similar principles.

KEY FORMULAE

Add (or cap) power:

Equivalent viewing power = (M) (add power)

Effective magnification:

$$M_{25} = \frac{F}{4}$$

Angular magnification produced by telescopes:

$$M_{ang} = -\frac{F_2}{F_1}$$

$$M_{ang} = \frac{1}{1 - dF_1}$$

$$M_{ang} = \frac{\text{entrance pupil diameter}}{\text{exit pupil diameter}}$$

FURTHER READING

Bailey IL. Locating the image in stand magnifiers. _Optom Monthly_. 1981a;72(6):22.

Bailey IL. The use of fixed focus stand magnifiers. _Optom Monthly_. 1981b;72(8):37.

Bailey IL. Locating the image in stand magnifiers—an alternative method. _Optom Monthly_. 1983;74:487.

Bailey IL. Magnification of the problem of magnification. _Optician_. 1984;185:16.

Cole RG. Predicting the low vision reading add. _J Am Optom Assoc_. 1993;64:19.

Kestenbaum A, Sturman RM. Reading glasses for patients with very poor vision. _Arch Ophthalmol_. 1956;56:451–470.

Nowakowski RW. _Primary Low Vision Care_. Norwalk, CT: Appleton & Lange, 1994.

Schwartz SH. _Visual Perception: A Clinical Orientation_, 4th ed. New York: McGraw-Hill, 2010.

SELF-ASSESSMENT PROBLEMS

1. A Keplerian telescope consists of a +10.00 D objective and a +25.00 D eyepiece. (a) What is the angular magnification provided by the telescope? (b) What is the tube length of the telescope?

2. A patient with 5.00 D of myopia wishes to view a distant object using a telescope that has a +8.00 D objective and –40.00 D ocular. She is not wearing a correction and adjusts the telescope's tube length to compensate for her ametropia. (a) What angular magnification does she experience? (b) What is the adjusted tube length?

3. An emmetrope uses the telescope in Prob. 2 (focused for infinity) to view an object located 100.0 cm anterior to the objective lens. (a) How much accommodation is required to focus the object onto the retina? (b) What is the power of the lens cap that should be prescribed if your goal is for the patient not to accommodate?

4. When looking through a +2.50 bifocal add, a patient can read 6 M print at a distance of 40.0 cm. She desires to read 2 M print. (a) What is the dioptric power of the magnifier that will allow her to read 2 M print if the print is at the focal point of the magnifier and she views through the distance correction? (b) When viewing through the distance portion of her spectacles, at what distance should she be from the magnifier in order to obtain maximum magnification? (c) The patient occasionally must resolve print that is slightly smaller than 2 M. How can she obtain greater magnification with the magnifier that you prescribed in part (a) of this problem?

5. When looking through his bifocal add, your patient is able to read 8 M print at a distance of 40.0 cm. Using a magnifying glass that was given to him as a gift, he can read 1 M print if the print is held at the focal point of the magnifying lens while he views through the distance portion on his spectacles. (a) What is the dioptric power of the magnifying glass? (b) What is effective magnification of the lens?

6. A patient who has adequate near vision with a +5.00 D magnifying lens would like to be fit with a spectacle-mounted telemicroscope so she can use both hands to type on the keyboard of a computer. (a) If the telescope has an angular magnification of 2.0×, what is the dioptric power of the lens cap that you should prescribe? (b) How far should the cap be from the computer screen? (c) What is a limitation of the telemicroscope?

7. If a patient has a distance visual acuity of 20/200, what power magnifying lens would allow her to read 2 M print? (Assume the print will be held at the focal point of the lens.)

8. When looking through his +2.50 add, a 75-year-old patient can read 4 M print. He would like to read 2 M print by resting a handheld electronic magnifier upon the print while looking though his bifocal add. (a) What is the minimum magnification the magnifier should be set at? (b) At what distance should it be held?

9. A patient can read 3 M print when it is held 40.0 cm from his spectacles. You prescribe a stand magnifier that contains a +10.00 D lens. The lens is at a fixed distance of 6.0 cm from the reading material. How close must the patient's eye be to the plus lens for him to read 1 M print?

Retinal Image Size

The size of the image that falls upon the retina is influenced by the nature of the patient's refractive error and the manner in which it is corrected. Retinal image size is of clinical importance because clear, comfortable, and functional binocular vision requires the fusion of the images formed on the two eye's retinas. When the images are sufficiently unequal in size, fusion becomes difficult and the patient may manifest asthenopic and other symptoms. A difference between the retinal image size (or shape) of the two eyes is referred to as **aniseikonia**.

SPECTACLE MAGNIFICATION

Both the refractive power and shape of a spectacle lens may affect retinal image size. Plus lens power causes angular magnification, while minus lens power causes minification. The change in retinal image size due to lens refractive power is referred to as the **power factor**.

Lens shape also affects retinal image size. For our discussion, shape is defined as front surface power, thickness, and index of refraction. All these contribute to the **shape factor** magnification produced by a lens.

The power and shape factors are independent from one another. Consider two equally powered lenses (e.g., two +5.00 DS lenses). Because of their equal powers, both have the same power factor. If refractive power was the only consideration, both lenses would produce the same magnification. But if the two lenses had different shapes, meaning that the front surface powers, thicknesses, or indices of refraction were different, they would cause unequal magnification because they have unequal shape factors.

In trying to understand the shape factor, it may be helpful to recall that a telescope, when focused for infinity, has no refractive power, yet produces angular magnification. It's possible to make a miniature Galilean telescope from a spectacle lens that has a plus front and minus back surface. Since this spectacle-telescope does not have any refractive power, it does not cause power magnification (the power factor is 1.0×), but it does have magnification due to its shape. A lens (such as the one we just described), which has no refractive power, but does produce angular magnification, is sometimes referred to as a **size lens**.

Spectacle magnification (M_{spect}) can be expressed as follows:

$$M_{spect} = (M_{power})\,(M_{shape})$$

where M_{power} is the power factor, and M_{shape} is the shape factor.

The power factor is calculated with the following formula:

$$M_{power} = \frac{1}{1 - dF_v}$$

where d is the vertex distance and F_v is the back vertex power.

The formula for the shape factor is

$$M_{shape} = \frac{1}{1 - \left(\dfrac{t}{n}\right) F_1}$$

where t is the lens thickness, n is the lens's index of refraction, and F_1 is the power of the front surface.

Putting this all together, we have

$$\boldsymbol{M_{spect} = (M_{power})(M_{shape})}$$

or

$$\boldsymbol{M_{spect} = \left(\frac{1}{1 - dF_v}\right) \left(\frac{1}{1 - \left(\dfrac{t}{n}\right) F_1}\right)}$$

Let's see how we can use this formula. A polycarbonate lens has a power of +5.00 D and a front surface refractive power of +2.00 D. If the lens has a center thickness of 4.0 mm and the vertex distance is 14 mm, what is the magnification produced by the lens?

It's straightforward to substitute in the formula for spectacle magnification as follows:

$$M_{spect} = \left(\frac{1}{1 - dF_v}\right) \left(\frac{1}{1 - \left(\dfrac{t}{n}\right) F_1}\right)$$

$$M_{spect} = \left(\frac{1}{1 - (0.014\text{ m})(+5.00\text{ D})}\right) \left(\frac{1}{1 - \left(\dfrac{0.004\text{ m}}{1.586}\right)(+2.00\text{ D})}\right)$$

$$M_{spect} = (1.08)(1.01) = 1.09\times$$

The spectacle magnification produced by the lens is 1.09×. Of this, 1.08× is due to the power of the lens and 1.01× is due to its shape.

As we mentioned previously, two lenses with the same refractive power may have different spectacle magnifications. *Let's consider another lens that has a power of +5.00 DS, but has a front surface power of +15.00 DS. We'll assume that the lens is made of the same material and has the same center thickness and vertex distance. What magnification is produced by this lens?*

$$M_{\text{spect}} = \left(\frac{1}{1 - dF_v}\right)\left(\frac{1}{1 - \left(\frac{t}{n}\right)F_1}\right)$$

$$M_{\text{spect}} = \left(\frac{1}{1 - (0.014 \text{ m})(+5.00 \text{ D})}\right)\left(\frac{1}{1 - \left(\frac{0.004 \text{ m}}{1.586}\right)(+15.00 \text{ D})}\right)$$

$$M_{\text{spect}} = (1.08)(1.04) = 1.12$$

Although each of these +5.00 DS lenses has a power factor of 1.08×, they produce different spectacle magnification because the shape factors are different (1.01× vs. 1.04×). The lens that has the more curved front surface results in more magnification. **When two lenses of equal power are made of the same material and have the same thickness and vertex distance, the lens with the more curved front surface will produce greater magnification. (Keep in mind that almost all spectacle lenses have a plus front surface.[1])**

Now that we've discussed the magnification produced by spectacle lenses, you might be curious about contact lenses. How do contact lenses affect image size? First consider the power factor. Since the vertex distance is zero, the power factor is 1.0×. As to the shape factor, contact lenses are very thin, making the shape factor approximately 1.0×. So for clinical purposes, contact lenses do not affect the retinal image size.

We've learned the basics of spectacle magnification and are just about ready to see how spectacle lenses affect the retinal image size when used to correct ametropia.

---

1. A lens clock is used clinically to measure the **base curve**, which is on the front surface of a spectacle lens. If the front surface is toric, the weaker (less curved) meridian is the base curve. It's important to keep in mind that a lens clock is calibrated for a refractive index of 1.53. This means that the base curve does not equal the surface refractive power unless the lens material is crown glass (which has an index very close to 1.53). Further details can be found in *Brooks CW, Borish IM*. A System for Ophthalmic Dispensing. *St. Louis: Butterworth-Heinemann, 2007.*

But before delving into this important issue, we first need to discuss retinal image size in uncorrected ametropia.

RETINAL IMAGE SIZE IN UNCORRECTED AMETROPIA

As we learned in Chapter 7, ametropia is due to a mismatch between the eye's refractive power and its axial length. The retinal image size in uncorrected ametropia depends on whether the ametropia is axial or refractive in nature.

The reduced eye has a length of 22.22 mm. When the eye is longer than this, it is said to have **axial myopia**, and when it is shorter, **axial hyperopia. Most myopia is axial in nature.** If the eye is more powerful than the reduced eye, which has a power of +60.00 D, the condition is called **refractive myopia**, and when the eye is weaker than +60.00 D, the condition is **refractive hyperopia.** Either myopia or hyperopia can have a mixture of axial and refractive components.

Let's first look at axial ametropia. Figure 13-1 shows three axial lengths that would be expected in hyperopia, emmetropia, and myopia. Suppose the eye is viewing an arrow. A light ray emerging from the tip of the arrow passes undeviated through the eye's nodal point and contributes to the retinal image. Note that as the eye's axial length increases, the size of the retinal image also increases. **This tells us that in uncorrected axial myopia, retinal image size is larger than in emmetropia and that in uncorrected axial hyperopia, it is smaller than in emmetropia.**

Now let's see what happens to retinal image size in uncorrected refractive ametropia. As illustrated in Figure 13-2A, the eye has a fixed length. When the refractive power of the eye increases (as in myopia) or decreases (as in hyperopia), the image becomes blurred, but its size does not change. Think of a projector that focuses an arrow on a screen. If we adjust the focus so that the image is blurred, as in Figure 13-2B, the blurred image, as measured from the centers of the blur circles, is the same size as the focused image. It doesn't matter if

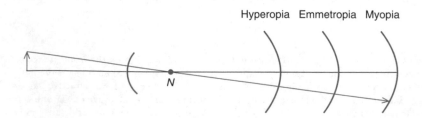

Figure 13-1. In axial ametropia, the retinal image size increases as the eye's axial length increases.

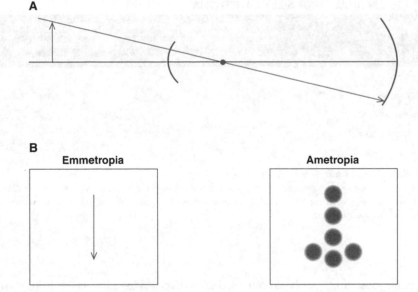

Figure 13-2. A. In refractive ametropia, image blur is not due to the axial length being too short or long. **B.** Refractive ametropia results in a blurred retinal image, but does not affect the image size.

the projector lens is made too strong or too weak. **The take home message is that in uncorrected refractive ametropia, the image is the same size as in emmetropia.**

RETINAL IMAGE SIZE IN CORRECTED AMETROPIA

Before talking about retinal image size in corrected ametropia, let's recap what we've learned so far about spectacle magnification and retinal image size in *uncorrected* ametropia:

- A plus spectacle lens causes magnification.
- A minus spectacle lens causes minification.
- A contact lens causes no magnification (or minification).
- In axial myopia, the retinal image is larger than in emmetropia and in axial hyperopia, it is smaller than in emmetropia.
- In refractive myopia and hyperopia, the retinal image is the same size as in emmetropia.

TABLE 13-1. RETINAL IMAGE SIZE IN AMETROPIA

| | Retinal Image Size When the Ametropia Is | | |
Condition	Uncorrected (mm)	Corrected with a Contact Lens (mm)	Corrected with a Spectacle Lens* (mm)
Emmetropia	x	x	x
Axial myopia	>x	>x	x
Refractive myopia	x	x	<x**
Axial hyperopia	<x	<x	x
Refractive hyperopia	x	x	>x**

*Spectacle lens located at anterior focal point of eye.

**The retinal image size in uncorrected refractive myopia and hyperopia is the same as in emmetropia. Correction of refractive myopia with a spectacle lens causes minification, while correction of refractive hyperopia with a spectacle lens causes magnification.

What does this imply about retinal image size in *corrected* ametropia? We can assume that the retinal image size will be about the same as in emmetropia when:

- Axial ametropia is corrected with spectacles (A minus lens minifies the enlarged image found in uncorrected axial myopia and a plus lens magnifies the diminished image found in uncorrected axial hyperopia.)
- Refractive ametropia is corrected with contact lenses (The retinal image size in uncorrected refractive myopia and hyperopia is the same as in emmetropia, and a contact lens doesn't change this.)

For the retinal image in corrected axial ametropia to be exactly the same size as in the emmetropic eye, the spectacle lenses should be positioned at the anterior focal point of the eye, which is 16.7 mm (i.e., 1000/60.00 D = 16.7 mm) anterior to the reduced eye's front surface. This is referred to as **Knapp's law**. In clinical practice, it is not necessary for the vertex distance to be exactly 16.7 mm. Retinal image size in uncorrected and corrected ametropia is summarized in Table 13-1.

What are the clinical implications of all this? Consider **anisometropia**, a relatively prevalent condition in which the two eyes have different refractive errors. Depending on the magnitude and nature of the anisometropia (axial or refractive) and the manner in which it is corrected (spectacles or contact lenses), the retinal images in the two eyes may be different sizes, a condition we previously referred to as aniseikonia.

Let's look at an example. *A patient has the following refractive error:*

OD   −2.00 DS
OS   −5.00 DS

Through a clinical procedure called keratometry, which is discussed in the following chapter, we determine that the corneas of the two eyes have the same power. Is the anisometropia axial or refractive in nature? Which eye has a larger image? If our goal is to equalize retinal image size, should we prescribe spectacles or contact lenses?

Since the corneas of the two eyes have the same power, we can assume that the anisometropia is axial in nature. The left eye has a longer axial length, making its uncorrected retinal image larger than the right eye's. Correction with spectacle lenses would minify the images of both eyes, but since the left lens is more minus, it would cause more minification. As a result, both eyes would have image sizes equal to that found in emmetropia.

Does this mean that we should not consider prescribing contact lenses for this patient?[2] Not really. The visual system is remarkably adaptable, and patients with axial anisometropia generally do well with contact lenses. If a patient with significant axial anisometropia cannot adapt to contact lenses, however, it is possible that their symptoms are related to aniseikonia.

We'll do one more case. A patient has no visual discomfort when she wears contact lenses, but has never felt comfortable wearing her current polycarbonate spectacles, which have the following powers:

> OD   −5.00 DS
> OS   −2.50 DS

Both of these lenses have front curvatures of +2.00 D and center thicknesses of 1.5 mm. Keratometry readings reveal that the right cornea is about 4.00 diopters stronger than the left. Assuming that the spectacle lens powers are appropriate and that the patient's symptoms are due to aniseikonia, how could we design her new spectacle lenses to minimize the symptoms?

This is a case of refractive anisometropia. When not wearing any correction or while wearing contact lenses, the retinal images are equal in size. Wearing spectacles, however, causes the right eye's retinal image to be smaller than the left eye's image. Assuming a vertex distance of 14 mm, the power factor for the right lens is

$$\text{Power factor} = \frac{1}{1 - dF_v}$$

$$\text{Power factor} = \frac{1}{1 - (0.014 \text{ m})(-5.00 \text{ D})} = 0.935\times$$

---

2. Contact lenses would *not* affect the difference in image size between the two eyes.

For the left lens, the power factor is

$$\text{Power factor} = \frac{1}{1 - (0.014 \text{ m})(-2.50 \text{ D})} = 0.966\times$$

When both lenses have a front surface curvature of +2.00 D and a center thickness of 1.5 mm, the shape factor for each lens is

$$\text{Shape factor} = \left(\frac{1}{1 - \left(\frac{t}{n} \right) F_1} \right)$$

$$\text{Shape factor} = \left(\frac{1}{1 - \left(\frac{0.0015}{1.586} \right) + 2.00 \text{ D}} \right) = 1.00\times$$

Since the total spectacle magnification is the product of the power and shape factors, a front surface power of +2.00 D and a center thickness of 1.5 mm result in magnification of 0.935× for the right eye and 0.966× for the left eye.

We can compensate for this difference by changing the shape factor for the right lens. By increasing its curvature and thickness, we can increase its magnification relative to the left lens.[3] Let's select a front surface curvature of +10.00 D and a thickness of 5.0 mm for the right lens. The shape factor is

$$\text{Shape factor} = \left(\frac{1}{1 - \left(\frac{0.005}{1.586} \right) + 10.00 \text{ D}} \right) = 1.03\times$$

The total spectacle magnification for the right lens is

$$M_{\text{spect}} = (M_{\text{power}})(M_{\text{shape}})$$

$$M_{\text{spect}} = (0.935)(1.03) = 0.963\times$$

With this design, the spectacle magnification of the right lens (0.963×) is very close to that produced by the flatter, thinner left lens, thereby all but eliminating the aniseikonia. The right lens, however, would look much different than the left lens, and this may not be cosmetically acceptable to the patient. When the shape of a lens is intentionally manipulated to affect retinal image size, the lens is sometimes referred to as an **iseikonic lens.**

In many cases it's not necessary to design an iseiknonic lens that fully compensates for the difference in retinal image sizes. Modestly adjusting front surface power and thickness may be sufficient to relieve symptoms. For example, in the current case we could try increasing the right lens front surface power to +5.00 D

---

3. While changing the thickness and front surface power can significantly affect the shape factor, changing the index of refraction has little effect.

(from +2.00 D) and the center thickness to 3.0 mm (from 1.5 mm). This solution would be more cosmetically acceptable. We could also try to minimize the power factor by making sure the vertex distance is as short as possible.

SUMMARY

The retinal image size depends on the nature of the ametropia (axial or refractive) and how it is corrected (contact lenses or spectacles). In uncorrected axial myopia, the retinal image is larger than in emmetropia, while in uncorrected axial hyperopia, it is smaller than in emmetropia. Correction with a contact lens does not alter this, whereas correction with a spectacle lens makes the retinal images in axial myopia and hyperopia about the same size as in emmetropia. In comparison, the retinal image sizes in uncorrected refractive myopia and hyperopia are both equal to that in emmetropia. Again, correction with a contact lens does not alter this, whereas a minus spectacle lens used to correct refractive myopia makes the image smaller than in emmetropia, and a plus spectacle lens used to correct refractive hyperopia makes the image larger than in emmetropia.

The correction of anisometropia may result in aniseikonia. In the case of axial anisometropia, one would expect that correction with spectacles would be preferable to contact lenses, but this often is not the case. When prescribing spectacles for refractive anisometropia, it's sometimes necessary to minimize the difference in spectacle magnification between the two eyes. This may require special lens designs in which front surface power and lens thickness are selected for this purpose. Commonly, however, modest adjustments in front surface power and thickness, while minimizing vertex distance, are sufficient.

KEY FORMULAE

Spectacle magnification:

$$M_{spect} = (M_{power})(M_{shape})$$

$$M_{spect} = \left(\frac{1}{1 - dF_v}\right)\left(\frac{1}{1 - \left(\frac{t}{n}\right)F_1}\right)$$

SELF-ASSESSMENT PROBLEMS

1. What is the spectacle magnification produced by a −6.50 DS polycarbonate spectacle lens that has a front surface power of +3.00 D and a center thickness of 2.00 mm? (Assume a vertex distance of 12.0 mm.)

2. Your patient has the following spectacle prescription (vertex distance of 14.0 mm):

OD   −6.00 DS
OS   −3.00 DS

(a) Assuming that both lenses are made of CR 39 and have front surface powers of +2.00 D and center thicknesses of 2.00 mm, what is the spectacle magnification for each lens? (b) The anisometropia is refractive, and the corrected patient experiences symptoms of aniseikonia. If you wish to remedy this by increasing the thickness of the right lens to 4.00 mm, what surface power should you prescribe for this lens? (c) Is this a reasonable solution for the patient?

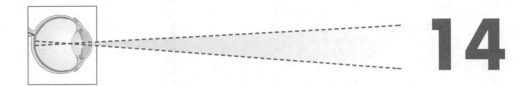

Reflection

14

Light rays that are incident upon a surface can be transmitted, absorbed, or reflected. In this chapter, we consider reflection that is produced by **specular surfaces**—smooth (shiny) surfaces such as mirrors. As illustrated in Figure 14-1, the angle of reflection for a mirror is equal to the angle of incidence. Referred to as the **law of reflection**, all angles are measured with respect to the normal to the surface.

Not all surfaces are specular. **Perfectly diffusing surfaces,**[1] such as a black-board, have the same brightness regardless of the angle from which they are viewed. Unlike specular surfaces, they do not appear shiny or glossy. In geometrical optics, we are concerned with only specular surfaces.

RAY TRACING: CONCAVE, CONVEX, AND PLANE MIRRORS

Concave Mirrors

Like converging spherical refracting surfaces and lenses, concave mirrors have plus power and converge light. Figure 14-2 shows parallel light rays—traveling from left to right—incident on a converging mirror. After reflection, the rays are traveling in the reverse direction and intersect at what we'll call the mirror's secondary focal point, F'.

The **center of curvature** for the mirror in Figure 14-2 is labeled "C." Dotted lines that emanate from the center of curvature are **radii of curvature**. Each of these is, by definition, normal to the mirror's surface. Note that the law of reflection is followed, meaning that the angle of reflection for each light ray is equal to the angle of incidence. As with a spherical refracting surface, the optical axis of a mirror includes the center of curvature and focal point.

---

1. A perfectly diffusing surface is also referred to as a **cosine** or **Lambert surface.**

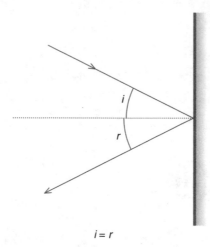

i = r

Figure 14-1. For a specular surface, such as a mirror, the angle of reflection (*r*) equals the angle of incidence (*i*). Both angles are specified with respect to the normal to the surface (*dotted line*).

Similar to lenses, ray tracing can be used to locate the image formed by a mirror. In Figure 14-3A, we see how four rays are used to locate an image. Ray 1 emerges from the object parallel to the optical axis and is reflected through the secondary focal point. Ray 2 strikes the mirror at the optical axis; the angles of incidence and reflection are symmetrical with regard to the optical axis. The third ray passes through the secondary focal point and is reflected parallel to the optical axis. Finally, ray 4 passes

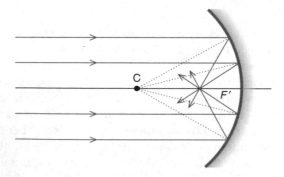

Figure 14-2. Parallel light rays, incident upon a converging mirror, are focused at the mirror's secondary focal point, *F'*. The dotted lines are radii that extend from the center of curvature (C) to the mirror's surface. The radii are normal to the surface of the mirror.

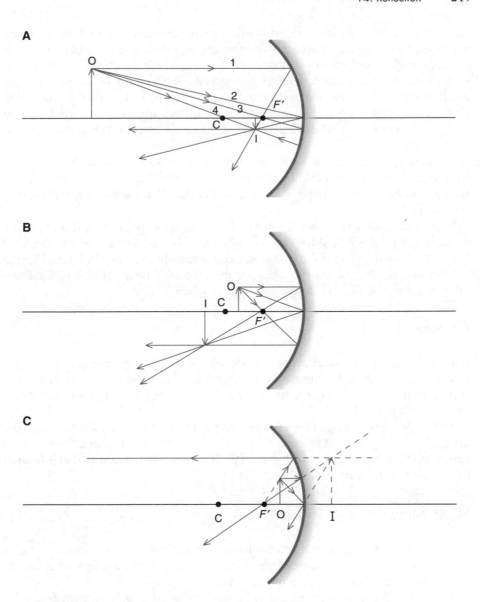

Figure 14-3. Ray tracing can be used to locate the image formed by a mirror. **A.** An object (O) located beyond a converging mirror's center of curvature (which is at 2*f*) length results in a real, inverted, and minified image (I). **B.** An object located between the center of curvature and focal point of a converging mirror results in a real, inverted, and magnified image. **C.** An object located within the converging mirror's focal length results in a virtual, erect, and magnified image.

through the center of curvature, strikes the mirror perpendicular to its surface, and is reflected back through the center of curvature (i.e., since the angle of incidence is zero, the angle of reflection is also zero). In this case, where the object is farther away than the center of curvature, the reflected rays intersect to form a real, inverted, and minified image that is located to the left of the mirror. (As is the case with refracting surfaces and lenses, the real images formed by mirrors are always inverted and can be focused on a screen, while virtual images are always erect and cannot be focused on a screen.)

A real image produced by a concave mirror is not always minified. As we can see from Figure 14-3B, when the object is situated between the center of curvature and the focal point, the inverted real image is larger than the object (and to the left of the mirror).

In the two examples we just discussed, the object is located farther from the mirror than the focal point. What happens when the object is located within the focal length of the mirror? As is the case with a converging lens, an object located within the focal length results in a virtual, erect, and magnified image (Fig. 14-3C). For a mirror, the virtual image is to the right of its surface.

Convex Mirrors

Like diverging spherical refracting surfaces and lenses, convex mirrors have minus power and diverge light. Figure 14-4A shows parallel light rays incident upon a convex mirror. After reflection, these rays appear to emerge from the mirror's secondary focal point, F'.

As can be seen in Figure 14-4B, the same four rays that are used to locate the image formed by a concave mirror can be used to locate the image formed by a convex mirror. A convex mirror forms a minified, erect, virtual image that is located to the right of the mirror.

Plane Mirrors

A plane mirror is flat, meaning that it has an infinite radius of curvature. Unlike a concave or convex mirror, it does not change the vergence of the light that is incident upon it and therefore has a power of zero.

Figure 14-5A shows an object that is located in front of a plane mirror. By applying the law of reflection to each of the light rays, we can locate the image. Note that the image is virtual and located to the right of the mirror at the same distance from the mirror as the object. If, for example, the object is 3.0 m in front of the mirror, the virtual image is 3.0 m behind the mirror.

What is the magnification produced by a plane mirror? In Figure 14-5B, the object is an arrow. As you can see, the separation of the top and bottom points of the arrow is equal to the separation of the images of these two points. The image produced by a plane mirror is the same size and orientation (erect) as the object (i.e., the magnification is +1.0×).

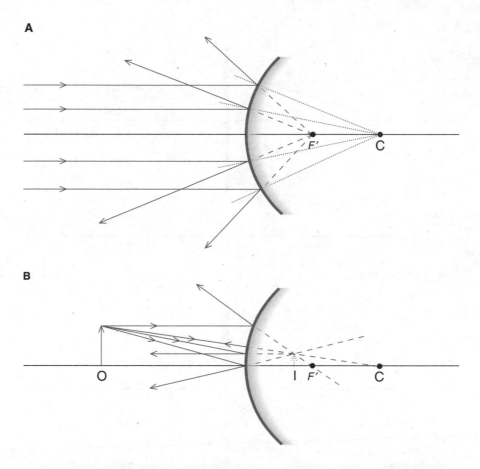

Figure 14-4. A. Parallel rays, incident upon a convex mirror, appear to emerge from the secondary focal point, *F′*. The dotted lines that extend from the center of curvature are radii of curvature; they are perpendicular to the mirror's surface. **B.** Ray tracing shows that the image formed by this convex mirror is virtual, erect, and minified. The virtual image is located behind the mirror.

POWER OF MIRRORS

It is relatively straightforward to adapt the principles and formulae that apply to spherical refracting surfaces to mirrors.[2] To do so, we must recognize that there is only one medium (usually air), and that after reflection, the direction of the rays is reversed.

---

2. Whereas the branch of optics dealing with refraction is referred to as **dioptrics**, the branch dealing with mirrors is **catoptrics**.

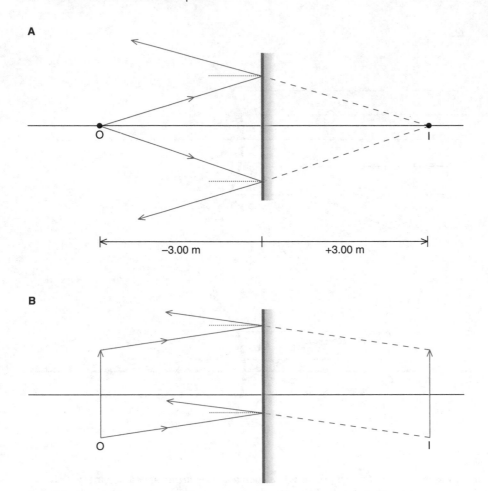

Figure 14-5. A. The image formed by a plane mirror is virtual and located the same distance from the mirror as the object. **B.** The image formed by a plane mirror is the same size as the object.

Recall from Chapter 2 that the power of a spherical refracting surface can be determined with the following relationship:

$$F = \frac{n' - n}{r}$$

Referring back to Figures 14-3 and 14-4, we see that both the incident and reflected rays exist in the primary medium and that the direction of the rays is reversed after reflection. To use our linear sign convention, this reversal in direction can be accounted for as follows:

$$n' = -n$$

Substituting, we have

$$F = \frac{-n - n}{r}$$

$$F = \frac{-2n}{r}$$

If the mirror is in air ($n = 1$), then

$$\mathbf{F = \frac{-2}{r}}$$

As with a spherical refracting surface, the power of a mirror can be calculated directly from its focal length. Recall that the relationship between the power of a spherical refracting surface and its secondary focal length is

$$F = \frac{n'}{f'}$$

But for a mirror,

$$n' = -n$$

Thus, the relationship between the power of a mirror and the secondary focal length is

$$F = \frac{-n}{f'}$$

If the mirror is in air, then

$$\mathbf{F = \frac{-1}{f'}}$$

Another useful relationship can be derived by equating the previous power formulae

$$\frac{-2}{r} = \frac{-1}{f'}$$

or

$$\mathbf{r = 2f'}$$

This relationship tells us that the radius of curvature of a mirror is equal to twice its focal length.

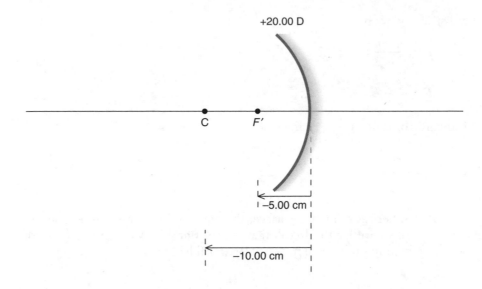

Figure 14-6. A mirror with a radius of curvature of −10.00 cm has a secondary focal length of −5.00 cm and a power of +20.00 D.

Let us look at an example. *A concave mirror has a radius of curvature of 10.00 cm. Where is the focal point located with respect to the mirror's surface? What is the mirror's power?*

As can be seen in Figure 14-6, the center of curvature of a concave mirror is to the left of its surface. Using the linear sign convention that we have employed throughout this book (in which distances are measured from surfaces), this is designated as a negative distance. The focal length is calculated as follows:

$$r = 2f'$$

$$-10.00 \text{ cm} = 2f'$$

$$f' = -5.00 \text{ cm}$$

The focal point is located 5.00 cm to the left of the mirror's surface. The mirror's power is

$$F = \frac{-1}{f'}$$

$$F = \frac{-1}{-0.05 \text{ m}}$$

$$F = +20.00 \text{ D}$$

THE VERGENCE RELATIONSHIP

As with spherical refracting surfaces and lenses, the vergence relationship can be used to locate the image produced by a mirror and to determine its magnification. We need to keep in mind, however, that after reflection the direction of the light is reversed.

Consider this example. An object is located 80.00 cm in front of a concave mirror that has a radius of curvature of 33.33 cm. The object is 5.00 cm in height. Where is the image located? Is the image real or virtual? Is it erect or inverted? What is its height?

The solution to this problem is illustrated in Figure 14-7. Since the center of curvature is located to the left of the mirror's surface, this distance is negative. The power of the converging mirror is

$$F = \frac{-2}{r}$$

$$F = \frac{-2}{-0.3333 \text{ m}}$$

$$F = +6.00 \text{ D}$$

This makes sense because we know that all concave mirrors have positive power.

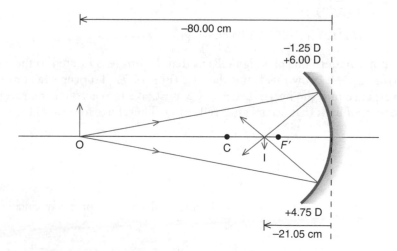

Figure 14-7. Formation of a real, minified, and inverted image by a converging mirror. The paraxial relationship can be used to determine the location and size of the image. For this and following diagrams in this chapter, the object vergence and mirror power are given at the top of the mirror and the image vergence is given below the mirror. See the text for details.

Recall from Chapter 3 that the vergence for an object situated in air is calculated as follows:

$$L = \frac{1}{l}$$

$$L = \frac{1}{-0.80 \text{ m}}$$

$$L = -1.25 \text{ D}$$

To determine the image vergence, we use the vergence relationship

$$L' = L + F$$

$$L' = -1.25 \text{ D} + 6.00 \text{ D}$$

$$L' = +4.75 \text{ D}$$

Since the vergence is positive, the image is real and must be located, as can be seen in Figure 14-7, to the *left* of the mirror. (Recall that converging light rays form a real image that can be focused on a screen. Such an image can be formed only to the left of a concave mirror's surface.) Suppose we determine image distance with the same formula we use for a lens situated in air. In this case,

$$L' = \frac{1}{l'}$$

$$l' = \frac{1}{+4.75 \text{ D}}$$

$$l' = +0.2105 \text{ m} \quad \text{or} \quad +21.05 \text{ cm}$$

This is not correct! The plus sign tells us that the image is located to the right of the mirror, but we know this is not the case (Fig. 14-7). To properly convert the image vergence into the image distance, we must take into account the reversal in the direction of light that occurs after reflection. Therefore, for mirrors,

$$L' = \frac{-1}{l'}$$

Returning to the sample problem, the image distance is properly calculated as follows:

$$l' = \frac{-1}{+4.75 \text{ D}}$$

$$l' = -21.05 \text{ cm}$$

The real image is formed 21.05 cm to the left of the mirror.

Now let's calculate the lateral magnification. From Chapter 3, recall that

$$M_L = \frac{L}{L'}$$

Therefore,

$$M_L = \frac{-1.25 \text{ D}}{+4.75 \text{ D}}$$

$$M_L = -0.26\times$$

The image is minified and inverted. Its size is

$$(-0.26)(5.00 \text{ cm}) = -1.30 \text{ cm}$$

As with lenses, we can also calculate magnification using linear distances. But because the light rays reverse direction after reflection, we must insert a minus sign into the equation:

$$\mathbf{M_L} = \frac{-l'}{l}$$

For our example, we have

$$M_L = -\frac{-21.05 \text{ cm}}{-80.00 \text{ cm}}$$

$$M_L = -0.26\times$$

For this same mirror, locate the image if the object is located 10.0 cm in front of the mirror. Is the image real or virtual? Is it erect or inverted? What is the magnification?

Before performing any calculations, it's helpful to note that the object is located within the focal distance ($f' = -100/6.00$ D $= -16.67$ cm). As is the case for a converging lens, this results in an image that is virtual, erect, and magnified.

The object vergence is

$$L = \frac{1}{l}$$

$$L = \frac{1}{-0.10 \text{ cm}}$$

$$L = -10.00 \text{ D}$$

The image vergence is determined with the paraxial equation

$$L' = L + F$$

$$L' = -10.00 \text{ D} + 6.00 \text{ D}$$

$$L' = -4.00 \text{ D}$$

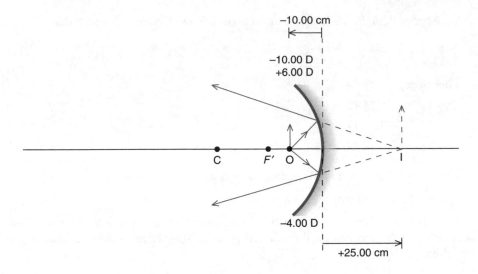

Figure 14-8. Formation of a virtual, magnified, and erect image by a converging mirror. See the text for details.

The negative vergence confirms that the image is virtual. As can be seen in Figure 14-8, which illustrates the solution to this problem, it is formed by diverging rays and must be located to the right of the mirror. Its exact location is determined as follows:

$$L' = \frac{-1}{l'}$$

$$l' = \frac{-1}{-4.00 \text{ D}}$$

$$l' = 0.25 \text{ m} \quad \text{or} \quad +25.0 \text{ cm}$$

What is the magnification? Using the vergence formula for lateral magnification, we have

$$M_L = \frac{L}{L'}$$

$$M_L = \frac{-10.00 \text{ D}}{-4.00 \text{ D}}$$

$$M_L = +2.50\times$$

This confirms that the virtual image is erect and magnified.

Now consider an object located 20.00 cm in front of a convex mirror whose focal length is 25.00 cm. Where is the image located? Is the image real or virtual? Is it erect or inverted? What is the magnification?

The first thing to recognize is that this convex mirror, like a diverging surface or lens, forms an image that is virtual, erect, and minified. Since the secondary focal point is located to the right of the mirror, it is designated with a positive sign (Fig. 14-9). The mirror's power is calculated as

$$F = \frac{-1}{f'}$$

$$F = \frac{-1}{0.25 \text{ m}}$$

$$F = -4.00 \text{ D}$$

Since the object is located 20.00 cm to the left of the mirror, the object vergence is −5.00 D. The image vergence is determined with the vergence relationship as follows:

$$L' = L + F$$

$$L' = -5.00 \text{ D} + (-4.00 \text{ D})$$

$$L' = -9.00 \text{ D}$$

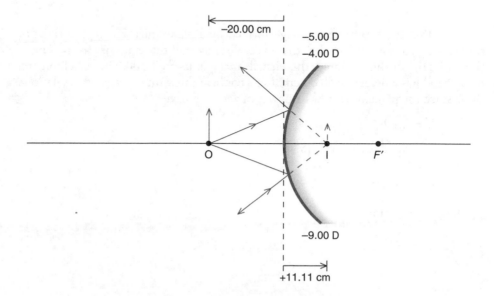

Figure 14-9. Formation of a virtual, minified, and erect image by a diverging mirror. See the text for details.

The negative image vergence confirms that the image is virtual. Where is it located? From Figure 14-9 and our understanding of mirrors, we know that the virtual image must be located to the right of the mirror. The distance is

$$L' = \frac{-1}{l'}$$

$$l' = \frac{-1}{-9.00 \text{ D}}$$

$$l' = +0.111 \text{ m} \quad \text{or} \quad +11.1 \text{ cm}$$

The magnification is

$$M_{\text{L}} = \frac{L}{L'}$$

$$M_{\text{L}} = \frac{-5.00 \text{ D}}{-9.00 \text{ D}}$$

$$M_{\text{L}} = +0.56\times$$

This confirms that the virtual image is erect and minified.

Before we move on, let's do one more problem. *An object 60.00 cm in height is located 200.00 cm from a plane mirror. Where is the image, and what is the magnification?*

Recall that the erect virtual image formed by a plane mirror is to the right of the mirror at a distance equal to the object distance and the same size as the object (Fig. 14-5B). In this example, the virtual image is located 200.00 cm behind the mirror and has a height of 60.00 cm. Let's confirm this with the vergence relationship. Since the plane mirror has a power of zero, we have

$$L' = L + F$$

$$L' = \left(\frac{1}{-2.00 \text{ m}}\right) + 0.00 \text{ D}$$

$$L' = -0.50 \text{ D}$$

The image distance is

$$L' = \frac{-1}{l'}$$

$$l' = \frac{-1}{-0.50 \text{ D}}$$

$$l' = +2.00 \text{ m} \quad \text{or} \quad +200 \text{ cm}$$

TABLE 14-1. IMAGE FORMATION BY MIRRORS

	Object Location*	Nature of Image**	Image Orientation	Image Size
Plus (concave)	$2f$	Real	Inverted	Equal to object
Plus (concave)	$>2f$	Real	Inverted	<Object
Plus (concave)	$>f$ but $<2f$	Real	Inverted	>Object
Plus (concave)	$<f$	Virtual	Erect	>Object
Minus (convex)	Anywhere	Virtual	Erect	<Object
Plano	Anywhere	Virtual	Erect	Equal to object

*$2f = r$

** Real images are located on the same side of the mirror as the object, while virtual images are located on the other side.

The magnification is

$$M_L = \frac{L}{L'}$$

$$M_L = \frac{-0.50 \text{ D}}{-0.50 \text{ D}}$$

$$M_L = +1.00\times$$

These calculations confirm our conclusions from Figure 14-5: for a plane mirror, image distance is equal to object distance, and the image and object are the same height.

Table 14-1 summarizes image formation by mirrors. Note the similarities to thin lenses.

REFLECTIONS AND ANTIREFLECTION COATINGS

A transparent surface can both transmit and reflect light. Take, for instance, a typical window. The window transmits light—you can see through it and someone on the other side of the window can see you. If you look closely, however, you may also see your reflection in the window—it acts as a mirror.

As the refractive index of a surface increases, the amount of light that is reflected increases. For light rays that are perpendicular to a transparent surface, the fraction of light (R) that is reflected is given by the following relationship:

$$R = \left[\frac{n' - n}{n' + n}\right]^2$$

where n is the refractive index of the medium surrounding the surface (generally air) and n' is the refractive index of the surface.

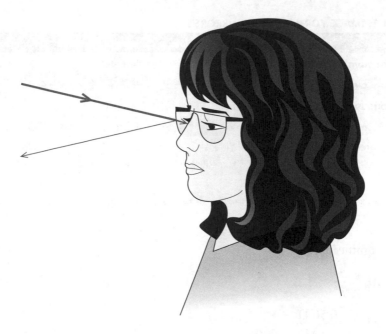

Figure 14-10. Although most of the light incident upon a spectacle lens is transmitted, a small fraction is reflected off the surface.

According to this formula, a CR-39 plastic lens (index of 1.498) reflects about 4.0% of the light incident on its front surface, while a polycarbonate lens ($n = 1.586$) reflects 5.1%.

Not only do the reflections off the front surface of a spectacle lens reduce the amount of light that is transmitted by the lens, they may also be noticeable to people looking at the patient (Fig. 14-10). Stray light that hits the back (ocular) surface of a lens may be reflected into the patient's eye and seen by the patient as annoying and distracting images.

Bothersome reflections can be reduced by applying a thin, transparent **antireflection coating** to the lens surface. A coating is maximally effective for only one wavelength. As can be seen in Figure 14-11, destructive interference occurs when light rays reflected by the surfaces of the lens and coating are 180 degrees out of phase. For this to happen, light reflected off the *lens* front surface must travel one-half wavelength farther than light reflected by the *coating* front surface. Consequently, the coating must be an odd number of quarter wavelengths thick (i.e., one-quarter, three-quarters, etc., wavelengths thick).

To obtain maximum destructive interference, the amount of light reflected from the lens and coating surfaces should be equal. This occurs when

$$\left[\frac{1 - n_c}{1 + n_c}\right]^2 = \left[\frac{n_c - n_L}{n_c + n_L}\right]^2$$

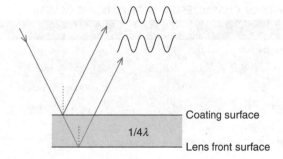

Figure 14-11. An antireflective coating, because of its thickness, causes destructive interference between light rays that are reflected off the coating front surface and lens front surface.

where n_L is the index of the lens and n_c is the index of the coating.

This relationship can be simplified to

$$n_c = \sqrt{n_L}$$

Let's apply this formula. *A CR-39 lens requires an antireflection coating. What should be the refractive index of the coating?*

$$n_c = \sqrt{n_L}$$
$$n_c = \sqrt{1.498}$$
$$n_c = 1.22$$

For a CR-39 lens, the antireflection coating should have a refractive index of 1.22.

If you were to look at this coating, it would appear purplish. Why is this? As discussed in the following chapter, a lens's refractive index is specified for light of 589 nm, which appears yellow. This is the wavelength for which destructive reflective interference will be maximized. Wavelengths shorter (which appear blue) and longer (which appear red) are reflected off the lens and combine to form a purplish color. In clinical practice these reflections can be minimized by applying additional layers of antireflective coatings of other indices.

PURKINJE IMAGES

The four primary optical interfaces of the eye—the anterior and posterior surfaces of the cornea and lens—not only refract, but also reflect, light. When you shine a penlight onto a patient's eye, you see a bright reflection off the anterior surface of the

TABLE 14-2. SUMMARY OF CHARACTERISTICS OF PURKINJE IMAGES

Number	Source	Location* (mm)	Nature	Brightness**
I	Anterior cornea	3.9	Virtual, erect	1
II	Posterior cornea	3.8	Virtual, erect	2
III	Anterior lens	10.6	Virtual, erect	3
IV	Posterior lens	4.0	Real, inverted	3

*Location with respect to the corneal apex.
**Comparative brightness is given, with the brightest image designated by "1."

cornea. The reflection is bright because of the relatively large difference between the indices of air and the cornea ($n = 1.376$). Under optimal viewing conditions, it is also possible to see considerably dimmer reflections from the other three ocular surfaces. These four reflected images are called **Purkinje** (or **Purkinje–Sanson**) images.

Table 14-2 lists the four Purkinje images and their characteristics, and Figure 14-12 shows their approximate locations. Since the first three images are formed by convex reflecting surfaces, they are virtual and erect, but because Purkinje image IV is formed by the concave posterior surface of the lens, it is real and inverted. The size and location of Purkinje image III, whose origin is the anterior surface of the crystalline lens, changes during accommodation. As the anterior lens surface's radius of curvature decreases during accommodation, Purkinje image III decreases in size and moves closer to this surface.

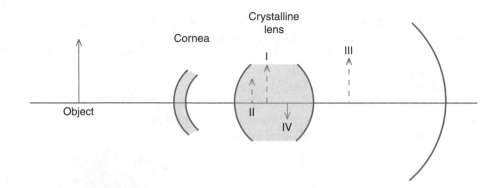

Figure 14-12. Approximate locations of the Purkinje images. Purkinje images I, II, III, and IV are formed, respectively, by the cornea anterior surface, cornea posterior surface, lens anterior surface, and lens posterior surface. All of the images are virtual except for Purkinje image IV, which is formed by the concave posterior lens surface.

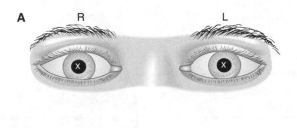

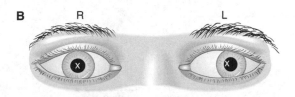

Figure 14-13. In the Hirschberg test, the position of Purkinje image I (with respect to the center of the pupil) in one eye is compared to its position in the fellow eye. This test is clinically useful for diagnosing strabismus (an eye turn), particularly in nonresponsive patients. **A.** The patient's two eyes are aligned with the fixation light. As a result, Purkinje image I, which is represented by **X**, is located in the same position in each eye. **B.** This patient has left eye exotropia—the left eye turns outward; consequently, the left eye's Purkinje image is located closer to the nasal edge of the pupil. The outward turning of the eye causes Purkinje image I to move with respect to the pupil. The absolute position of the image itself does not significantly move; rather, the eye rotates.

Purkinje image I has many important clinical applications, including keratometry and corneal topography, which are discussed later in this chapter. The clinician views Purkinje image I when measuring **angle kappa** to determine the amount of eccentric fixation and performing the **Hirschberg test** to measure the angle of strabismus (Fig. 14-13).

We can locate the first Purkinje image by treating the anterior cornea surface as a mirror. Let's assume that the light source is at infinity, and the anterior cornea radius of curvature is 7.80 mm.[3] First, we'll calculate its reflective power as follows:

$$F = \frac{-2}{r}$$

$$F = \frac{-2}{0.0078}$$

$$F = -256.41 \text{ D}$$

---

3. Note that we use the anterior *cornea* surface radius of curvature. We do not use 5.55 mm, which is the radius of curvature of the *front surface of the reduced eye*.

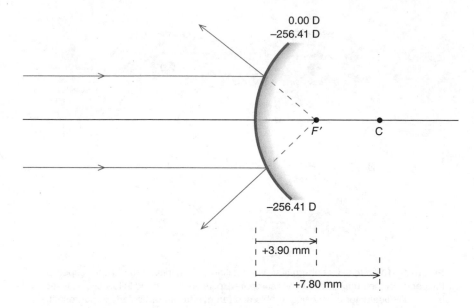

Figure 14-14. The vergence relationship can be used to calculate the location of Purkinje image I by treating the anterior cornea surface as a mirror.

Since the light source is at infinity, it has a vergence of zero. As illustrated in Figure 14-14, we can use the vergence relationship to locate the *reflected* image.

$$L' = L + F$$

$$L' = 0 - 256.41 \text{ D}$$

$$L' = -256.41 \text{ D}$$

The reflected image is virtual, and its distance from the corneal surface is

$$L' = \frac{-1}{l}$$

$$l' = \frac{-1}{-256.41 \text{ D}}$$

$$l' = +0.0039 \text{ m} \quad \text{or} \quad +3.90 \text{ mm}$$

Purkinje image I is located 3.90 mm to the right of the corneal surface.

There is another way to approach this problem. Since the object is at infinity, the image must be located at the secondary focal point of the mirror. The secondary focal length can be determined from the radius of curvature as follows:

$$r = 2f'$$

$$+7.80 \text{ mm} = 2f'$$

$$f' = +3.90 \text{ mm}$$

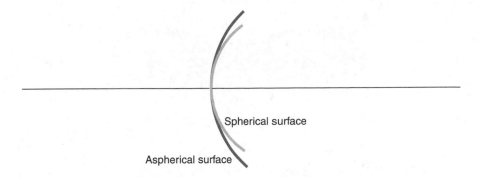

Figure 14-15. The cornea does not have a single radius of curvature—it is aspherical. Its center (axial region) is more curved than its periphery (paraxial region). The light curve represents a spherical surface and the darker curve, an aspherical surface.

Determining the location of the other Purkinje images is a bit more complicated because we need to take into account both reflection and refraction. Appendix B shows how we can locate Purkinje image III using the concept of an equivalent mirror.

CORNEAL TOPOGRAPHY

For the purposes of fitting contact lenses, evaluating the cornea prior to and following surgical or laser refractive procedures, and diagnosing certain conditions (e.g., keratoconus[4]), it is important to know the topography of the cornea. Contrary to the schematic eye that we discussed in Chapter 7, the cornea is actually an **aspherical**, not a spherical, structure: it does not have a single radius of curvature (Fig. 14-15). Rather, the center (i.e., paraxial region) of the cornea is more curved than is its periphery.[5]

Corneal topographers—clinical instruments that are used to determine the shape of the cornea—often utilize Purkinje image I. Luminous rings of known diameters are reflected off the cornea (Fig. 14-16A). The dimensions of each ring are compared to the dimensions of its reflected image to calculate the corneal radii of curvature from center to periphery. This information is presented in a topographic map with various colors used to designate curvature.

In with-the-rule corneal toricity, where the corneal vertical meridian is stronger than the horizontal, the vertical dimensions of the rings will be less than the

---

4. **Keratoconus** is a degenerative corneal disease in which the central cornea becomes progressively steeper and thinner. It is treated with custom contact lenses and/or penetrating keratoplasty.

5. As we will learn in Chapter 15, the flattening of the periphery of the cornea reduces the eye's spherical aberration.

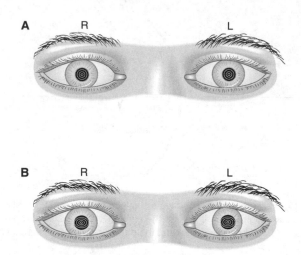

Figure 14-16. Commonly used corneal topographers work by shining luminous rings of known dimensions onto the cornea and measuring the dimensions of the reflected images (Purkinje image I). **A.** For a cornea that has no toricity, the reflected rings are circular in shape. **B.** In with-the-rule astigmatism, the steeper vertical corneal meridian causes the vertical dimension of the image to be minified with respect to the horizontal dimension. As a result, the virtual image is a horizontal ellipse.

horizontal dimensions. As a result, the reflected rings will look like a horizontal ellipse (Fig 14-16B). The opposite appearance is seen if the cornea manifests against-the-rule toricity—the reflected image looks like a vertical ellipse.

For certain clinical applications, it is not necessary to obtain a detailed topographic map of the cornea. In **keratometry**, the radii of curvature for the two principal meridians are determined at a given corneal eccentricity.[6] The dimensions of luminous objects—known as **mires** and depicted in Figure 14-17—are compared with the dimensions of their reflected corneal images, thereby allowing determination of radii of curvature for the principal meridians. Assuming an index of refraction of 1.3375, the keratometer converts these radii to dioptric values. The keratometer is particularly useful for the fitting of contact lenses. Appendix C provides an introduction to this topic.

Both corneal and lenticular toricity can contribute to the total amount of ocular astigmatism. The amount of ocular astigmatism can be predicted from keratometry readings by using Javal's rule. Although not commonly used for clinical purposes, Javal's rule is of historical interest and discussed in Appendix D.

---

6. The two principal meridians, which are orthogonal to each other, are the cornea's most curved and least curved meridians (Chapter 9).

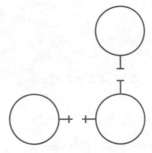

Figure 14-17. In keratometry, luminous objects (called mires) are reflected off the cornea. Since the dimensions of the mires are known, the radii of curvature for the corneal principal meridians can be calculated.

SUMMARY

Similar to spherical refractive surfaces and lenses, mirrors can change the vergence of light rays that are incident upon them. When using the vergence relationship for mirrors, it is necessary to take into account that the direction of light is reversed after reflection.

A refracting surface, such as a surface of a spectacle lens, can reflect light. Bothersome reflections can be reduced through the use of antireflection coatings.

Reflections off the eye's four primary refracting surfaces are referred to as Purkinje images. Purkinje image I, formed by the anterior surface of the cornea, has numerous clinical applications, including corneal topography, keratometry, and the Hirschberg test.

KEY FORMULAE

Relationship between a mirror's radius of curvature and its power:

$$F = \frac{-2}{r}$$

Relationship between a mirror's focal length and its power:

$$F = \frac{-1}{f'}$$

Relationship between a mirror's focal length and radius of curvature:

$$r = 2f'$$

Image location for a mirror:

$$L' = \frac{-1}{l'}$$

Magnification for a mirror:

$$M_L = \frac{-l'}{l}$$

Fraction of light reflected off a refractive surface:

$$R = \left[\frac{n' - n}{n' + n}\right]^2$$

Index of coating needed to minimize reflections:

$$n_c = \sqrt{n_L}$$

SELF-ASSESSMENT PROBLEMS

1. An object is located 5.00 cm anterior to a concave mirror that has a radius of curvature of 30.00 cm. (a) Locate the image. (b) Is the image real or virtual? (c) If the object is 2.00 cm in height, what is the height of the image?

2. For the mirror in Problem 1, the object is located at a distance of 20.00 cm. (a) Locate the image. (b) Is the image real or virtual? (c) If the object is 2.00 cm in height, what is the height of the image?

3. An object is located 25.00 cm anterior to a convex mirror that has a focal length of +15.00 cm. (a) Locate the image. (b) Is the image real or virtual? (c) If the object is 2.00 cm in height, what is the height of the image?

4. A real image is located 40.00 cm from a +30.00 D mirror. Locate the object.

5. A virtual image is located 10.00 cm from a –30.00 D mirror. Locate the object.

6. An object is located 20.00 cm anterior to a +15.00 D lens. This lens is located 3.00 cm anterior to a mirror that has a radius of curvature of +2.00 cm. (a) Locate the image. (b) What is the magnification of the optical system?

7. A light is located 10.00 cm anterior to the cornea of the eye. Assuming that the anterior surface of the cornea has a radius of 7.80 mm, locate the first Purkinje image.

8. A circular light is located 7.00 cm anterior to the cornea of the eye. If the first Purkinje image is oval in shape with its long axis vertical, is the corneal toricity with-the-rule or against-the-rule?

9. (a) What percentage of light is reflected by the front surface of a lens that is made from a high-index plastic material ($n = 1.74$)? (b) Answer the same question for a CR-39 lens. (c) For which lens would an antireflection coating be most important? Why? (d) What should be the index of refraction of the antireflection coating for the higher-index lens?

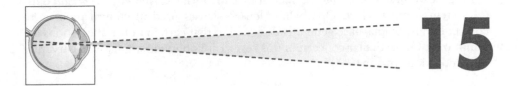

Aberrations

Virtually all optical systems have aberrations that degrade the quality of the image they create. If an aberration can be produced with a single wavelength of light, it is referred to as a **monochromatic aberration**. In comparison, **chromatic aberrations** occur only with polychromatic light, which is composed of multiple wavelengths.[1] Aberrations are an important consideration in the design of spectacle lenses and the correction of refractive errors.

THE PARAXIAL ASSUMPTION AND SEIDEL ABERRATIONS

The paraxial equation (i.e., vergence relationship) is very useful because it allows us to readily locate the images produced by spherical optical systems. It is only accurate, however, for light rays that make a sufficiently small angle of incidence with the refracting surface, commonly referred to as **paraxial rays** because they are close to the optical axis. For these rays, we can make an assumption that $\sin \theta = \theta$ (in radians). This paraxial assumption, which is made in the derivation of the paraxial equation (refer to Appendix E for the derivation), becomes less accurate as the angle of incidence increases. A better estimate of $\sin \theta$ is given by the following expansion:

$$\sin\theta = \theta - \left(\frac{\theta^3}{3!}\right) + \left(\frac{\theta^5}{5!}\right) - \left(\frac{\theta^7}{7!}\right) + \cdots$$

When the third-order approximation $[\theta - (\theta^3/3!)]$ is used, image formation differs from what is predicted by the paraxial equation in five ways. These interrelated deviations, which are referred to as **Seidel**, or **classic**, **aberrations**, are spherical aberration, coma, oblique (sometimes called radial or marginal) astigmatism, curvature of field (power error), and distortion.

---

1. White light is polychromatic.

Because of these *monochromatic* aberrations, the image formed by a *spherical* optical system is not perfect. Ophthalmic lenses—lenses used in clinical practice to correct for ametropia—are generally designed so that certain of the aberrations are minimized. Of particular concern in this regard are oblique astigmatism, curvature of field, and distortion.

Longitudinal Spherical Aberration

Spherical lenses suffer from **positive (undercorrected) longitudinal spherical aberration**, meaning that light rays striking the periphery of the lens (nonparaxial rays) are focused closer to the lens than those striking near its center (paraxial rays).[2] As can be seen in Figure 15-1, positive longitudinal spherical aberration is present in both plus and minus lenses.

The amount of longitudinal spherical aberration is dependent on, among other factors, the radii of curvatures of the front and back surfaces of a lens. These can be used to calculate the **Coddington shape factor**, σ, which is related to the amount of spherical aberration.[3]

$$\sigma = \left(\frac{r_2 + r_1}{r_2 - r_1}\right)$$

where r_1 is the front surface's radius of curvature and r_2 is the back (ocular) surface's radius of curvature.

Figure 15-2 shows longitudinal spherical aberration plotted as a function of the shape factor for various lenses all of which have the *same* power. As you can see, longitudinal spherical aberration is *minimized* for lenses with approximately planoconvex shapes that are oriented so that the front surface is more convex. (The orientation of the lens is critical—turning it around so that the front surface is flat increases spherical aberration.)

Is longitudinal spherical aberration an important consideration in the design of spectacle lenses? Because peripheral rays that emerge from a spectacle lens are blocked by the iris, preventing them from reaching the retina and participating in image formation, longitudinal spherical aberration in spectacle lenses generally does not significantly reduce retinal image quality.

If longitudinal spherical aberration in spectacle lenses does not typically reduce retinal image quality, what accounts for the popularity of aspheric front surfaces in high plus prescriptions? Whereas a plus spherical surface has a single radius of curvature, the radius of curvature of a plus aspheric surface lens increases from the lens's center to periphery (i.e., the surface becomes flatter). This is schematically

---

2. Nonspherical lenses, where the periphery of the lens is flatter than its center, may suffer from negative (overcorrected) spherical aberration. In this case, the paraxial rays are focused closer to the lens than are the nonparaxial rays.

3. The Coddington shape factor (sometimes called the bending factor) should not be confused with the shape factor in Chapter 13. The latter is applicable to magnification, not spherical aberration.

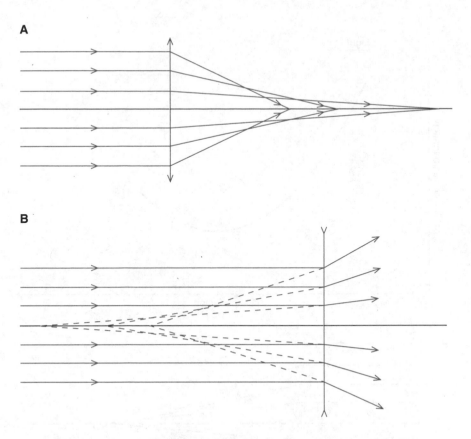

Figure 15-1. A. Positive (undercorrected) longitudinal spherical aberration in a converging lens. Note that peripheral rays are more refracted than central rays. **B.** Positive (undercorrected) longitudinal spherical aberration in a diverging lens. Again, note that the peripheral rays are more refracted than central rays. For illustrative purposes, the spherical aberration in these diagrams is exaggerated.

illustrated in Figure 15-3. An aspheric front surface improves the cosmetic appearance of a plus lens not only by allowing it to be made thinner, but also because the flatter front surface results in less spectacle magnification; this reduces the magnified appearance of the patient's eyes that may occur with plus lenses.

The unaccommodated eye typically (but not always) manifests positive spherical aberration, which tends to increase with age (Guirao et al., 2000). The spherical aberration would be even greater if not for the aspheric nature of the cornea—the periphery of the cornea is flatter than its center (Chapter 14). As the eye accommodates, the amount of positive spherical aberration decreases (Ivanoff, 1956).

The eye's spherical aberration may have clinical implications for nighttime vision. Under dim lighting conditions the pupil dilates, exposing the retina to nonparaxial light rays. These light rays may be focused in front of the retina, making

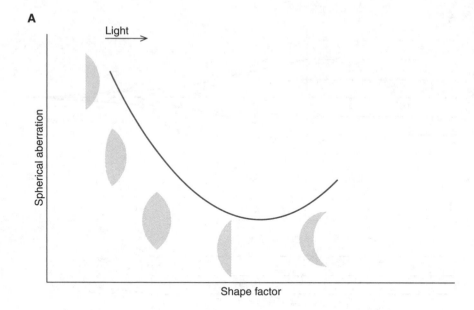

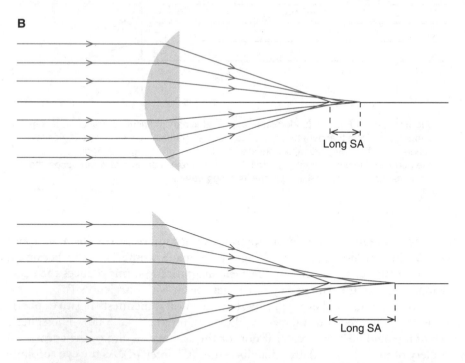

Figure 15-2. A. Longitudinal spherical aberration as a function of the shape factor. The graph shows that this aberration can be minimized with an approximately planoconvex design in which the front surface is convex. Coma is also minimized with this lens design. **B.** For a planoconvex lens, longitudinal spherical aberration is minimized when light rays are incident on the convex surface of the lens, but not on the plano surface.

Figure 15-3. An aspherical surface can be used to reduce lens thickness.

the eye myopic. This can be one contributing factor to **night myopia**—myopia that is present only under low illumination.[4] Clinically, consideration should be given to prescribing lenses with slightly more minus power (or less plus power) for those patients who do considerable nighttime driving.

Coma

Both spherical aberration and coma occur because the refractive power of a spherical surface is not uniform. When light rays are parallel to the optical axis, the result is spherical aberration. Coma, in comparison, results when the light rays are oblique with respect to the optical axis. Such rays may originate from objects that do not fall along the optical axis. Because of coma, an off-axis point source results in an image with a comet-like shape as illustrated in Figure 15-4. When the tip of the comet is pointed toward the optical axis, the coma is said to be positive, and when it is pointed away, the coma is negative. The asymmetrical nature of coma is especially detrimental to image formation. While coma is most often associated with

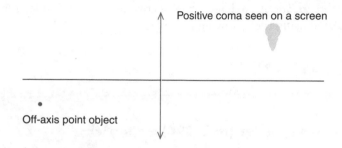

Figure 15-4. Coma results when an off-axis point source is imaged by a spherical lens.

---

4. Empty-field accommodation probably contributes to night myopia.

off-axis objects, it can also occur with on-axis objects when the optical components are noncentered and tilted with respect to each other. This is the case in the eye, where coma may be a major foveal aberration.

Like spherical aberration, coma increases as the diameter of the ray pencil increases. If an aperture is placed close to a lens and the diameter of the aperture is decreased, the amounts of coma and spherical aberration decrease.

Coma is similar to spherical aberration in the manner it is dependent on the lens shape factor. It can be minimized by making the curvatures of the lens surfaces similar to those that also reduce spherical aberration (Fig. 15-2). As with spherical aberration, coma is usually not a concern in the design of spectacle lenses because peripheral spectacle lens rays are generally blocked by the eye's iris.

Oblique Astigmatism

As discussed in Chapter 9, we can think of a point source as emitting both horizontally and vertically diverging light rays. If the point source is on the optical axis of a spherical lens, the angle of incidence for the horizontally diverging rays is equal to the angle of incidence for the vertically diverging rays. If the point source is off-axis, however, the horizontally diverging rays strike the surface of the lens at a different angle than the vertically diverging rays. This occurs even if the rays emerging from the off-axis object pass through the center of the lens. The result is oblique astigmatism (also called radial or marginal astigmatism).

Since oblique astigmatism can occur when light rays emerging from an off-axis object pass through the center of a lens, it is of clinical significance in the design of spectacle lenses. Correct selection by the surfacing laboratory of the front surface power can minimize this aberration.

Even when oblique astigmatism is minimized through proper selection of the front surface power, it can still be problematic when the lens is tilted with respect to the eye. For example, as illustrated in Figure 15-5, wrap-around sunglasses may be tilted with respect to the horizontal plane of the face (i.e., horizontal frontal plane.) This is referred to as face-form; it induces cylinder whose *axis* is 090 degrees and sign (plus or minus) is the same as tilted lens. Face-form also affects the power in the vertical *meridian* of the lens. The effective lens power induced by face form can be calculated using the following formulae:

$$F_{@090} = F\left(1 + \frac{\sin^2\theta}{2n}\right)$$

and

Induced cylinder (axis 090) = $F(\tan^2\theta)$

where $F_{@090}$ is the induced power in the vertical meridian, F is the power of the original spherical lens, θ is the face-form angle, n is the lens's index of refraction, and the *induced cylinder* has an axis of 090 degrees.

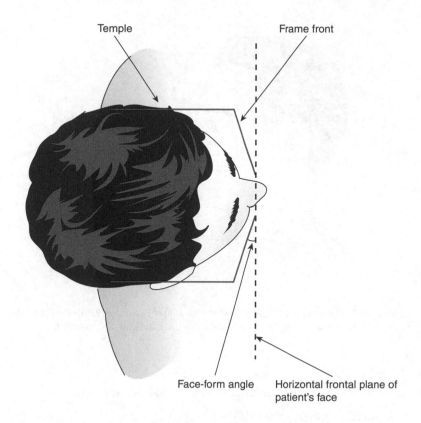

Temple   Frame front

Face-form angle   Horizontal frontal plane of
                      patient's face

Figure 15-5. Face-form results when the frame front is rotated with respect to the face's horizontal frontal plane. The axis of the induced cylinder is 090 degrees. Large amounts of face-form are common in wrap-around sunglasses.

To see how lens tilt can be clinically significant, let's take an example. *A patient with a prescription of −6.00 DS selects a frame with a face-form angle of 20 degrees. If the lens is made of polycarbonate, what is the effective power that the patient experiences?*

First let's calculate the power in the vertical meridian

$$F_{@090} = F\left(1 + \frac{\sin^2\theta}{2n}\right)$$

$$F_{@090} = -6.00\ \mathrm{D}\left(1 + \frac{\sin^2(20)}{2(1.586)}\right)$$

$$F_{@090} = -6.22\ \mathrm{D}$$

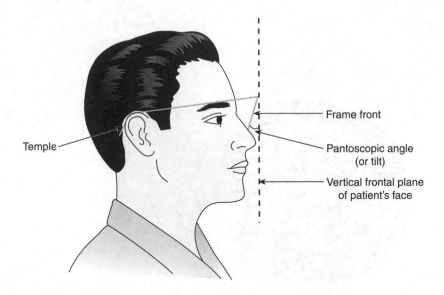

Figure 15-6. Pantoscopic tilt results when the frame is rotated with respect to the face's vertical frontal plane. The axis of the induced cylinder is 180 degrees.

Now, we'll determine the amount of induced cylinder at axis 090

Induced cylinder = F $(\tan^2\theta)$

Induced cylinder = -6.00 D$[\tan^2(20)]$

Induced cylinder = -0.80 D

These calculations tell us that when a -6.00 DS polycarbonate lens is placed in a frame with 20 degrees of face-form, the effective lens power is $-6.22 - 0.80 \times$ 090. This is clinically significant and must be accounted for when the lenses are made. Generally, the dispenser or fabricator of the glasses will make calculations and adjust the prescription to compensate for face-form prior to making the lenses.

Not only can lenses be tilted with respect to the horizontal frontal plane, they can also be tilted with respect to the vertical frontal plane. This occurs when a frame has pantoscopic tilt as illustrated in Figure 15-6. The induced cylinder has an *axis* of 180 degrees and the same sign (plus or minus) as the tilted lens. **The calculations are similar to those for face-form wrap except that (1) $F_{@180}$, rather than $F_{@090}$, is determined and (2) the induced cylinder has an axis of 180 degrees.**

What is the effective power of a -8.00 DS polycarbonate lens that is mounted in a frame that has a pantoscopic tilt of 15 degrees?

First let's calculate the power in the horizontal meridian

$$F_{@180} = F\left(1 + \frac{\sin^2\theta}{2n}\right)$$

$$F_{@180} = -8.00 \text{ D}\left(1 + \frac{\sin^2(15)}{2(1.586)}\right)$$

$$F_{@180} = -8.17 \text{ D}$$

Now, we'll calculate the induced cylinder at axis 180

Induced cylinder (axis 180) $= F(\tan^2\theta)$

Induced cylinder $= -8.00 \text{ D}[\tan^2(15)]$

Induced cylinder $= -0.57 \text{ D}$

When a −8.00 DS lens is in a frame with a pantoscopic tilt of 15 degrees, the effective power experienced by the patient is $-8.17 - 0.57 \times 180$.

Note that pantoscopic tilt increases a minus lens's minus power. It is for this reason that undercorrected myopic patients sometimes intentionally tilt their spectacles to improve distance vision.

Curvature of Field

Not all points on the extended object in Figure 15-7 are the same distance from the spherical converging lens. If you measure with a ruler, you'll see that the arrow's tip

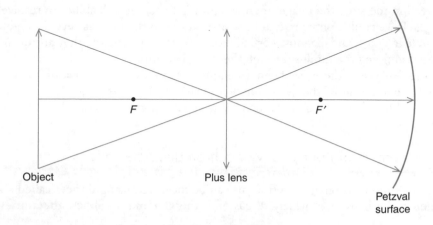

Figure 15-7. The image plane for a flat object is curved, resulting in curvature of field. The off-axis components of the object (the tip and base of the arrow) are further from the lens than the on-axis components. Consequently, the image distance is less for the tip and base.

and base are farther from the lens than the arrow's center. Consequently, the *image* distances for the arrow tip and base are less than that for the arrow center. This results in an image plane that is not flat, but curved, hence the term, curvature of field.[5] Since off-axis rays that pass through the center of a lens can cause curvature of field, this aberration is clinically important in the design of spectacle lenses. It can be minimized by the proper selection of the lens front surface power.

Distortion

The central and peripheral regions of a spherical lens do not produce the same amount of lateral magnification. For an extended source, this results in distortion, of which there are two basic types: **barrel distortion**, which is found with minus lenses, and **pincushion distortion**, which is found with plus lenses (Fig. 15-8). Barrel distortion occurs because *minification* in the periphery of a minus lens is greater than in its center, while pincushion distortion results from greater *magnification* in the periphery of a plus lens compared to its center. Distortion is a consideration in the design of spectacle lenses.

WAVEFRONT SENSING AND ADAPTIVE OPTICS

The eye's monochromatic aberrations can degrade the image that is focused on the retina, thereby limiting the ability to resolve detail. If these aberrations could be corrected, it may be possible to improve visual acuity to better than the typical 20/20 or 20/15.[6]

Monochromatic aberrations limit the clinician's ability to examine the fundus[7] because it must be viewed through the imperfect optics of the patient's eye. Optical aberrations degrade the image, thereby limiting the clinician's ability to resolve its details. If we could compensate for the aberrations in the patient's eye, it might be possible to detect and diagnose certain diseases earlier (i.e., before they are apparent when examining the fundus through the eye's aberrations).

In recent years, there has been a heightened interest in the measurement and possible correction of the eye's monochromatic aberrations. The aberrations are measured by determining how much a wavefront of light is distorted by the optics of the eye.

Measurement of the Eye's Monochromatic Aberrations

The eye's monochromatic aberrations can be measured using devices called aberrometers. Perhaps most widely discussed is the **Hartmann–Shack aberrometer,**

---

5. This curved image plane is sometimes called a **Petzval surface**.
6. The improvement of visual acuity beyond 20/10 or so is limited by the packing density of foveal cones.
7. The fundus consists of the retina and other posterior ocular structures as seen with an ophthalmoscope or other instrument.

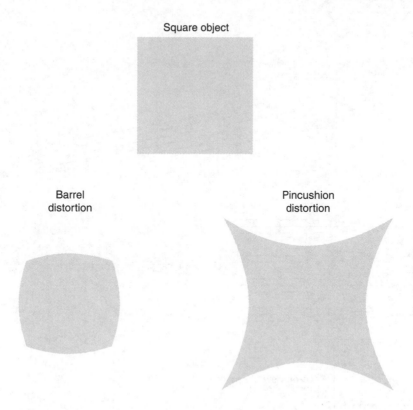

Square object

Barrel
distortion

Pincushion
distortion

Figure 15-8. Barrel distortion can occur with minus spherical lenses, while pincushion distortion is found with plus spherical lenses. Note that viewing through a minus lens produces a minified image relative to the square object, while viewing through a plus lens results in magnification.

which is schematically illustrated in Figure 15-9A (Liang et al., 1994). This apparatus focuses a point of light on the retina, which, in turn, serves as a point source object for the eye's optical system. The light rays emanating from the point source travel back out through the eye's optical system, forming a pattern that reveals the eye's monochromatic aberrations.

Let's discuss this in more detail.[8] All eyes have aberrations, but for the purposes of this explanation, think of a theoretical eye that has none. The rays emitted by the retinal point source emerge from the eye parallel to each other. These parallel light rays are incident upon an array consisting of many tiny lenslets. As can be seen in Figure 15-9B, the lenslets focus the parallel light rays onto a sensor, forming a regular grid of points.

---

8. For a more detailed and very lucid description of the Hartmann–Shack aberrometer, see Thibos (2000).

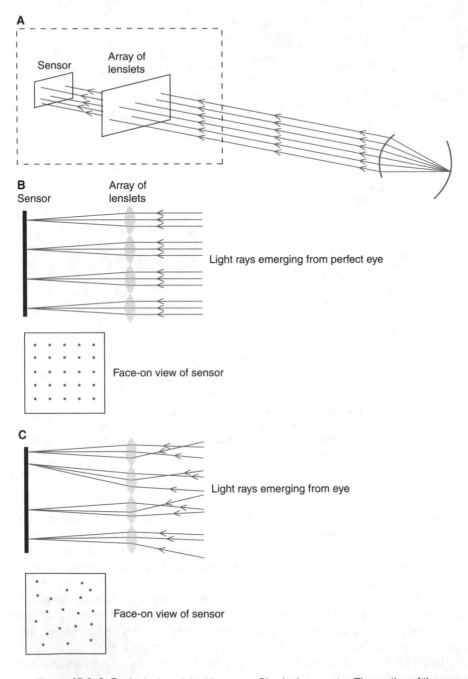

Figure 15-9. A. Basic design of the Hartmann–Shack aberrometer. The portion of the aberrometer enclosed by the dashed lines is illustrated in more detail in (B) and (C). **B.** Lenslets focus the parallel light rays that emerge from an eye without aberrations (a perfect eye) onto a sensor, forming a regular grid of points. **C.** Because of aberrations, the rays that actually emerge from the eye do not form a regular grid pattern.

TABLE 15-1. **ZERNIKE POLYNOMIALS AND THEIR SEIDEL ABERRATION EQUIVALENTS**

Zernike Polynomial*	Seidel Aberration
Second order	Ametropia (defocus and astigmatism)
Third order	Coma and other aberrations
Fourth order	Spherical and other aberrations
Fifth to tenth orders	Irregular aberrations**

* Data from Liang and Williams (1997).

** Irregular aberrations are not present in spherical surfaces.

In reality, the rays emerging from an actual eye are not perfectly parallel to each other, and the resulting pattern formed by the lenslets is not a regular grid. This is depicted in Figure 15-9C. The manner in which the pattern deviates from a regular grid reveals the nature of the eye's aberrations and is quantified as **Zernike polynomials** (i.e., second order, third order, etc.). It is now common to characterize the eye's aberrations as Zernike polynomials rather than as Seidel aberrations. Table 15-1 gives some of the Zernike polynomials and the equivalent Seidel aberrations.

There is another way to conceptualize the nonparallel light rays in Figure 15-9C. Recall from Chapter 1 that light rays are perpendicular to wavefronts. As can be seen in Figure 15-10A, a point source produces wavefronts that become flatter as they move farther away from the source. When a wavefront is infinitely far from a source, it is flat. (Consequently the light rays are parallel to each other.) This flat wavefront results in a regular grid on the Hartmann–Shack wavefront sensor as indicated in Figure 15-10B.

What does the wavefront that emerges from the eye look like? Due to aberrations, the wavefront emerges distorted and/or irregular, forming an irregular grid pattern (Fig. 15-10C).

Supernormal Vision

When a person's pupil is greater than 3 mm in diameter, aberrations can interfere with the ability to resolve detail (Liang and Williams, 1997). Compensation for the eye's aberrations may result in improved contrast sensitivity and resolution, a condition referred to as supernormal vision. In the laboratory, it is possible to compensate for aberrations with a **deformable mirror**, schematically illustrated in Figure 15-11. By adjusting the mirror's surface topography, we can compensate for the distortions in the wavefront, thereby minimizing aberrations—a process referred to as **adaptive optics**.[9]

It is conceivable that custom contact lenses or laser procedures could be used to improve vision beyond the typical 20/20 or 20/15 (Applegate, 2000). Laser

---

9. Not only the Seidel aberrations (which are spherical) but also nonspherical (i.e., *irregular*) aberrations can be corrected.

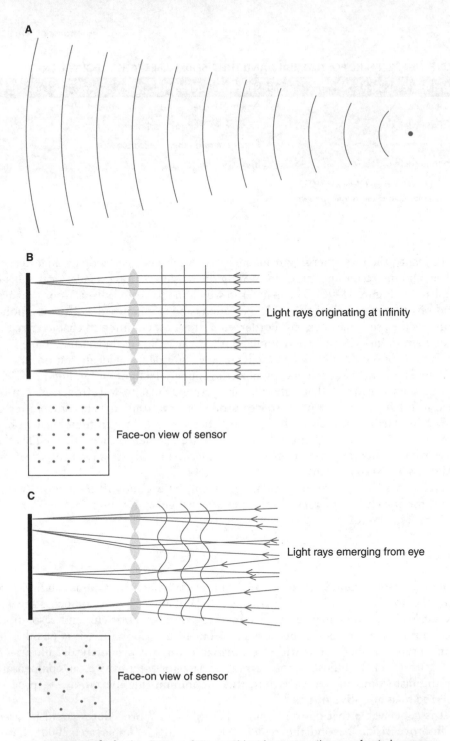

Figure 15-10. A. As the distance from an object increases, the wavefronts become flatter. When the object is located at infinity, the wavefronts are flat. **B.** Flat wavefronts from light originating at infinity cause a regular grid pattern to be formed on the sensor of the Hartmann–Shack aberrometer. **C.** The aberrations of the eye cause the wavefronts that emerge from the eye to be distorted. These distorted wavefronts result in an irregular grid pattern.

A

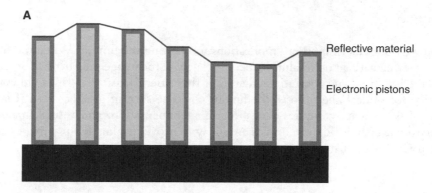

Reflective material

Electronic pistons

B

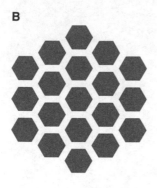

FIGURE 15-11. **A.** Profile of a deformable mirror. Miniaturized pistons control the orientation of small sections of the mirror. **B.** Face-on view of a deformable mirror showing the smaller mirror sections that constitute it. These can be controlled independently of each other.

procedures as normally performed at this time, however, often increase the eye's monochromatic aberrations rather than decreasing them. Nonetheless, it is now possible to measure the eye's aberrations prior to a laser procedure and then to customize the ablation pattern.[10] The goal is to minimize the aberrations introduced by the laser procedure or to even reduce the aberrations to a level lower than before the procedure. While this is conceivable, the long-term stability of these corrections depends on the physical properties of the cornea. The cornea is not a stable, uniform material such as plastic or glass—it is a living tissue that is neither uniform in its composition nor perfectly stable. Consequently, the stable, long-term correction of aberrations through corneal shaping will be challenging.

10. The eye's total aberrations are a combination of corneal aberrations and internal optical aberrations, particularly those of the crystalline lens. Therefore, to measure the eye's total aberrations prior to a corneal laser procedure, a wavefront sensing device—not corneal topography—should be used (Artal et al., 2001).

Imaging the Fundus

Adaptive optics has important implications for viewing the fundus. When the fundus is viewed with an ophthalmoscope, the clarity of the image seen by the clinician is limited by the same aberrations that limit the patient's vision. If we could compensate for optical aberrations, the fundus could be seen in greater detail (Liang et al., 1997). Adaptive optics allows for this compensation, and retinal imaging devices that include adaptive optics are likely to prove invaluable for patient care. The basic design of such an apparatus is given in Figure 15-12.

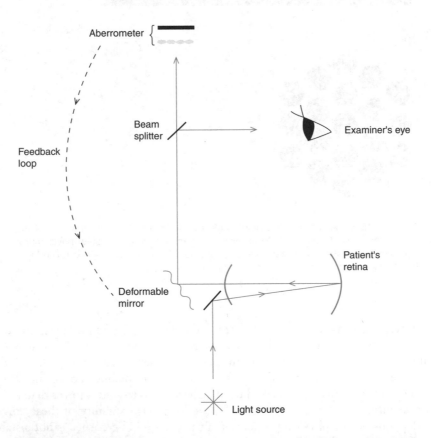

Figure 15-12. Instruments that incorporate adaptive optics can be used to obtain high-resolution images of internal ocular structures. Light is reflected off a plane mirror into the eye, illuminating the retina. This light is subsequently reflected off the retina onto a deformable mirror which, in turn, reflects the light through a beam splitter that sends half of it to the Hartmann–Shack aberrometer and the other half to the examiner's eye. The aberrometer provides feedback to the deformable mirror, and this feedback is used to adjust the deformable mirror such that aberrations are minimized. An examiner obtains a high-resolution view of the retina when the aberrations are minimized. (This schematic diagram is a simplification.)

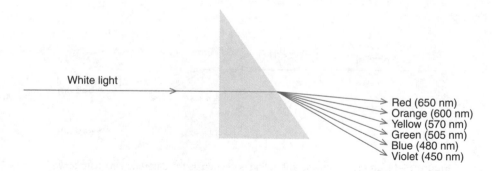

Figure 15-13. Because refractive index varies with the wavelength of light, a prism separates white light into a spectrum. Shorter wavelengths are more refracted than longer wavelengths. One nanometer (nm) is equal to 10^{-9} m.

CHROMATIC ABERRATION

While the aberrations we've discussed so far can be produced with a single wavelength of light, chromatic aberration occurs only with polychromatic light, a mixture of different wavelengths. The transmission speed within a refractive medium depends upon the wavelength, with shorter wavelengths travelling more slowly than longer wavelengths. Consequently, the refractive index, which is the ratio of the speed of light in a vacuum to that in a given medium, is different for each wavelength. Shorter wavelengths, which have a higher index of refraction, are more refracted than longer wavelengths.

Figure 15-13 shows white light—a combination of different wavelengths—incident upon a prism. Because the index of refraction and, consequently, the amount that light is refracted, depends on wavelength, the emergent light forms a spectrum of colors.[11] This separation of white light into its component elements by a prism (or other optical element) is referred to as chromatic **dispersion**.

Dispersive Power and Constringence

As a general rule, a single refractive index is specified for a refractive medium. For instance, the refractive index for CR-39 is typically given as 1.498. This index is for a specific wavelength, namely 589 nm. As we have just learned, however, the refractive index is different for other wavelengths, resulting in a spectrum of colors when the incident light is white.

To quantify the amount of dispersion produced by a prism or lens, we use three wavelengths: 486, 589, and 656 nm. The refractive indices for these wavelengths

---

11. The color of light is dependent on its wavelength. Wavelength is a physical property, and color is a perception. See Schwartz (2010) for an introductory discussion of color perception.

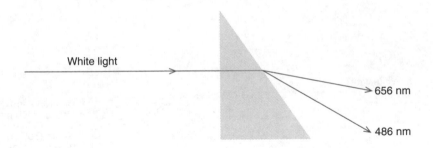

Figure 15-14. Lateral chromatic aberration is defined as the difference in prism power for wavelengths of 486 and 656 nm.

are designated as n_f, n_d, and n_c, respectively.[12] The **dispersive power (ω)** is given by

$$\omega = \frac{n_f - n_c}{n_d - 1}$$

As this value increases, the dispersion of the prism or lens increases.

As given below, the reciprocal of the dispersive power is defined as the **constringence** (also called the **Abbe number or v**) of the refracting element[13]:

$$v = \frac{1}{\omega} = \frac{n_d - 1}{n_f - n_c}$$

As the Abbe number increases, dispersion decreases. Lens manufacturers use the Abbe number to specify the chromatic aberration of their products, with higher numbers indicating smaller amounts of this aberration. It is important to note that the Abbe number and refractive index are not necessarily correlated. For instance, the Abbe number for polycarbonate, which has an index of 1.586, is 30, whereas the Abbe number for Essilor Thin&Lite® , which has an index of 1.74, is 33 (Brooks and Borish, 2007). Although Thin&Lite® has a higher refractive index than polycarbonate, it results in less chromatic aberration.

Lateral (Transverse) Chromatic Aberration

Let's look at the chromatic aberration produced by prisms in more detail. In Figure 15-14, we show the refraction that occurs for 486 nm (which appears blue)

---

12. These wavelengths are absent in sunlight that reaches the surface of the earth, creating dark lines in the solar spectrum that are called **Fraunhofer lines**.
13. The Abbe number has no units.

and 656 nm (which appears red). What is the power of this prism? The answer is that it depends on the refractive index, which, in turn, depends on the wavelength of light. If the prism were made of CR-39, we might say that its index is 1.498. This value is correct, but only for a wavelength of 589 nm, which is the wavelength that is used in the ophthalmic industry to specify index of refraction. The index is different for 486 and 656 nm, resulting in chromatic aberration.

The chromatic aberration produced by a prism is referred to as lateral chromatic aberration, transverse chromatic aberration, or chromatic power. We can define it as the difference in prismatic power for wavelengths of 486 and 656 nm as indicated in Figure 15-14. More formally, we have

Lateral CA = $P_f - P_c$

where Lateral CA is the lateral chromatic aberration, P_f is the prismatic power for 486 nm, and P_c is the prismatic power for 656 nm.

Lateral chromatic aberration can also be calculated using the Abbe number and prism power for light of 589 nm (P_d) with the following formula:

Lateral CA $= \dfrac{P_d}{v}$

Do lenses manifest lateral chromatic aberration? Recall from Chapter 10 that lenses have not only dioptric power (i.e., they change the vergence of incident light), they also have prismatic power, which increases with increasing distance from the optical center of the lens. Figure 15-15 illustrates lateral chromatic aberration in a lens.

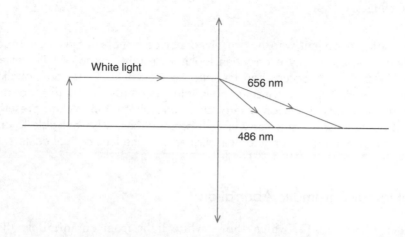

Figure 15-15. Because a lens has prismatic power, it suffers from lateral chromatic aberration. As the lens's prismatic power increases toward the periphery of the lens, the lateral chromatic aberration also increases.

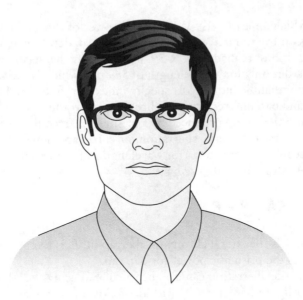

Figure 15-16. The patient is not looking through the optical centers of the lenses, but above them. Depending on the lens material's Abbe number, strength of the prescription, and distance from the optical center, this may result in lateral chromatic aberration that reduces visual acuity.

Lateral chromatic aberration is an important consideration when prescribing lens materials with low Abbe numbers, such as polycarbonate. As the patient looks through more peripheral regions of the lens, the prismatic power increases, resulting in greater lateral chromatic aberration. This may be seen by the patient as colored fringes.

Occasionally, a patient who has received polycarbonate lenses may report a reduction in visual acuity even when looking straight ahead. As illustrated in Figure 15-16, this can occur when the optical centers of the lenses are not aligned with the patient's pupils, forcing the patient to view through a noncentral region of the lens that has significant lateral chromatic aberration. When prescribing polycarbonate lenses, particularly in high prescriptions, it is advisable to ensure that the patient's pupils are not too misaligned with the lens optical centers.

Longitudinal Chromatic Aberration

Consider Figure 15-17, which shows white light from an infinitely distant object incident upon a converging lens. Because the lens's index of refraction is different for each of the wavelengths constituting white light, its focal length is

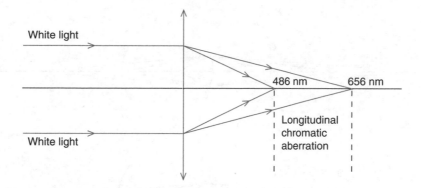

Figure 15-17. Longitudinal chromatic aberration is defined as the difference in dioptric power for wavelengths of 486 and 656 nm.

different for each. The difference in dioptric power for wavelengths of 486 and 656 nm is defined as the lens's longitudinal chromatic aberration. Stated as an equation,

Longitudinal CA $= F_f - F_c$

where Longitudinal CA is the longitudinal chromatic aberration, F_f is the dioptric power for 486 nm, and F_c is the dioptric power for 656 nm.

Longitudinal chromatic aberration can also be calculated using the Abbe number and dioptric power for light of 589 nm (F_d) with the following formula:

Longitudinal CA $= \dfrac{F_d}{v}$

While longitudinal chromatic aberration is generally not a concern in spectacle lenses, it is a consideration for the design of lenses used in optical instruments. Achromatic doublets, in which plus and minus lenses of different indices are fused together, are frequently used to reduce longitudinal chromatic aberration. Appendix F discusses the design of these lenses.

Chromatic Aberration in the Human Eye

For electromagnetic radiation ranging from 380 to 760 nm, the human eye exhibits about 2.50 D of longitudinal chromatic aberration, corresponding to a

A

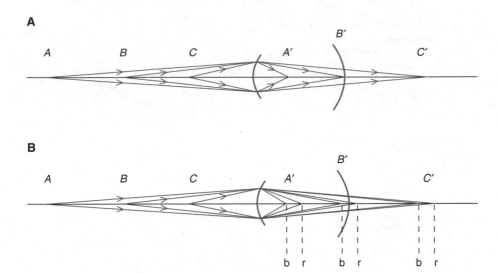

B

Figure 15-18. **A.** Points *A*, *B*, and *C* result in the images *A'*, *B'*, and *C'*. **B.** Upon closer inspection, we see that each of the images (*A'*, *B'*, and *C'*) suffers from longitudinal chromatic aberration. For the image *C'*, blue (b) is focused closer to the retina, and for the image *A'*, red (r) is focused closer to the retina. The visual system may use this information to determine if accommodation should be increased (as is required to focus on *C*) or decreased (as is required to focus on *A*).

linear distance of 0.93 mm (Kruger et al., 1993). Although we are not normally aware of longitudinal chromatic aberration, it is thought to be a stimulus to accommodation.

In Figure 15-18A, an eye is focused on point *B*. The image of point *A* (i.e., *A'*) is anterior to the retina and produces the same amount of retinal blur as the image of point *C* (i.e., *C'*), which is posterior to the retina. Suppose the subject wishes to change his or her fixation to point *A*. Since this point's image (*A'*) has the same amount of retinal blur as *C'*, how does the accommodative system know if it should increase or decrease its power?

Figure 15-18B shows the longitudinal chromatic aberration present in the images *A'*, *B'*, and *C'*. For *C'*, the shorter wavelengths are focused closer to the retina than the longer wavelengths. For *A'*, the longer wavelengths are focused closer to the retina. If the accommodative system were able to use this information, it could accommodate in the correct direction (i.e., increase its power for the near object and decrease its power for the far object). Research suggests that chromatic aberration may be a cue to accommodation. For instance, the ability to accommodate accurately is impaired under monochromatic conditions (Aggarwala et al., 1995).

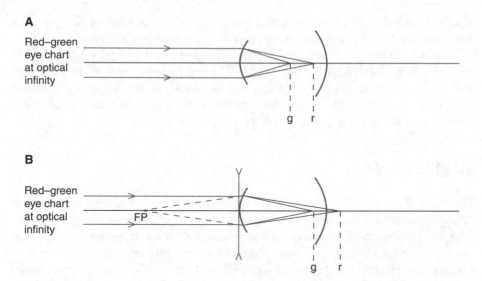

Figure 15-19. When a patient views a red–green acuity chart, images on the green background (g) are focused in front of those on the red background (r). **A.** In a myopic eye (or an emmetropic eye viewing through a plus lens), the optotypes on both the red and green backgrounds are focused in front of the retina. Since red is imaged closer to the retina, letters on this background appear clearer. **B.** The goal of the red–green refraction technique is to straddle the retina with the green and red images such that they are positioned equally distant from the retina and the optotypes on both backgrounds are equally clear to the patient. This occurs when the appropriate correction—in this case a minus lens to correct the myopia—is in place.

The Red–Green Refraction Technique[14]

This commonly used refraction procedure takes advantage of the eye's longitudinal chromatic aberration. When a patient views a visual acuity chart that is green on one side and red on the other side, the green image is focused anterior to the red image. If the patient is myopic, both the green and red images are focused anterior to the retina and both will appear blurred (Fig. 15-19A). The optotypes on the red background, however, appear less blurred because they are focused closer to the retina than the optotypes on the green background.

When the duochrome test is performed in the clinic, plus lenses may be placed in front of the patient's eye to ensure that both the green and red images fall anterior to the retina.[15] Under these conditions, the optotypes on the red background

---

14. This is also called the duochrome or bichrome refraction technique.
15. Since the images in an uncorrected myopic eye fall anterior to the retina, it is not necessary to add plus lenses. For an emmetropic or hyperopic eye, however, plus lenses must be placed in front of the eye so that the images are focused anterior to the retina.

appear clearer than those on the green background. The amount of plus power is then decreased (or the amount of minus power is increased) in a stepwise fashion (0.25 or 0.50 D per step) until the letters on the green background are just slightly clearer than those on the red background.[16] The lens power is subsequently adjusted so that the letters on the green background and those on the red background are equally clear (Fig. 15-19B). When this occurs, the green and red images straddle the retina, with each the same distance (dioptrically) from the retina.

SUMMARY

The paraxial (vergence) equation, which is probably the most important equation in this book, makes the assumption that incident light rays make a small angle with the refractive surface. While this approximation is useful for solving many optical problems, it does not account for image quality. More accurate assumptions allow us to describe aberrations that degrade image quality. Traditionally referred to as Seidel aberrations, it is now common to express them as Zernike polynomials. Oblique astigmatism, curvature of field, and distortion are important considerations in the design of spectacle lenses.

While Seidel aberrations are present in monochromatic light, chromatic aberration is manifested only with polychromatic light. It results from differences in refractive index for different wavelengths of light. Lateral chromatic aberration, which is due to prismatic power, can reduce visual acuity when a patient views through an off-axis point of a lens with a low Abbe number.

KEY FORMULAE

Bending factor for spherical aberration:

$$\sigma = \frac{r_2 + r_1}{r_2 - r_1}$$

Oblique astigmatism (face-form):

$$F_{@090} = F\left(1 + \frac{\sin^2\theta}{2n}\right)$$

Induced cylinder (axis 090) $= F(\tan^2\theta)$

Oblique astigmatism (pantoscopic tilt):

$$F_{@180} = F\left(1 + \frac{\sin^2\theta}{2n}\right)$$

Induced cylinder (axis 180) $= F(\tan^2\theta)$

---

16. The mnemonic **RAM GAP** reminds the examiner that if the red letters are clearest to add **minus** power, and if the **green** are clearest to add **plus** power.

Dispersive power:

$$\omega = \frac{n_f - n_c}{n_d - 1}$$

Constringence:

$$v = \frac{1}{\omega} = \frac{n_d - 1}{n_f - n_c}$$

Lateral chromatic aberration:

$$\text{Lateral } CA = P_f - P_c$$

$$\text{Lateral } CA = \frac{P_d}{v}$$

Longitudinal chromatic aberration:

$$\text{Longitudinal } CA = F_f - F_c$$

$$\text{Longitudinal } CA = \frac{F_d}{v}$$

REFERENCES

Aggarwala KR, Nowbotsing S, Kruber PB. Accommodation to monochromatic and white-light targets. _Invest Vis Sci._ 1995;13:2595.

Applegate RA. Limits to vision: can we do better than nature? _J Refract Surg._ 2000; 16:S547.

Artal P, Guirao A, Berrio E, Williams DR. Compensation of corneal aberrations by internal optics of the human eye. _J Vis._ 2001;1:1.

Brooks, CW, Borish IM. _System for Ophthalmic Dispensing_, 3rd ed. St. Louis: Butterworth-Heinemann, 2007.

Guirao A, Redondo M, Artal P. Optical aberrations of the human eye as a function of age. _J Opt Soc Am A._ 2000;17:1697.

Ivanoff A. About the spherical aberration of the eye. _J Opt Soc Am._ 1956;46:901.

Kruger PB, Mathews S, Aggarwala KR, Sanchez N. Chromatic aberration and ocular focus: Fincham revisited. _Vis Res._ 1993;33:1397.

Liang J, Grimm B, Goetz S, Bille JF. Objective measurement of wave aberrations of the human eye with the use of a Hartmann–Shack wave-front sensor. _J Opt Soc Am A._ 1994;11:1949.

Liang J, Williams DR. Aberrations and retinal image quality of the normal human eye. _J Opt Soc Am A._ 1997;14:2873.

Liang J, Williams DR, Miller DT. Supernormal vision and high-resolution retinal imaging through adaptive optics. _J Opt Soc Am A._ 1997;14:2884.

Schwartz, SH. _Visual Perception: A Clinical Orientation_, 4th ed. New York: McGraw-Hill, 2010.

Thibos LN. Principles of Hartmann–Shack aberrometry. _J Refract Surg._ 2000;16:S563.

SELF-ASSESSMENT PROBLEMS

1. An emmetropic subject, whose pupil has been pharmacologically dilated, views a distant point source through an opaque disk that has two vertically-aligned small holes (each hole is about 1 mm in diameter) drilled through it.[17] The two holes are separated by about 8 mm. (a) Will the patient see a single point source or two points? Why? (b) What happens when the subject places her finger in front of the top hole? Explain.

2. Does a spherical rigid contact lens neutralize the eye's Seidel aberrations? Explain your answer.

3. (a) Determine the shape factor for a +5.00 DS equiconvex CR-39 lens. (Assume an index of 1.50 for CR-39.) (b) For a +5.00 DS lens to have minimal spherical aberration, what shape should it be? (c) Which surface of the lens should face the patient's eye? (d) For the answer to C, what is the shape factor for the lens?

4. What prescription does a patient experience when wearing a +4.00 DS polycarbonate lens that has a 25 degree face-form wrap?

5. Your patient is best corrected with −8.00 DS spectacle lenses. If the pantoscopic tilt is 15 degrees, what power does she experience? (The lens is polycarbonate.)

---

17. This disk is referred to as a Scheiner disk.

Answers to Self-Assessment Problems

CHAPTER 1
Basic Terms and Concepts

1. $n \sin\theta = n' \sin\theta'$
   $(1.33) \sin\theta = (1.00) \sin 45°$
   $\theta = 32.1°$

2. $n \sin\theta = n' \sin\theta'$
   $(1.00) \sin 25° = (1.33) \sin\theta'$
   $\theta' = 18.53°$

   If the ray was not deviated:

   $\tan 25° = \dfrac{d}{200.0 \text{ cm}}$

   $d = 93.26$ cm

   But because the ray is refracted:

   $\tan 18.53° = \dfrac{d}{200.0 \text{ cm}}$

   $d = 67.04$ cm

   Therefore, the deviation of the ray is

   $93.26 - 67.04$ cm $= 26.22$ cm

3. At the first interface:

   $n \sin\theta = n' \sin\theta'$
   $(1.00) \sin 30° = 1.52 \sin\theta'$
   $\theta' = 19.2°$

At the second interface:

$n \sin\theta = n' \sin\theta'$

$(1.52) \sin 19.2° = (1.00) \sin\theta'$

$\theta' = 30.0°$

4. $n \sin\theta = n' \sin\theta'$

$(1.72) \sin\theta = (1.00) \sin 90°$

$\theta = 35.5°$

5. $n \sin\theta = n' \sin\theta'$

$(2.42) \sin\theta = (1.33) \sin 90°$

$\theta = 33.3°$

CHAPTER 2
Refraction at Spherical Surfaces

1. (a) Positive

   (b) $F = \dfrac{n' - n}{r}$

   $F = \dfrac{1.52 - 1.00}{+0.15 \text{ m}}$

   $F = +3.47 \text{ D}$

   (c) $F = \dfrac{n'}{f'}$

   $+3.47 = \dfrac{(100)(1.52)}{f'}$

   $f' = +43.8 \text{ cm}$

   F' is 43.80 cm to the right of the surface.

2. (a) Negative.

   (b) $F = \dfrac{n' - n}{r}$

   $F = \dfrac{1.52 - 1.00}{-0.20 \text{ m}}$

   $F = -2.60 \text{ D}$

(c) $F = \dfrac{n'}{f'}$

$-2.60 \text{ D} = \dfrac{(100)(1.52)}{f'}$

$f' = -58.46 \text{ cm}$

F' is located 58.46 cm to the left of the surface.

3. (a) Positive
   (b) Negative
   (c) Positive
   (d) Negative

4. (a) $F = \dfrac{n'}{f'}$

$-10.00 \text{ D} = \dfrac{(100)(1.52)}{f'}$

$f' = -15.2 \text{ cm}$

F' is 15.2 cm to the left of the diverging surface.

$F = -\dfrac{n}{f}$

$-10.00 \text{ D} = \dfrac{-(100)(1.00)}{f}$

$f' = +10.0 \text{ cm}$

F is 10.0 cm to the right of the diverging surface.

$F = \dfrac{n' - n}{r}$

$-10.00 = \dfrac{1.52 - 1.00}{r}$

$r = -0.052 \text{ m}$ or -5.2 cm

The center of curvature is 5.2 cm to the left of the surface.

(b) The image distance is about 7.2 cm to the left of the surface. The image height is about 1.6 cm.

(c) The magnification is +1.6 cm/+3.0 cm ≈ +0.5×.

(d) The image is erect. Because it is formed by diverging light rays, it is virtual. The image can be seen, but cannot be focused on a screen.

5. (a) $F = \dfrac{n'}{f'}$

$+10.00\text{ D} = \dfrac{(100)(1.52)}{f'}$

$f' = +15.2\text{ cm}$

F' is 15.2 cm to the right of the converging surface.

$F = -\dfrac{n}{f}$

$+10.00\text{ D} = -\dfrac{(100)(1.00)}{f}$

$f = -10.0\text{ cm}$

F is 10.0 cm to the left of the converging surface

$F = \dfrac{n' - n}{r}$

$+10.00 = \dfrac{1.52 - 1.00}{r}$

$r = +0.052\text{ m}\quad\text{or}\quad +5.2\text{ cm}$

The center of curvature is 5.2 cm to the right of the surface.

(b) Image distance is about 30.4 cm to the right of the surface. The image height is about 2.0 cm.

(c) The magnification is $-2.0\text{ cm}/+2.0\text{ cm} \approx -1.0\times$.

(d) The image is inverted. Because it is formed by converging light rays that could be focused onto a screen, it is real.

6. (a) The image appears closer to the surface.

(b) The diverging light rays that are emitted by the rock are further diverged at the surface of the pond (at the water–air interface). The rays appear to come from a point that is less than 3.0 m from the surface. Because the image is formed by diverging light rays, it is virtual (see Fig. 3-8).

CHAPTER 3
The Vergence Relationship

1. (a) $F = \dfrac{n' - n}{r}$

$-10.00 = \dfrac{1.586 - 1.00}{r}$

$r = -0.059\text{ m}\quad\text{or}\quad -5.9\text{ cm}$

(b) $F = \dfrac{n'}{f'}$

$-10.00 \text{ D} = \dfrac{1.586}{f'}$

$f' = -0.159 \text{ m} \quad \text{or} \quad -15.9 \text{ cm}$

2. (a) $F = \dfrac{(n' - n)}{r}$

$+20.00 \text{ D} = \dfrac{(1.50 - 1.00)}{r}$

$r = +0.025 \text{ m} \quad \text{or} \quad +2.5 \text{ cm}$

(b) $F = -\dfrac{n}{f}$

$+20.00 \text{ D} = -\dfrac{1.00}{f}$

$f = -0.050 \text{ m} \quad \text{or} \quad -5.0 \text{ cm}$

3. (a) $F = \dfrac{(n' - n)}{r}$

$F = \dfrac{(1.52 - 1.00)}{+0.15 \text{ m}}$

$F = +3.47 \text{ D}$

(b) $F = \dfrac{n'}{f'}$

$+3.47 \text{ D} = \dfrac{1.52}{f'}$

$f' = +0.438 \text{ m} \quad \text{or} \quad +43.8 \text{ cm}$

4. $F = \dfrac{(n' - n)}{r}$

$F = \dfrac{(1.586 - 1.000)}{-0.125 \text{ m}}$

$F = -4.69 \text{ D}$

5. (a) $L' = L + F$

$$L' = \left(\frac{1.00}{-0.20 \text{ m}}\right) + (-10.00 \text{ D})$$

$$L' = -15.00 \text{ D}$$

$$L' = \frac{n'}{l'}$$

$$-15.00 \text{ D} = \frac{1.52}{l'}$$

$$l' = -0.101 \text{ m} \quad \text{or} \quad -10.1 \text{ cm}$$

$$M = \frac{L}{L'}$$

$$M = \frac{-5.00 \text{ D}}{-15.00 \text{ D}}$$

$$M = +0.33\times$$

$$(6.00 \text{ mm})(+0.33\times) = +2.00 \text{ mm}$$

(b) Virtual.

(c) Erect.

6. (a) $L' = L + F$

$$L' = \left(\frac{1.00}{-0.20 \text{ m}}\right) + (+10.00 \text{ D})$$

$$L' = +5.00 \text{ D}$$

$$L' = \frac{n'}{l'}$$

$$+5.00 \text{ D} = \frac{1.52}{l'}$$

$$l' = +0.304 \text{ m} \quad \text{or} \quad +30.4 \text{ cm}$$

$$M = \frac{L}{L'}$$

$$M = \frac{-5.00 \text{ D}}{+5.00 \text{ D}}$$

$$M = -1.00\times$$

$$(10.00 \text{ mm})(-1.00\times) = -10.00 \text{ mm}$$

(b) Real.

(c) Inverted.

7. (a) $L' = L + F$

$$L' = \left(\frac{1.00}{-0.050 \text{ m}}\right) + (+10.00 \text{ D})$$

$$L' = -10.00 \text{ D}$$

$$L' = \frac{n'}{l'}$$

$$-10.00 \text{ D} = \frac{1.52}{l'}$$

$$l' = -0.152 \text{ m} \quad \text{or} \quad -15.2 \text{ cm}$$

$$M = \frac{L}{L'}$$

$$M = \frac{-20.00 \text{ D}}{-10.00 \text{ D}}$$

$$M = +2.00\times$$

$$(10.00 \text{ mm})(+2.00\times) = +20.00 \text{ mm}$$

(b) Virtual.

(c) Erect.

8. Since the image is virtual, it must be located to the left of the surface.

$$L' = L + F$$

$$\frac{1.52}{-0.05 \text{ m}} = L + 15.00 \text{ D}$$

$$L = -45.40 \text{ D}$$

$$L = \frac{n}{l}$$

$$-45.40 \text{ D} = \frac{1.00}{l}$$

$$l = -0.022 \text{ m} \quad \text{or} \quad -2.2 \text{ cm}$$

9. Since the image is real, it must be located to the right of the surface.

$$L' = L + F$$

$$\frac{1.52}{+0.20 \text{ m}} = L + 15.00 \text{ D}$$

$$L = -7.40 \text{ D}$$

$$L = \frac{n}{l}$$

$$-7.40 \text{ D} = \frac{1.00}{l}$$

$$l = -0.135 \text{ m} \quad \text{or} \quad -13.5 \text{ cm}$$

10. The water surface is flat (infinite radius of curvature), giving it a power of zero. The object is located in water at a distance of −3.00 m from the surface. We need to locate the image, which is formed by rays existing in air.

$$L' = L + F$$

$$L' = \left(\frac{1.33}{-3.00 \text{ m}}\right) + 0.00 \text{ D}$$

$$L' = -0.44 \text{ D}$$

$$L' = \frac{n'}{l'}$$

$$-0.44 \text{ D} = \frac{1.00}{l'}$$

$$l' = -2.27 \text{ m}$$

The virtual image of the rock is located 2.27 m below the surface of the pond. Consequently, the rock appears to be 2.27 m below the surface of the pond.

11. This problem can be confusing because it is easy to incorrectly use the linear sign convention. For instance, if you draw a diagram that shows the pupil to the right of the cornea, you must assume that light travels from right to left; this is not consistent with our linear sign convention. Alternatively, you could draw the diagram with the pupil to the left of the cornea and then use the linear sign convention. This is the approach we will take to solve this problem.

The first step is to determine the power of the cornea. We treat the cornea as a spherical refracting surface that separates the aqueous from water. The cornea is assumed to have no thickness and no index of refraction. It simply gives shape to the aqueous–air interface. Its power is as follows:

$$F = \frac{(n' - n)}{r}$$

$$F = \frac{(1.000 - 1.333)}{-0.0078 \text{ m}}$$

$$F = +42.69 \text{ D}$$

The object (the pupil) is located in the aqueous and is 3.60 mm from the cornea:

$$L' = L + F$$

$$L' = \left[\frac{(1000)(1.333)}{-3.60 \text{ mm}}\right] + 42.69 \text{ D}$$

$$L' = -327.59 \text{ D}$$

$$L' = \frac{n'}{l'}$$

$$-327.59 \text{ D} = \frac{(1000)(1.000)}{l'}$$

$$l' = -3.05 \text{ mm}$$

When you look into someone's eye, you see a virtual image of the pupil that is located nearer to the cornea (3.05 mm) than the actual pupil (3.60 mm).

12. $M = \dfrac{L}{L'}$

$$M = \frac{-370.28 \text{ D}}{-327.59 \text{ D}}$$

$$M = +1.13\times$$

$$(4.00 \text{ mm})(+1.13\times) = +4.52 \text{ mm}$$

The (virtual) image of the pupil that you see when looking into the eye is larger than the actual pupil.

CHAPTER 4
Thin Lenses

1. (a) $F_1 = \dfrac{(n' - n)}{r}$

$$F_1 = \frac{(1.52 - 1.00)}{+0.08}$$

$$F_1 = +6.50 \text{ D}$$

$$F_2 = \frac{(n' - n)}{r}$$

$$F_2 = \frac{(1.00 - 1.52)}{-0.06 \text{ m}}$$

$$F_2 = +8.67 \text{ D}$$

For a thin lens:

$$F_T = F_1 + F_2$$
$$F_T = +6.50 \text{ D} + 8.67 \text{ D}$$
$$F_T = +15.17 \text{ D}$$

(b) $F = \dfrac{1.00}{f'}$

$$15.17 \text{ D} = \frac{(100)(1.00)}{f'}$$

$$f' = +6.59 \text{ cm}$$

The secondary focal point is located 6.59 cm to the right of the lens. Since the primary focal length of a thin lens is equal to the secondary focal length (in absolute values), the primary focal point is 6.59 cm to the left of the lens.

(c) Biconvex

2. (a) $L' = L + F$

$$L' = \left[\frac{(100)(1.00)}{-15.00 \text{ cm}}\right] + 20.00 \text{ D}$$

$$L' = +13.33 \text{ D}$$

$$L' = \frac{n'}{l'}$$

$$+13.33 \text{ D} = \frac{(100)(1.00)}{l'}$$

$$l' = +7.50 \text{ cm}$$

$$M = \frac{L}{L'}$$

$$M = \frac{-6.67 \text{ D}}{+13.33 \text{ D}}$$

$$M = -0.50\times$$

Since the index of refraction is the same on both sides of the thin lens, magnification can also be calculated as

$$M = \frac{l'}{l}$$

$$M = \frac{+7.50 \text{ cm}}{-15.00 \text{ cm}}$$

$$M = -0.50\times$$

$$(13.00 \text{ mm})(-0.50\times) = -6.50 \text{ mm}$$

(b) Real because it is formed by converging light.

(c) Inverted.

3. (a) $L' = L + F$

$$L' = \left[\frac{(100)(1.00)}{-5.00 \text{ cm}}\right] + 10.00 \text{ D}$$

$$L' = -10.00 \text{ D}$$

$$L' = \frac{n'}{l'}$$

$$-10.00 \text{ D} = \frac{(100)(1.00)}{l'}$$

$$l' = -10.00 \text{ cm}$$

$$M = \frac{L}{L'}$$

$$M = \frac{-20.00 \text{ D}}{-10.00 \text{ D}}$$

$$M = +2.00\times$$

$$(30.00 \text{ mm})(+2.00\times) = +60.00 \text{ mm}$$

(b) Virtual, because it is formed by diverging light.

(c) Erect.

4. (a) $L' = L + F$

$$L' = \left[\frac{(100)(1.00)}{-10.00 \text{ cm}}\right] + (-30.00 \text{ D})$$

$$L' = -40.00 \text{ D}$$

$$L' = \frac{n'}{l'}$$

$$-40.00 \text{ D} = \frac{(100)(1.00)}{l'}$$

$$l' = -2.50 \text{ cm}$$

$$M = \frac{L}{L'}$$

$$M = \frac{-10.00 \text{ D}}{-40.00 \text{ D}}$$

$$M = +0.25\times$$

$$(30.00 \text{ mm})(+0.25\times) = +7.50 \text{ mm}$$

(b) Virtual.

(c) Erect.

5. $L' = L + F$

$$\frac{(100)(1.00)}{+50.00 \text{ cm}} = L + (+25.00 \text{ D})$$

$$L = -23.00 \text{ D}$$

$$L = \frac{n}{l}$$

$$-23.00 \text{ D} = \frac{(100)(1.00)}{l}$$

$$l = -4.35 \text{ cm}$$

When an object is located 4.35 cm to the left of this plus lens, a real image is focused 50.00 cm to the right of the lens.

6. $L' = L + F$

$$\frac{(100)(1.00)}{-50.00 \text{ cm}} = L + (+25.00 \text{ D})$$

$L = -27.00 \text{ D}$

$$L = \frac{n}{l}$$

$$-27.00 \text{ D} = \frac{(100)(1.00)}{l}$$

$l = -3.70 \text{ cm}$

When an object is located 3.70 cm to the left of this plus lens, a virtual image is formed 50.00 cm to the left of the lens. Since the object is located within the focal length of this thin plus lens, the image is virtual and magnified.

7. $L' = L + F$

$$\frac{(100)(1.00)}{-10.00 \text{ cm}} = L + (-5.00 \text{ D})$$

$L = -5.00 \text{ D}$

$$L = \frac{n}{l}$$

$$-5.00 \text{ D} = \frac{(100)(1.00)}{l}$$

$l = -20.00 \text{ cm}$

When an object is located 20.00 cm to the left of this negative lens, a virtual image is formed 10.00 cm to the left of the lens.

8. $(x)(x') = f^2$

$(0.25 \text{ m})(0.40 \text{ m}) = f^2$

$f = 0.32 \text{ m}$

$$F = \frac{n}{f'}$$

$$F = \frac{1.00}{+0.32 \text{ m}}$$

$F = +3.13 \text{ D}$

CHAPTER 5
Optical Systems with Multiple Surfaces

1. (a) *Power of first surface*:

$$F_1 = \frac{(n' - n)}{r}$$

$$F_1 = \frac{(1.52 - 1.00)}{+0.05 \text{ m}}$$

$$F_1 = +10.40 \text{ D}$$

Power of the second surface:

$$F_2 = \frac{(n' - n)}{r}$$

$$F_2 = \frac{(1.00 - 1.52)}{-0.025 \text{ m}}$$

$$F_2 = +20.80 \text{ D}$$

Refraction at first surface:

$$L' = L + F$$

$$L' = \left[\frac{(1.00)(100)}{-25.00 \text{ cm}}\right] + 10.40 \text{ D}$$

$$L' = -4.00 \text{ D} + 10.40 \text{ D}$$

$$L' = +6.40 \text{ D}$$

$$L' = \frac{n'}{l'}$$

$$+6.40 \text{ D} = \frac{(1.52)(100)}{l'}$$

$$l' = +23.75 \text{ cm}$$

This real image is located 23.75 cm to the right of the first surface and 20.75 cm to the right of the second surface (i.e., $23.75 - 3.00 \text{ cm} = 20.75 \text{ cm}$). It serves as a virtual object for the second surface. Keep in mind that the rays that form this virtual object exist in the glass.

Refraction at second surface:

$$L' = L + F$$

$$L' = \left[\frac{(1.52)(100)}{+20.75 \text{ cm}}\right] + 20.80 \text{ D}$$

$$L' = +7.33 \text{ D} + 20.80 \text{ D}$$

$$L' = +28.13 \text{ D}$$

The light rays that form this real image exist in air.

$$L' = \frac{n'}{l'}$$

$$+28.13 \text{ D} = \frac{(1.00)(100)}{l'}$$

$$l' = +3.55 \text{ cm}$$

The image is located 3.55 cm to the right of the second lens surface.

(b) Total lateral magnification = (M_L for first surface)(M_L for second surface)

$$\text{Total lateral magnification} = \left(\frac{-4.00 \text{ D}}{+6.40 \text{ D}}\right)\left(\frac{+7.33 \text{ D}}{+28.13 \text{ D}}\right)$$

Total lateral magnification = $-0.17\times$
$(30.00 \text{ mm})(-0.17\times) = -5.10 \text{ mm}$

(c) Since the final image is formed by converging light rays, it is real.

(d) The final real image is inverted. This is indicated by the negative sign that is given for the total magnification.

(e) Biconvex

2. (a) *Power of first surface*:

$$F_1 = \frac{(n' - n)}{r}$$

$$F_1 = \frac{(1.52 - 1.00)}{+0.12 \text{ m}}$$

$$F_1 = +4.33 \text{ D}$$

Power of second surface:

$$F_2 = \frac{(n' - n)}{r}$$

$$F_2 = \frac{(1.00 - 1.52)}{-0.07 \text{ m}}$$

$$F_2 = +7.43 \text{ D}$$

Refraction at first surface:

$$L' = L + F$$

$$L' = \left[\frac{(1.00)(100)}{-3.00 \text{ cm}}\right] + 4.33 \text{ D}$$

$$L' = -33.33 \text{ D} + 4.33 \text{ D}$$

$$L' = -29.00 \text{ D}$$

$$L' = \frac{n'}{l'}$$

$$-29.00 \text{ D} = \frac{(1.52)(100)}{l'}$$

$$l' = -5.24 \text{ cm}$$

This virtual image is located 5.24 cm to the left of the first surface and 7.74 cm (i.e., 5.24 + 2.50 cm = 7.74 cm) to the left of the second surface. The rays that form this image exist in glass. It serves as the object for the second surface.

Refraction at second surface:

$$L' = L + F$$

$$L' = \left[\frac{(1.52)(100)}{-7.74 \text{ cm}}\right] + 7.43 \text{ D}$$

$$L' = -19.64 \text{ D} + 7.43 \text{ D}$$

$$L' = -12.21 \text{ D}$$

The light rays that form this virtual image exist in air.

$$L' = \frac{n'}{l'}$$

$$-12.21 \text{ D} = \frac{(1.00)(100)}{l'}$$

$$l' = -8.19 \text{ cm}$$

The image is located 8.19 cm to the left of the second lens surface.

(b) Total lateral magnification = (M_L for first surface)(M_L for second surface)

$$\text{Total lateral magnification} = \left(\frac{-33.33 \text{ D}}{-29.00 \text{ D}}\right)\left(\frac{-19.64 \text{ D}}{-12.21 \text{ D}}\right)$$

Total lateral magnification = +1.85×
(30.00 mm)(+1.85×) = +55.5 mm

(c) The final image is formed by diverging light rays—it is to the left of the second surface. Therefore, the final image is virtual.

(d) This virtual image is erect as indicated by the plus sign for magnification.

(e) Biconvex.

3. (a) *Power of first surface*:

$$F_1 = \frac{(n' - n)}{r}$$

$$F_1 = \frac{(1.52 - 1.00)}{+0.15 \text{ m}}$$

$$F_1 = +3.47 \text{ D}$$

Power of second surface:

$$F_2 = \frac{(n' - n)}{r}$$

$$F_2 = \frac{(1.00 - 1.52)}{+0.15 \text{ m}}$$

$$F_2 = -3.47 \text{ D}$$

Refraction at first surface:

$$L' = L + F$$

$$L' = \left[\frac{(1.00)(100)}{-40.00 \text{ cm}} \right] + 3.47 \text{ D}$$

$$L' = -2.50 \text{ D} + 3.47 \text{ D}$$

$$L' = +0.97 \text{ D}$$

$$L' = \frac{n'}{l'}$$

$$+0.97 \text{ D} = \frac{(1.52)(100)}{l'}$$

$$l' = +156.70 \text{ cm}$$

This real image is located 156.70 cm to the right of the first surface and 153.70 cm (i.e., 156.70 − 3.00 cm = 153.70 cm) to the right of the second surface. It serves as a virtual object for the second surface. Keep in mind that the rays that form this virtual object exist in the glass.

Refraction at second surface:

$$L' = L + F$$

$$L' = \left[\frac{(1.52)(100)}{+153.70 \text{ cm}} \right] + (-3.47 \text{ D})$$

$$L' = +0.99 \text{ D} + (-3.47 \text{ D})$$

$$L' = -2.48 \text{ D}$$

The rays that form this virtual image exist in air.

$$L' = \frac{n'}{l'}$$

$$-2.48 \text{ D} = \frac{(1.00)(100)}{l'}$$

$$l' = -40.32 \text{ cm}$$

The image is located 40.32 cm to the left of the second lens surface.

(b) Total lateral magnification = (M_L for first surface)(M_L for second surface)

$$\text{Total lateral magnification} = \left(\frac{-2.50 \text{ D}}{+0.97 \text{ D}}\right)\left(\frac{+0.99 \text{ D}}{-2.48 \text{ D}}\right)$$

Total lateral magnification = +1.03×
(30.00 mm)(+1.03×) = +30.90 mm

(c) Since the final image is formed by diverging light rays, it is virtual.

(d) The final virtual image is erect as indicated by the positive sign of the magnification.

(e) Meniscus

4. (a) *Refraction at first lens*:

$$L' = L + F$$

$$L' = \left[\frac{(1.00)(100)}{-30.00 \text{ cm}}\right] + (-10.00 \text{ D})$$

$$L' = -3.33 \text{ D} + (-10.00 \text{ D})$$

$$L' = -13.33 \text{ D}$$

$$L' = \frac{n'}{l'}$$

$$-13.33 \text{ D} = \frac{(1.00)(100)}{l'}$$

$$l' = -7.50 \text{ cm}$$

This virtual image is located 7.50 cm to the left of the first lens and 10.00 cm (i.e., 7.50 + 2.50 cm = 10.00 cm) to the left of the second lens. Keep in mind that the rays that form this image exist in *air*. It serves as an object for the second lens.

Refraction at second lens:

$$L' = L + F$$

$$L' = \left[\frac{(1.00)(100)}{-10.00\ \text{cm}}\right] + 1.00\ \text{D}$$

$$L' = -10.00\ \text{D} + 1.00\ \text{D}$$

$$L' = -9.00\ \text{D}$$

$$L' = \frac{n'}{l'}$$

$$-9.00\ \text{D} = \frac{(1.00)(100)}{l'}$$

$$l' = -11.11\ \text{cm}$$

The virtual image is located 11.11 cm to the left of the second lens.

(b) Total lateral magnification = (M_L for first lens)(M_L for second lens)

$$\text{Total lateral magnification} = \left(\frac{-3.33\ \text{D}}{-13.33\ \text{D}}\right)\left(\frac{-10.00\ \text{D}}{-9.00\ \text{D}}\right)$$

Total lateral magnification = +0.28×
(45.00 mm)(+0.28×) = +12.60 mm

(c) Since the final image is formed by diverging light rays, it is virtual.

(d) The final virtual image is erect. This is indicated by the positive sign that is given for the total magnification.

CHAPTER 6
Thick Lenses

1. (a) This is the same lens as in Problem 1 of Chapter 5. We have already calculated the following:

$$F_1 = +10.40\ \text{D}$$
$$F_2 = +20.80\ \text{D}$$

Equivalent power:

$$F_e = F_1 + F_2 - \left(\frac{t}{n}\right)F_1 F_2$$

$$F_e = 10.40\ \text{D} + 20.80\ \text{D} - \left(\frac{0.030\ \text{m}}{1.52}\right)(+10.40\ \text{D})(+20.80\ \text{D})$$

$$F_e = +26.93\ \text{D}$$

Calculation of f_e and f_e'

$$F_e = \frac{n'}{f_e'}$$

$$+26.93 \text{ D} = \frac{(1.00)(100)}{f_e'}$$

$$f_e' = +3.71 \text{ cm}$$

This distance is measured *from* the secondary principal plane, H'.

Since the lens is surrounded by air, f_e is equal to -3.71 cm. This distance is measured *from* the primary principal plane, H.

Location of principal planes:

$$\overline{A_1 H} = \frac{\left(\dfrac{t}{n}\right) F_2}{F_e}$$

$$\overline{A_1 H} = \frac{\left(\dfrac{0.030 \text{ m}}{1.52}\right)(+20.80 \text{ D})}{+26.93 \text{ D}} \ (100 \text{ cm/m})$$

$$\overline{A_1 H} = +1.52 \text{ cm}$$

$$\overline{A_2 H'} = \frac{-\left(\dfrac{t}{n}\right) F_1}{F_e}$$

$$\overline{A_2 H'} = \frac{-\left(\dfrac{0.030 \text{ m}}{1.52}\right)(+10.40 \text{ D})}{+26.93 \text{ D}} \ (100 \text{ cm/m})$$

$$\overline{A_2 H'} = -0.76 \text{ cm}$$

Calculation of F_n and F_v:

We can calculate F_n and F_v using the thick lens formulae:

$$F_n = \frac{F_2}{1 - cF_2} + F_1$$

$$F_n = \frac{+20.80 \text{ D}}{1 - \left(\dfrac{0.030 \text{ m}}{1.52}\right)(+20.80 \text{ D})} + 10.40 \text{ D}$$

$$F_n = +45.69 \text{ D}$$

$$F_v = \frac{F_1}{1 - cF_1} + F_2$$

$$F_v = \cfrac{+10.40}{1 - \left(\cfrac{0.030 \text{ m}}{1.52}\right)(+10.40 \text{ D})} + 20.80 \text{ D}$$

$$F_v = +33.89 \text{ D}$$

(b) When treating the lens as an equivalent lens, distances are measured from the principal planes. The equivalent lens exists in air. As in the case of a thin lens, we ignore the lens index of refraction. If the object is located 25.00 cm from the front surface of the lens, then it is located 26.52 cm (i.e., 25.00 + 1.52 cm = 26.52 cm) in front of the primary principal plane. Substituting, we have:

$$L' = L + F_e$$

$$L' = \left[\frac{(100)(1.00)}{-26.52 \text{ cm}}\right] + 26.93 \text{ D}$$

$$L' = +23.16 \text{ D}$$

$$L' = \frac{n'}{l'}$$

$$+23.16 \text{ D} = \frac{(100)(1.00)}{l'}$$

$$l' = +4.32 \text{ cm}$$

This real image is located 4.32 cm to the right of the second principal plane or 3.56 cm (i.e., 4.32 − 0.76 cm = 3.56 cm) to the right of the second lens surface.

$$M = \frac{L}{L'}$$

$$M = \frac{-3.90 \text{ D}}{+23.16 \text{ D}}$$

$$M = -0.17\times$$

$$(30.00 \text{ mm})(-0.17\times) = -5.1 \text{ mm}$$

This real image is inverted.

(c) See the solution to Problem 1 in Chapter 5. Due to rounding, the equivalent lens approach gives a slightly different answer than the surface-by-surface approach for the image distance (measured from the back surface of the lens).

2. (a) Calculate powers of two surfaces:

$$F_1 = \frac{(n' - n)}{r_1}$$

$$F_1 = \frac{(1.52 - 1.00)}{+0.025 \text{ m}}$$

$$F_1 = +20.80 \text{ D}$$

$$F_2 = \frac{(n' - n)}{r_2}$$

$$F_2 = \frac{(1.00 - 1.52)}{+0.075 \text{ m}}$$

$$F_2 = -6.93 \text{ D}$$

Equivalent power:

$$F_e = F_1 + F_2 - \left(\frac{t}{n}\right) F_1 F_2$$

$$F_e = 20.80 \text{ D} + (-6.93 \text{ D}) - \left(\frac{0.010 \text{ m}}{1.52}\right)(+20.80 \text{ D})(-6.93 \text{ D})$$

$$F_e = +14.82 \text{ D}$$

Calculation of f_e and f_e':

$$F_e = \frac{n'}{f_e'}$$

$$+14.82 \text{ D} = \frac{(1.00)(100)}{f_e'}$$

$$f_e' = +6.75 \text{ cm}$$

Since the lens is surrounded by air, f_e is equal to -6.75 cm. The secondary equivalent focal length is measured from the secondary principal plane, and the primary equivalent focal length is measured from the primary principal plane.

Location of principal planes:

$$\overline{A_1 H} = \frac{\left(\frac{t}{n}\right) F_2}{F_e}$$

$$\overline{A_1 H} = \frac{\left(\frac{0.010 \text{ m}}{1.52}\right)(-6.93 \text{ D})}{+14.82 \text{ D}} (100 \text{ cm/m})$$

$$\overline{A_1 H} = -0.31 \text{ cm}$$

$$\overline{A_2 H'} = \frac{-\left(\dfrac{t}{n}\right) F_1}{F_e}$$

$$\overline{A_2 H'} = \frac{-\left(\dfrac{0.010 \text{ m}}{1.52}\right)(+20.80 \text{ D})}{+14.82 \text{ D}} \quad (100 \text{ cm/m})$$

$$\overline{A_2 H'} = -0.92 \text{ cm}$$

Calculation of F_n and F_v

We can calculate F_n and F_v using the thick lens formulae:

$$F_n = \frac{F_2}{1 - cF_2} + F_1$$

$$F_n = \frac{-6.93 \text{ D}}{1 - \left(\dfrac{0.010 \text{ m}}{1.52}\right)(-6.93 \text{ D})} + 20.80 \text{ D}$$

$$F_n = +14.17 \text{ D}$$

$$F_v = \frac{F_1}{1 - cF_1} + F_2$$

$$F_v = \frac{+20.80}{1 - \left(\dfrac{0.010 \text{ m}}{1.52}\right)(+20.80 \text{ D})} + (-6.93 \text{ D})$$

$$F_v = +17.17 \text{ D}$$

(b) In treating the lens as an equivalent lens, distances are measured from the principal planes. As in the case of a thin lens, we ignore the lens's index of refraction. If the object is located 15.00 cm from the front surface of the lens, then it is located 14.69 cm (i.e., 15.00 − 0.31 cm = 14.69 cm) in front of the primary principal plane. Substituting, we have:

$$L' = L + F_e$$

$$L' = \left[\frac{(100)(1.00)}{-14.69 \text{ cm}}\right] + 14.82 \text{ D}$$

$$L' = -6.81 \text{ D} + 14.82 \text{ D}$$

$$L' = +8.01 \text{ D}$$

$$L' = \frac{n'}{l'}$$

$$+8.01 \text{ D} = \frac{(100)(1.00)}{l'}$$

$$l' = +12.48 \text{ cm}$$

This real image is located 12.48 cm to the right of the secondary principal plane or 11.56 cm (i.e., 12.48 − 0.92 cm = 11.56 cm) to the right of the second lens surface.

$$M = \frac{L}{L'}$$

$$M = \frac{-6.81 \text{ D}}{+8.01 \text{ D}}$$

$$M = -0.85\times$$

$$(10.00 \text{ mm})(-0.85\times) = -8.50 \text{ mm}$$

This real image is inverted.

(c) *At the first surface*:

$$L' = L + F$$

$$L' = \left[\frac{(100)(1.00)}{-15.00 \text{ cm}}\right] + 20.80 \text{ D}$$

$$L' = -6.67 \text{ D} + 20.80 \text{ D}$$

$$L' = +14.13 \text{ D}$$

The light rays that form this image exist in glass:

$$L' = \frac{n'}{l'}$$

$$+14.13 \text{ D} = \frac{(100)(1.52)}{l'}$$

$$l' = +10.75 \text{ cm}$$

This image is located 10.75 cm to the right of the first surface and 9.75 cm (i.e., 10.75 − 1.00 cm = 9.75 cm) to the right of the second surface. It serves as a virtual object for the second surface. The rays that form this virtual object exist in glass.

At the second surface:

$$L' = L + F$$

$$L' = \left[\frac{(100)(1.52)}{+9.75 \text{ cm}}\right] + (-6.93 \text{ D})$$

$$L' = +15.59 \text{ D} + (-6.93 \text{ D})$$

$$L' = +8.66 \text{ D}$$

The rays that form this image exist in air.

$$L' = \frac{n'}{l'}$$

$$+8.66 \text{ D} = \frac{(100)(1.00)}{l'}$$

$$l' = +11.55 \text{ cm}$$

Magnification:

Total lateral magnification = (M_L for first surface)(M_L for second surface)

$$\text{Total lateral magnification} = \left(\frac{-6.67 \text{ D}}{+14.13 \text{ D}}\right)\left(\frac{+15.59 \text{ D}}{+8.66 \text{ D}}\right)$$

Total lateral magnification = $-0.85\times$
$(10.00 \text{ mm})(-0.85\times) = -8.50 \text{ mm}$

Note that the surface-by-surface approach gives about the same answers as the equivalent lens approach.

CHAPTER 7
Ametropia

1. (a) $\dfrac{100(1.00)}{-6.00 \text{ D}} = -16.67 \text{ cm}$

   $-16.67 \text{ cm} + (-1.20 \text{ cm}) = -17.87 \text{ cm}$

   $\dfrac{(100)(1.00)}{-17.87 \text{ cm}} = -5.60 \text{ D}$

   To correct this myopic refractive error, the contact lens should have a power of -5.50 D.

   (b) $\dfrac{100(1.00)}{+6.00 \text{ D}} = +16.67 \text{ cm}$

   $16.67 \text{ cm} - 1.20 \text{ cm} = +15.47 \text{ cm}$

   $\dfrac{(100)(1.00)}{+15.47 \text{ cm}} = +6.47 \text{ D}$

   To correct this hyperopic refractive error, the contact lens should have a power of $+6.50$ D.

2. (a) $\dfrac{(100)(1.00)}{-7.00 \text{ D}} = -14.29 \text{ cm}$

   $-14.29 \text{ cm} - (-1.20 \text{ cm}) = -13.09 \text{ cm}$

   $\dfrac{(100)(1.00)}{-12.79 \text{ cm}} = -7.64 \text{ D}$

   To correct this myopic refractive error, the spectacle lens should have a power of -7.75 D.

(b) $\dfrac{(100)(1.00)}{+7.00\ \text{D}} = +14.29\ \text{cm}$

14.29 cm + 1.20 cm = +15.49 cm

$\dfrac{(100)(1.00)}{+15.49\ \text{cm}} = +6.46\ \text{D}$

To correct this hyperopic refractive error, the spectacle lens should have a power of +6.50 D.

3. (a) $L' = L + F$

$\left[\dfrac{(1000)(1.333)}{l'}\right] = -10.00\ \text{D} + 60.00\ \text{D}$

$l' = 26.67\ \text{mm}$

(b) $L' = L + F$

$\left[\dfrac{(1000)(1.333)}{+22.22\ \text{mm}}\right] = -10.00\ \text{D} + F$

$F = +70.00\ \text{D}$

4. The eye is corrected with a +5.00 D spectacle lens. What is the vergence this lens produces at the cornea?

$\dfrac{(100)(1.00)}{+5.00\ \text{D}} = +20.00\ \text{cm}$

20.00 cm − 1.50 cm = +18.50 cm

$\dfrac{(100)(1.00)}{+18.50\ \text{cm}} = +5.41\ \text{D}$

$L' = L + F$

$\left[\dfrac{(1000)(1.333)}{l'}\right] = +5.41\ \text{D} + 60.00\ \text{D}$

$l' = 20.38\ \text{mm}$

5. The patient's far point is 25.00 cm anterior to the eye, making her 4.00 D myopic as measured at the cornea. The appropriate spectacle correction is determined as follows:

−25.00 cm − (−1.50 cm) = −23.50 cm

$\dfrac{(100)(1.00)}{-23.50\ \text{cm}} = -4.26\ \text{D}$

To correct this myopic refractive error, the spectacle lens should have a power of −4.25 D.

6. The required vergence (at the spectacle plane) with the old correction in place is −1.00 D. Therefore, the patient's myopia will be corrected with −5.00 D spectacle lenses. The power of the contact lens required to correct the ametropia is determined as follows:

$$\frac{(100)(1.00)}{-5.00 \text{ D}} = -20.00 \text{ cm}$$

$$-20.00 \text{ cm} + (-1.50 \text{ cm}) = -21.50 \text{ cm}$$

$$\frac{(100)(1.00)}{-21.50 \text{ cm}} = -4.65 \text{ D}$$

A −4.75 D contact lens would correct the patient's ametropia.

7. When light rays with a vergence of zero are incident on the surface of an unaccommodated emmetropic eye, an image will be focused on the retina. This will occur when an object is at the primary focal point of a plus spectacle lens. Given that the object is located 15.00 cm from the cornea and the vertex distance is 1.2 cm, the lens power is calculated as follows:

$$15.00 \text{ cm} - 1.20 \text{ cm} = +13.80 \text{ cm}$$

$$\frac{(100)(1.00)}{+13.80 \text{ cm}} = +7.25 \text{ D}$$

To clearly see an object located 15.00 cm anterior to his cornea, this emmetrope (who cannot accommodate) may look through a +7.25 D spectacle lens.

8. $L' = L + F$

$$\left[\frac{(1000)(1.333)}{+24.22 \text{ mm}} \right] = \left[\frac{(1000)(1.000)}{l} \right] + 60.00 \text{ D}$$

$$l = -201.5 \text{ mm}$$

The object is located 20.15 cm anterior to front surface of the reduced eye.

CHAPTER 8
Accommodation

1. (a) $F_{FP} = L + F_A$

$$-3.50 \text{ D} = \left[\frac{(100)(1.00)}{-10.00 \text{ cm}} \right] + F_A$$

$$F_A = +6.50 \text{ D}$$

The uncorrected eye must accommodate 6.50 D.

(b) When corrected with a contact lens, the required accommodation is equal and opposite to the near stimulus vergence. Since the object is located

10.00 cm from the eye, the near stimulus vergence is −10.00 D, and the required accommodation is 10.00 D.

(c) First, find the power of the spectacle correction:

$$F = \frac{1}{f'}$$

$$-3.50 \text{ D} = \frac{(100)(1.00)}{f'}$$

$$f' = -28.57 \text{ cm}$$

$$-28.57 \text{ cm} - (-1.5 \text{ cm}) = -27.07 \text{ cm}$$

$$F = \frac{1}{f'}$$

$$F = \frac{(100)(1.00)}{-27.07 \text{ cm}}$$

$$F = -3.69 \text{ D}$$

Next, find the image produced by the spectacle lens:

$$L' = L + F$$

$$L' = \left[\frac{(100)(1.00)}{-8.50 \text{ cm}} \right] + (-3.69 \text{ D})$$

$$L' = -15.45 \text{ D}$$

$$L' = \frac{1}{l'}$$

$$-15.45 \text{ D} = \frac{(100)(1.00)}{l'}$$

$$l' = -6.47 \text{ cm}$$

The distance from the image to the eye is −7.97 cm [i.e., −6.47 cm + (−1.50 cm) = −7.97 cm].

Now determine the amount of accommodation required to focus the image on the retina:

$$F_{FP} = L + F_A$$

$$-3.50 \text{ D} = \left[\frac{(100)(1.00)}{-7.97 \text{ cm}} \right] + F_A$$

$$F_A = +9.05 \text{ D}$$

Wearing a spectacle correction, the patient must accommodate 9.05 D.

2. First, locate the image produced by the +4.00 D contact lens:

$$L' = L + F$$

$$L' = \left[\frac{(100)(1.00)}{-10.00 \text{ cm}}\right] + 4.00 \text{ D}$$

$$L' = -6.00 \text{ D}$$

$$L' = \frac{1}{l'}$$

$$-6.00 \text{ D} = \frac{(100)(1.00)}{l'}$$

$$l' = -16.67 \text{ cm}$$

Next, determine the amount of accommodation required to produce the far point vergence:

$$F_{FP} = L + F_A$$

$$+5.00 \text{ D} = \left[\frac{(100)(1.00)}{-16.67 \text{ cm}}\right] + F_A$$

$$F_A = +11.00 \text{ D}$$

This 5.00 D hyperopic eye, which is uncorrected by 1.00 D, must accommodate 11.00 D to focus the object onto the retina.

3. The patient can accommodate 5.00 D [(i.e., (100/20.00 cm) − 0 = 5.00 D)]. One-half of the patient's amplitude of accommodation is 2.50 D. When this emmetropic patient wears a contact lens to view an object at a distance of 15.00 cm, the vergence leaving the contact lens must be zero.

$$F_{FP} = L + F_A$$

$$00.00 \text{ D} = \left[\left(\frac{100}{-15.00 \text{ cm}}\right) + F_{\text{contact lens}}\right] + 2.50 \text{ D}$$

$$F_{\text{contact lens}} = +4.17 \text{ D}$$

The contact lens should have a power of +4.17 D. When wearing this contact lens, an object at a distance of 15.00 cm results in an image vergence of −2.50 D. The patient can see the object clearly by accommodating 2.50 D, which is one-half of his or her amplitude of accommodation.

4. $$F_{FP} = L + F_A$$

$$+2.00 \text{ D} = \left[\frac{(100)(1.00)}{-33.00 \text{ cm}}\right] + F_A$$

$$F_A = +5.00 \text{ D}$$

Therefore, the patient's total amplitude of accommodation is 10.00 D (i.e., 2×5.00 D $= 10.00$ D).

5. First determine the location of the image produced by the spectacle lens.

The object is located 8.80 cm in front of the lens [i.e., $(-10.00$ cm$) - (-1.20$ cm$) = -8.80$ cm].

$$L' = L + F$$

$$L' = \left[\frac{(100)(1.00)}{-8.80 \text{ cm}} \right] + (+6.00 \text{ D})$$

$$L' = -5.36 \text{ D}$$

$$L' = \frac{1}{l'}$$

$$-5.36 \text{ D} = \frac{(100)(1.00)}{l'}$$

$$l' = -18.64 \text{ cm}$$

This image is situated 19.84 cm [$(-18.64$ cm$) + (-1.2$ cm$) = -19.84$ cm] in front of the eye.

Next, determine the far-point vergence at the eye:

$$\frac{(100)(1.00)}{+6.00 \text{ D}} = +16.67 \text{ cm}$$

$$(+16.67 \text{ cm}) + (-1.2 \text{ cm}) = +15.47 \text{ cm}$$

$$\frac{(100)(1.00)}{+15.47 \text{ cm}} = +6.47 \text{ D}$$

The required accommodation is:

$$F_{FP} = L + F_A$$

$$+6.47 \text{ D} = \left[\frac{(100)(1.00)}{-19.84 \text{ cm}} \right] + F_A$$

$$F_A = +11.51 \text{ D}$$

6. Determine image location:

The object is located 5.00 cm in front of the lens [i.e., $(-15.00$ cm$) - (-10.00$ cm$) = -5.00$ cm].

$$L' = L + F$$

$$L' = \left[\frac{(100)(1.00)}{-5.00 \text{ cm}} \right] + (-4.00 \text{ D})$$

$$L' = -24.00 \text{ D}$$

$$L' = \frac{1}{l'}$$

$$-24.00 \text{ D} = \frac{(100)(1.00)}{l'}$$

$$l' = -4.17 \text{ cm}$$

This image is located 14.17 cm [i.e., –4.17 cm + (–10.00 cm) = –14.17 cm] anterior to the cornea.

The eye's refractive error, as measured in the spectacle plane, is –5.00 D. The far point vergence at the eye is calculated as follows:

$$\frac{(100)(1.00)}{-5.00 \text{ D}} = -20.00 \text{ cm}$$

$$(-20.00 \text{ cm}) + (-1.3 \text{ cm}) = -21.3 \text{ cm}$$

$$\frac{(100)(1.00)}{-21.3 \text{ cm}} = -4.69 \text{ D}$$

The required accommodation is:

$$F_{FP} = L + F_A$$

$$-4.69 \text{ D} = \left[\frac{(100)(1.00)}{-14.17 \text{ cm}}\right] + F_A$$

$$F_A = +2.37 \text{ D}$$

The eye must accommodate 2.37 D.

7. (a) *First, we determine the location of the image produced by the spectacle lens.*

$$L' = L + F$$

$$L' = \left[\frac{(100)(1.00)}{-18.50 \text{ cm}}\right] + (-6.00 \text{ D})$$

$$L' = -11.41 \text{ D}$$

$$L' = \frac{1}{l'}$$

$$-11.41 \text{ D} = \frac{(100)(1.00)}{l'}$$

$$l' = -8.77 \text{ cm}$$

The image is located 10.27 cm [(–8.77 cm) + (–1.5 cm) = –10.27 cm] in front of the eye.

Next, we determine the far point vergence at the eye.

The focal length of the spectacle lens:

$$F = \frac{1}{f'}$$

$$-6.00 \text{ D} = \frac{(100)(1.00)}{f'}$$

$$f' = -16.67 \text{ cm}$$

Since the vertex distance is 1.5 cm, the secondary focal length must be −18.17 cm [i.e., −16.67 cm + (−1.50 cm) = −18.17 cm]. The correction required in the corneal plane is:

$$F = \frac{1}{f'}$$

$$F = \frac{(100)(1.00)}{-18.17 \text{ cm}}$$

$$F = -5.50 \text{ D}$$

The accommodation is calculated as follows:

$$F_{FP} = L + F_A$$

$$-5.50 \text{ D} = \left[\frac{(100)(1.00)}{-10.27 \text{ cm}}\right] + F_A$$

$$F_A = +4.24 \text{ D}$$

When corrected with spectacles, the eye must accommodate 4.24 D to image an object at 20.00 cm upon the retina.

(b) In LASIK, the correction occurs in the plane of the cornea. Consequently, the required accommodation is the same as if the eyes were corrected with a contact lens. Since the near stimulus vergence is −5.00 D, the required accommodation is 5.00 D.

(c) Subsequent to LASIK, the former spectacle-wearing myopic patient must accommodate 18% more in order to see the near object [(5.00 − 4.24 D)/4.24 D = 0.18]. This must be taken into account when counseling the patient prior to surgery and when determining the amount of correction. Because of the patient's age (45 years old), correction with LASIK may precipitate (or make more apparent) presbyopic symptoms. It may be decided to slightly undercorrect one of the patient's eyes so that this eye can be used for viewing near objects. This is referred to as *monovision*. Many, but not all, patients adapt to a monovision correction.

CHAPTER 9
Cylindrical Lenses and the Correction of Astigmatism

1. (a) The vertical meridian has a power of -1.00 D and the horizontal meridian has a power of -2.00 D.

   (b) $-2.00 + 1.00 \times 180$

2. (a) The vertical meridian of the lens has a power of $+6.00$ D and the horizontal meridian has a power of $+4.00$ D. The image focused by the stronger vertical meridian will be closest to the lens.

   (b) Vertically diverging light rays emitted from the object are focused closest to the lens by the stronger vertical meridian. A horizontal line that has fuzzy left and right edges is formed in this plane because the object's horizontally diverging rays are not yet focused. The upper and lower edges of this horizontal line are in focus, however, because the vertical meridian is in focus.

   (c) $L' = L + F$

   $$L' = \left[\frac{(100)(1.00)}{-50.00 \text{ cm}}\right] + 6.00 \text{ D}$$

   $L' = +4.00 \text{ D}$

   $$L' = \frac{1}{l'}$$

   $$+4.00 \text{ D} = \frac{(100)(1.00)}{l'}$$

   $l' = +25.00 \text{ cm}$

   (d) At the plane where the weaker $+4.00$ D horizontal meridian is in focus, rays that are focused by the vertical meridian (at 25.00 cm) diverge to form a vertical line. The focused horizontal rays give this vertical line sharp right and left edges. The upper and lower edges of the vertical line are fuzzy, however, because the vertical meridian is out of focus. The location of this vertical line is given by:

   $L' = L + F$

   $$L' = \left[\frac{(100)(1.00)}{-0.50 \text{ cm}}\right] + 4.00 \text{ D}$$

   $L' = +2.00 \text{ D}$

   $$L' = \frac{(100)(1.00)}{l'}$$

   $l' = +50.00 \text{ cm}$

   (e) $50.00 - 25.00 \text{ cm} = 25.00 \text{ cm}$

(f) The circle of least confusion is centered *dioptrically* between the image plane of the vertical meridian and the image plane of the horizontal meridian. The dioptric distance from the lens is

$$\frac{4.00 \text{ D} + 2.00 \text{ D}}{2} = 3.00 \text{ D}$$

This means that the circle of least confusion is located 33.33 cm from the lens.

3. (a) The vertical meridian of the lens has a power of +5.00 D and the horizontal meridian has a power of +7.00 D. The image focused by the stronger horizontal meridian will be closest to the lens.

(b) A vertical line is formed closest to the lens. At the plane where the object's horizontally diverging light rays are focused by the stronger horizontal meridian, the vertical rays have not yet focused. These out-of-focus rays form a vertical line with fuzzy upper and lower edges. The right and left edges of this line are in focus, however, because the horizontal meridian is in focus.

(c) $L' = L + F$

$$L' = \left[\frac{(100)(1.00)}{-25.00 \text{ cm}}\right] + 7.00 \text{ D}$$

$$L' = +3.00 \text{ D}$$

$$L' = \frac{1}{l'}$$

$$+3.00 \text{ D} = \frac{(100)(1.00)}{l'}$$

$$l' = +33.33 \text{ cm}$$

(d) A horizontal line is formed further from the lens. At the plane where the object's vertically diverging light rays are focused by the weaker vertical meridian, the horizontal rays are out of focus—they are focused closer to the lens, at +33.33 cm. These out-of-focus rays form a horizontal line with fuzzy left and right edges. The upper and lower edges of this line are in focus, however, because the vertical meridian is in focus.

$$L' = L + F$$

$$L' = \left[\frac{(100)(1.00)}{-25.00 \text{ cm}}\right] + 5.00 \text{ D}$$

$$L' = +1.00 \text{ D}$$

$$L' = \frac{1}{l'}$$

$$+1.00 \text{ D} = \frac{(100)(1.00)}{l'}$$

$$l' = +100.00 \text{ cm}$$

(e) 100.00 − 33.33 cm = 66.66 cm

(f) The interval of Sturm is *dioptrically* centered between the image plane of the horizontal meridian and the image plane of the vertical meridian. The dioptric distance from the lens is

$$\frac{3.00\ D + 1.00\ D}{2} = 2.00\ D$$

This means that the circle of least confusion is located 50.00 cm from the lens.

4. (a) The vertical meridian of the lens has a power of +6.00 D and the horizontal meridian has a power of +5.00 D. Vertically diverging object rays are focused by the stronger vertical meridian to form a horizontal line. The line is located at

$$L' = L + F$$

$$L' = \left[\frac{(100)(1.00)}{-40.00\ cm}\right] + 6.00\ D$$

$$L' = +3.50\ D$$

$$L' = \frac{1}{l'}$$

$$+3.50\ D = \frac{(100)(1.00)}{l'}$$

$$l' = +28.57\ cm$$

(b) Horizontally diverging object rays are focused by the weaker horizontal lens meridian to form a vertical line. The line is located at

$$L' = L + F$$

$$L' = \left[\frac{(100)(1.00)}{-40.00\ cm}\right] + 5.00\ D$$

$$L' = +2.50\ D$$

$$L' = \frac{1}{l'}$$

$$+2.50\ D = \frac{(100)(1.00)}{l'}$$

$$l' = +40.00\ cm$$

(c) 40.00 − 28.57 cm = 11.43 cm

(d) $$\frac{3.50\ D + 2.50\ D}{2} = 3.00\ D$$

Therefore, the circle of least confusion is located 33.33 cm from the lens.

5. (a/b) The vertical meridian of the lens has a power of +4.00 D and the horizontal meridian has a power of +6.00 D. Horizontally diverging object rays are focused by the stronger horizontal meridian to form a vertical line. The line is located at

$$L' = L + F$$

$$L' = \left[\frac{(100)(1.00)}{-40.00 \text{ cm}} \right] + 6.00 \text{ D}$$

$$L' = +3.50 \text{ D}$$

$$L' = \frac{1}{l'}$$

$$+3.50 \text{ D} = \frac{(100)(1.00)}{l'}$$

$$l' = +28.57 \text{ cm}$$

Vertically diverging rays are focused by the weaker vertical lens meridian to form a horizontal line. The line is located at

$$L' = L + F$$

$$L' = \left[\frac{(100)(1.00)}{-40.00 \text{ cm}} \right] + 4.00 \text{ D}$$

$$L' = +1.50 \text{ D}$$

$$L' = \frac{1}{l'}$$

$$+1.50 \text{ D} = \frac{(100)(1.00)}{l'}$$

$$l' = +66.67 \text{ cm}$$

(c) 66.67 − 28.57 cm = 38.10 cm

(d) $\dfrac{3.50 \text{ D} + 1.50 \text{ D}}{2} = 2.50 \text{ D}$

Therefore, the circle of least confusion is located 40.00 cm to the right of the lens.

6. (a) −4.00 + 14.00 × 180; +10.00 − 14.00 × 090

   (b) pl + 10.00 × 180; +10.00 − 10.00 × 090

   (c) +5.00 − 8.00 × 180; −3.00 + 8.00 × 090

   (d) −6.00 + 8.00 × 180; +2.00 − 8.00 × 090

7. (a) Against-the-rule compound hyperopic.

   (b) With-the-rule compound myopic astigmatism.

   (c) With-the-rule mixed astigmatism.

8. Both meridians of the eye are focused anterior to the retina. The vertical bars are focused by the horizontal meridian. Since these bars are clearer than the horizontal bars, they (the vertical bars) are focused closest to the retina. The more blurred horizontal bars are focused by the stronger vertical meridian anterior to the vertical bars. The astigmatism is therefore with-the-rule.

9. (a) The power in the vertical meridian due to the spherical component of the lens is +5.00 D. The power in this meridian due to the cylindrical component is calculated as follows:

$$F_\theta = (F_{cyl})\sin^2\theta$$
$$F_\theta = (-3.00 \text{ D})\sin^2(60)$$
$$F_\theta = -2.25 \text{ D}$$

The total power in the vertical meridian is +2.75 D [i.e., (+5.00 D) + (−2.25 D) = +2.75 D].

(b) The spherical component of the lens contributes +4.50 D in the horizontal meridian. The cylindrical component contributes

$$F_\theta = (F_{cyl})\sin^2\theta$$
$$F_\theta = (+2.75 \text{ D})\sin^2(110)$$
$$F_\theta = +2.43 \text{ D}$$

The total power in the horizontal meridian is +6.93 D (i.e., 4.50 + 2.43 D = 6.93 D).

10. The spherical equivalent generally provides the best visual acuity.

$$\text{spherical equivalent} = \text{spherical correction} + \frac{\text{cylindrical correction}}{2}$$

$$\text{spherical equivalent} = -4.00 \text{ D} + \frac{-1.50}{2}$$

$$\text{spherical equivalent} = -4.75 \text{ D}$$

CHAPTER 10
Prisms

1. $d_{min} = \alpha(n - 1)$
   $4.69° = 8.00° (n - 1)$
   $n = 1.59$

The material is most likely polycarbonate.

2. $P = (100)\left(\dfrac{x}{y}\right)$

   $P = (100)\left(\dfrac{4.00 \text{ cm}}{500 \text{ cm}}\right)$

   $P = 0.8^{\Delta}$

3. $P = (100)\left(\dfrac{x}{y}\right)$

   $15.00^{\Delta} = (100)\left(\dfrac{2.00 \text{ cm}}{y}\right)$

   $y = 13.3 \text{ cm}$

4. $P = cF$

   $P = (0.50 \text{ cm})(8.00 \text{ D})$

   $P = 4.0^{\Delta}$

   Remember, when using Prentice's rule, c is in centimeters.

5. $P = cF$

   $2.0^{\Delta} = (c)(6.00 \text{ D})$

   $d = 0.33 \text{ cm, or } 3.3 \text{ mm}$

   Remember, when using Prentice's rule, c is in centimeters.

6. $P = cF$

   $P = (0.4 \text{ cm})(3.00 \text{ D})$

   $P = 1.2^{\Delta}$

   Since the optical center is nasal to the pupil and the horizontal meridian has plus power, the prism experienced is 1.2^{Δ} base in. There is no vertical decentration, so there is no vertical prism.

7. The lens is decentered both horizontally and vertically.

   The dioptric power in the horizontal meridian is 2.00 D.

   $P = cF$

   $P = (0.50)(2.00 \text{ D})$

   $P = 1.00^{\Delta}$

   The optical center is temporal to the pupil and horizontal meridian has negative power. Consequently, the prism experienced is 1.0^{Δ} base in.

   The dioptric power in the vertical meridian is 2.00 D.

   $P = cF$

   $P = (0.30)(2.00 \text{ D})$

   $P = 0.60^{\Delta}$

Because the eye is looking through the lower portion of a meridian that has plus power, the patient experiences 0.60$^\Delta$ base up.

8. $(100)(1.00)/{-13.00}$ cm $= -7.69$ D. The prism does not change the vergence of the light rays that are incident upon it.

CHAPTER 11
Depth of Field

1. Since the hyperfocal distance is 200.00 cm, the total depth of field is 1.00 D. If the near point of accommodation is 10.00 cm, the true amplitude of accommodation is 9.50 D (i.e., 10.00 − 0.50 D = 9.50 D).

2. First, we calculate the true amplitude of accommodation. The patient's range of clear vision (at near) corresponds to a dioptric range of 1.00 to 4.00 D. Since the depth of field is 1.00 D, the true amplitude of accommodation is 2.00 D (i.e., 3.00 − 1.00 D = 2.00 D). When looking through the distance prescription, the patient can accommodate 2.00 D. If the depth of field was zero, the patient could not resolve objects nearer than 50.00 cm. The near boundary of the patient's range of clear vision, however, is extended by one-half of the depth of field (i.e., 0.50 D). Therefore, the range of clear vision through the distance portion of the spectacles is from infinity to 40.00 cm (i.e., 2.50 D). [Due to depth of field, when the patient is focused at 50.00 cm (2.00 D) she can see clearly at 40.00 cm (2.50 D).]

3. The far point for an uncorrected 1.00 D myope is at −1.00 D. Due to depth of field, which is centered at a distance of 100.00 cm, the patient can see clearly out to a distance of 0.25 D or 400.00 cm (i.e., 1.00 − 0.75 D = 0.25 D).

4. Through the add, the patient can see clearly out to 50.00 cm. Since the depth of field is 0.50 D, the patient's add has a power of +2.25 D (i.e., 2.00 + 0.25 D = 2.25 D). In other words, when a +2.25 D lens focuses the eye at 44.44 cm, the patient's depth of field allows her to see out to 50.00 cm.

Another approach to solving this problem is to first determine the true amplitude of accommodation. The dioptric range of clear vision is from 2.00 to 5.00 D. Since 0.50 D of this range is due to depth of field, the patient's amplitude of accommodation is 2.50 D. If there were no depth of field, the patient would need an add of 2.50 D to see at 20.00 cm (5.00 − 2.50 D = 2.50 D). Taking into account depth of field, however, we know the power of the patient's add is only 2.25.

5. (a) The true amplitude of accommodation is

$(5.00\ \text{D} - 2.50\ \text{D}) - 0.75\ \text{D} = 1.75\ \text{D}$

(b) Without spectacles, the 4.00 D myopic patient's eyes are focused at 25.00 cm. Combined with accommodation and depth of field, the uncorrected patient has a near point of:

$$4.00 \text{ D} + 1.75 \text{ D} + \left(\frac{0.75}{2 \text{ D}}\right) = 6.13 \text{ D}$$

This corresponds to a linear distance of 16.33 cm.

CHAPTER 12
Magnification and Low Vision Devices

1. (a) $M_{ang} = -\dfrac{F_2}{F_1}$

$M_{ang} = -\dfrac{(+25.00 \text{ D})}{(+10.00 \text{ D})}$

$M_{ang} = -2.5\times$

If the Keplerian telescope contains an erecting element, the magnification is +2.5×.

(b) The focal length of the objective lens is 10.00 cm and the focal length of the eyepiece (ocular) is 4.00 cm. Therefore, the tube length is 14.00 cm (i.e., 10.00 + 4.00 cm = 14.00 cm).

2. (a) We can consider the ocular as consisting of a −5.00 D lens that corrects the patient's ametropia and a −35.00 D lens that contributes to the telescope. The angular magnification of the telescope is

$M_{ang} = -\dfrac{F_2}{F_1}$

$M_{ang} = -\dfrac{(-35.00 \text{ D})}{(+8.00 \text{ D})}$

$M_{ang} = +4.4\times$

(b) Tube length may be calculated as follows:

$M_{ang} = \dfrac{1}{1 - dF_1}$

$4.4 = \dfrac{1}{1 - d(+8.00 \text{ D})}$

$d = 0.097$ m, or 9.7 cm

Alternatively, we can calculate the focal lengths of the objective (100/8.00 D = 12.5 cm) and ocular (100/35.00 D = 2.86 cm) and subtract the ocular focal length from that of the objective.

3. (a) Image formation by the objective:

$$L' = L + F$$

$$\frac{(100)(1.00)}{l'} = \left[\frac{(100)(1.00)}{-100.00 \text{ cm}}\right] + 8.00 \text{ D}$$

$$l' = +14.29 \text{ cm}$$

Since the lenses are separated by 10.00 cm, this image is 4.29 cm to the right of the eyepiece. It serves as a virtual object for this lens.

$$L' = L + F$$

$$L' = \left[\frac{(100)(1.00)}{+4.29 \text{ cm}}\right] + (-40.00 \text{ D})$$

$$L' = -16.69 \text{ D; therefore the eye must accommodate 16.69 D}$$

(b) If the light entering the telescope has zero vergence, then the light leaving it will also have zero vergence. When viewing an object at a distance of 100.00 cm, a +1.00 D lens cap results in light rays of zero vergence entering the telescope.

4. (a) The patient could read the material if it were 3× closer to the eye (6 M/ 2 M = 3×), at a distance of 13.3 cm (40.0 cm/3 = 13.3 cm). This is the equivalent viewing distance. The patient could hold the material 13.3 cm from her eye or at the focal point of a lens that has a power (equivalent viewing power) of about +7.50 D (100/13.3 cm ~ 7.50 D).

(b) Since the reading material is held at the focal point of the magnifying lens, the retinal image size is the same regardless of the distance between the magnifying lens and the eye. The patient can hold the lens at the distance from the eye that she finds most comfortable.

(c) Increased magnification can be obtained if the patient looks through the magnifying lens with her add, *and* the distance between the add and the magnifier is less than the focal length of the magnifying lens.

5. (a) For the patient to read 1 M print, the print must be held 8× closer than the original reading distance of 40.0 cm. The equivalent viewing distance is therefore 5.0 cm (40.0 cm/8 = 5.0 cm), and the magnifying lens power is +20.00 D (100/5.0 cm = 20.0 D).

(b) The effective magnification is calculated as follows:

$$M_{25} = \frac{F}{4}$$

$$M_{25} = \frac{20.0 \text{ D}}{4}$$

$$M_{25} = 5.0\times$$

6. (a) The equivalent viewing distance for a +5.0 D lens is 20.0 cm. Since the telescope has an angular magnification of 2.0×, the reading material can be held twice as far away—at 40.0 cm—and still subtend the same angle. For the light rays that enter the telescope to be parallel, the reading material must be held at the focal point of a lens cap with a power of 2.5 D (i.e., 100/40.0 cm = 2.5 D).

   (b) The reading material should be at the focal point of the lens cap (i.e., at 40.0 cm).

   (c) Telemicroscopes have narrow fields of views, permitting the patient to view only a limited portion of the reading material.

7. Since the distance visual acuity is 20/200, the patient's MAR is 10 arcmin. Based on this MAR, we expect that 10 M print could be read at 1 m. For the patient to read 2 M print, the magnification must be 5×. This means that the effective viewing distance is 20.0 cm (i.e., 100.00 cm/5 = 20.00 cm). If held at the focal point of a +5.00 D lens (i.e., 100.00/ 20.00 cm = 5.00 D), the patient should be able to read the print.

8. (a) The reading distance for a 2.50 D add is 40.0 cm. Looking through the add, the patient can read 4 M print. To read 2 M print, the magnification would need to be 2×.

   (b) The device should rest on the print at a distance of 40.0 cm from the patient.

9. The required magnification is 3× (i.e., 3 M/1 M = 3×), making the equivalent viewing distance 13.33 cm (i.e., 40.00 cm/3 = 13.33 cm).

   The virtual image produced by the stand magnifier's lens is located as follows:

   $$L' = L + F$$

   $$\frac{(100)(1.00)}{l'} = \left[\frac{(100)(1.00)}{-6.00 \text{ cm}}\right] + 10.00 \text{ D}$$

   $$l' = -15.00 \text{ cm}$$

   The lateral magnification is

   $$M_L = \frac{l'}{l}$$

   $$M_L = \frac{-15.00 \text{ cm}}{-6.00 \text{ cm}}$$

   $$M_L = +2.5\times$$

   Because of the lateral magnification, the image can be located 33.33 cm from the eye (i.e., 2.5× farther away than the equivalent viewing distance, or 2.5 × 13.33 cm ~ 33.33 cm). Since the virtual image is located 15.0 cm from the plus lens, the patient's eye must be 18.33 cm (i.e., 33.33 − 15.00 cm = 18.33 cm) from the lens (or closer).

CHAPTER 13
Retinal Image Size

1. $M_{\text{spect}} = \left(\dfrac{1}{1 - dF_v}\right)\left(\dfrac{1}{1 - \left(\frac{t}{n}\right)F_1}\right)$

   $M_{\text{spect}} = \left(\dfrac{1}{1 - (0.012\text{ m})(-6.50\text{ D})}\right)\left(\dfrac{1}{1 - \left[\left(\frac{0.002\text{ m}}{1.586}\right)(+3.00\text{ D})\right]}\right)$

   $M_{\text{spect}} = (0.928)(1.00)$

   $M_{\text{spect}} = 0.928\times$

2. (a) *Right lens*:

   $M_{\text{spect}} = \left(\dfrac{1}{1 - dF_v}\right)\left(\dfrac{1}{1 - \left(\frac{t}{n}\right)F_1}\right)$

   $M_{\text{spect}} = \left(\dfrac{1}{1 - (0.014\text{ m})(-6.00\text{ D})}\right)\left(\dfrac{1}{1 - \left[\left(\frac{0.002\text{ m}}{1.498}\right)(+2.00\text{ D})\right]}\right)$

   $M_{\text{spect}} = (0.923)(1.00)$

   $M_{\text{spect}} = 0.923\times$

   Left lens:

   $M_{\text{spect}} = \left(\dfrac{1}{1 - dF_v}\right)\left(\dfrac{1}{1 - \left(\frac{t}{n}\right)F_1}\right)$

   $M_{\text{spect}} = \left(\dfrac{1}{1 - (0.014\text{ m})(-3.00\text{ D})}\right)\left(\dfrac{1}{1 - \left[\left(\frac{0.002\text{ m}}{1.498}\right)(+2.00\text{ D})\right]}\right)$

   $M_{\text{spect}} = (0.960)(1.00)$

   $M_{\text{spect}} = 0.960\times$

   (b) If the shape factor of the right lens were increased to 1.04× (i.e., 0.960/0.923 = 1.04×), the images in both eyes would be the same size. We calculate the front surface power of the 4.00 mm thick right lens as follows:

$$M_{shape} = \left(\frac{1}{1 - \left(\frac{t}{n}\right)F_1} \right)$$

$$1.04 = \left(\frac{1}{1 - \left[\left(\frac{0.004 \text{ m}}{1.498}\right)(F_1)\right]} \right)$$

$$F_1 = +14.40 \text{ D}$$

(c) Although this lens may correct for the aniseikonia, its steep front curve and thickness would make it cosmetically unacceptable.

CHAPTER 14
Reflection

1. (a) $F = \frac{-2}{r}$

$$F = \frac{-2}{-0.30 \text{ m}}$$

$$F = +6.67 \text{ D}$$

$$L' = L + F$$

$$L' = \left[\frac{(100)(1.00)}{-5.00 \text{ cm}} \right] + 6.67 \text{ D}$$

$$L' = -13.33 \text{ D}$$

$$L' = \frac{-1}{l'}$$

$$-13.33 \text{ D} = \frac{-(100)(1.00)}{l'}$$

$$l' = +7.51 \text{ cm}$$

(b) Since the image vergence is negative, the image is formed by diverging light rays and is virtual.

(c) $M = \frac{-l'}{l}$

$$M = \frac{-(+7.51 \text{ cm})}{-5.00 \text{ cm}}$$

$$M = +1.50\times$$

$$(+1.50)(+2.00 \text{ cm}) = +3.00 \text{ cm}$$

Alternatively, we could use vergence to calculate the magnification as follows:

$$M = \frac{L}{L'}$$

$$M = \frac{-20.00 \text{ D}}{-13.33 \text{ D}}$$

$$M = +1.50\times$$

$$(+1.50)(+2.00 \text{ cm}) = +3.00 \text{ cm}$$

The image is erect.

2. (a) $L' = L + F$

$$L' = \left[\frac{(100)(1.00)}{-20.00 \text{ cm}}\right] + 6.67 \text{ D}$$

$$L' = +1.67 \text{ D}$$

$$L' = \frac{-1}{l'}$$

$$+1.67 \text{ D} = \frac{-(100)(1.00)}{l'}$$

$$l' = -59.88 \text{ cm}$$

(b) Since the image vergence is positive, the image is formed by converging light rays and is real.

(c) $M = \frac{-l'}{l}$

$$M = \frac{-(-59.88 \text{ cm})}{-20.00 \text{ cm}}$$

$$M = -3.00\times$$

$$(-3.00)(+2.00 \text{ cm}) = -6.00 \text{ cm}$$

The image is inverted.

3. (a) $F = \frac{-1}{f'}$

$$F = \frac{-1}{+0.15 \text{ m}}$$

$$F = -6.67 \text{ D}$$

$$L' = L + F$$

$$L' = \left[\frac{(100)(1.00)}{-25.00 \text{ cm}}\right] + (-6.67 \text{ D})$$

$$L' = -10.67 \text{ D}$$

$$L' = \frac{-1}{l'}$$

$$-10.67 \text{ D} = \frac{-(100)(1.00)}{l'}$$

$$l' = +9.37 \text{ cm}$$

(b) Since the image vergence is negative, the image is formed by diverging light rays and is virtual.

(c) $M = \frac{-l'}{l}$

$$M = \frac{-(+9.37 \text{ cm})}{-25.00 \text{ cm}}$$

$$M = +0.37\times$$

$$(+0.037)(+2.00 \text{ cm}) = +0.74 \text{ cm}$$

The image is erect.

4. Since the image is real and 40.00 cm from the mirror, the image vergence is +2.50 D.

$$L' = L + F$$

$$+2.50 \text{ D} = L + 30.00 \text{ D}$$

$$L = -27.50 \text{ D}$$

$$L = \frac{1}{l}$$

$$-27.50 \text{ D} = \frac{(100)(1.00)}{l}$$

$$l = -3.64 \text{ cm}$$

Since the object vergence is negative, the object is real. It is located 3.64 cm to the left of the mirror.

5. Since the image is virtual and 10.00 cm from the mirror, the image vergence is −10.00 D.

$$L' = L + F$$

$$-10.00 \text{ D} = L + -30.00 \text{ D}$$

$$L = +20.00 \text{ D}$$

$$L = \frac{1}{l}$$

$$+20.00 \text{ D} = \frac{(100)(1.00)}{l}$$

$$l = +5.00 \text{ cm}$$

Since the object vergence is positive, the object is virtual (i.e., a virtual object). It is located 5.00 cm to the right of the mirror.

6. The light rays that emerge from the source are first refracted by the lens, then reflected by the mirror, and once again refracted by the lens.

Refraction at lens:

$$L' = L + F$$

$$L' = \left[\frac{(100)(1.00)}{-20.00 \text{ cm}} \right] + 15.00 \text{ D}$$

$$L' = +10.00 \text{ D}$$

$$L' = \frac{1}{l'}$$

$$+10.00 \text{ D} = \frac{(100)(1.00)}{l'}$$

$$l' = +10.00 \text{ cm}$$

This image is located 7.00 cm to the right of the mirror (i.e., 10.00 − 3.00 cm = 7.00 cm). It serves as a virtual object for the convex mirror:

$$L' = L + F$$

$$L' = L + \left(\frac{-2}{r} \right)$$

$$L' = \left(\frac{1.00}{+0.07 \text{ m}} \right) + \left(\frac{-2}{+0.02 \text{ m}} \right)$$

$$L' = 14.29 \text{ D} + (-100.00 \text{ D})$$

$$L' = -85.71 \text{ D}$$

$$L' = \frac{-1}{l'}$$

$$-85.71 \text{ D} = \frac{-(100)(1.00)}{l'}$$

$$l' = +1.17 \text{ cm}$$

The virtual image (formed by diverging rays) is located 1.17 cm to the right of the mirror and 4.14 cm to the right of the lens (1.17 + 3.00 cm = 4.17 cm). This image serves as a real object for the lens. (The light rays incident on the mirror are reflected back through the lens.) Since the reflected light rays travel from right to left, we cannot use our linear sign convention. Rather, we use absolute values.

$$L = \left| \frac{1}{l} \right|$$

$$L = \left| \frac{100}{4.17 \text{ cm}} \right|$$

Since we know that the light rays are diverging, they have negative vergence
$L = -23.98$ D

Substituting into the vergence equation, we have
$L' = L + F$
$L' = -23.93$ D $+ 15.00$ D
$L' = -8.98$ D

This virtual image must be located on the same side of the lens as the object. It is located 11.13 cm to the *right* of the lens. (We didn't use our linear sign convention to determine the image location because the light rays are traveling from right to left.)

Alternatively, we can construct an equivalent mirror and use this mirror to determine the image distance. This approach is discussed in Appendix B.

7. $P = \dfrac{-2}{r}$

$P = \dfrac{-2}{+0.0078 \text{ m}}$

$P = -256.41$ D

$L' = L + F$

$L' = \left[\dfrac{(100)(1.00)}{-10.00 \text{ cm}} \right] + (-256.41 \text{ D})$

$L' = -266.41$ D

$L' = \dfrac{-1}{l'}$

$-266.41 \text{ D} = \dfrac{-(1.00)(1000)}{l'}$

$l' = +3.75$ mm

Purkinje image I is located 3.75 mm to the right of the cornea. (Recall that in Chapter 14 we determined that when the object is at infinity, Purkinje image I is located 3.90 mm to the right of the cornea.)

8. Relative to the vertical meridian, the horizontal meridian of the cornea minifies the image. Therefore the horizontal meridian is stronger and the patient has against-the-rule corneal toricity.

9. $R = \left[\dfrac{(n' - n)}{(n' + n)} \right]^2$

(a) $R = \left[\dfrac{(1.74 - 1.00)}{(1.74 + 1.00)} \right]^2$

$R = 0.073$

Percentage reflected is 7.3%.

(b) $R = \left[\dfrac{(1.498 - 1.000)}{(1.498 + 1.000)}\right]^2$

$R = 0.04$

Percentage reflected is 4.0%.

(c) The higher index lens because more light is reflected by its surface.

(d) $n_c = \sqrt{n_L}$

$n_c = \sqrt{1.74}$

$n_c = 1.32$

CHAPTER 15
Aberrations

1. (a) Due to positive spherical aberration, the subject will see two point images.

   (b) When the subject occludes the top hole, the upper image disappears. The rays entering the top hole are focused on the inferior portion of the retina and are seen as the upper image.

2. No, because Seidel aberrations are present in spherical optical systems.

3. (a) If we ignore the thickness of the lens, we can assume that both the front and back surfaces of the lens have a power of +2.50 DS. The radius of curvature for the front surface is

   $F = \dfrac{(n' - n)}{r}$

   $F + 2.50 \, \text{DS} = \dfrac{(1.50 - 1.00)}{r}$

   $r = +0.20 \, \text{m} \quad \text{or} \quad +20.00 \, \text{cm}$

   Therefore $r_1 = +20.00$ cm and $r_2 = -20.00$ cm.

   $\sigma = \dfrac{(r_2 + r_1)}{(r_2 - r_1)}$

   $\sigma = \dfrac{(-20.00 \, \text{cm} + 20.00 \, \text{cm})}{(-20.00 \, \text{cm} - 20.00 \, \text{cm})}$

   $\sigma = 0$

   (b) Approximately plano-convex.

   (c) The front surface should be convex and the back (ocular) surface should be plano.

(d) With a plus front surface and plano back surface, the bending factor will always be -1.0. For example, if the front surface has a radius of $+10.00$ cm, then

$$\sigma = \frac{(r_2 + r_1)}{(r_2 - r_1)}$$

$$\sigma = \frac{(0.00 \text{ cm} + 10.00 \text{ cm})}{(0.00 \text{ cm} - 10.00 \text{ cm})}$$

$$\sigma = -1.00$$

4. $F_{@090} = F\left(1 + \dfrac{\sin^2\theta}{2n}\right)$

$F_{@090} = +4.00 \text{ D}\left(1 + \dfrac{\sin^2(25)}{2(1.586)}\right)$

$F_{@090} = +4.23 \text{ D}$

Induced cylinder (axis 090) $= F(\tan^2\theta)$

Induced cylinder (axis 090) $= (+4.00 \text{ D}) [\tan^2(25)]$

Induced cylinder (axis 090) $= +0.87 \text{ D}$

The power experienced by the patient when wearing a $+4.00$ DS polycarbonate lens with a 25-degree face-form angle is $+4.23 + 0.87 \times 090$.

5. $F_{@180} = F\left(1 + \dfrac{\sin^2\theta}{2n}\right)$

$F_{@180} = -8.00 \text{ D}\left(1 + \dfrac{\sin^2(15)}{2(1.586)}\right)$

$F_{@180} = -8.17 \text{ D}$

Induced cylinder (axis 180) $= F(\tan^2\theta)$

Induced cylinder (axis 180) $= (-8.00 \text{ D}) [\tan^2(15)]$

Induced cylinder (axis 0180) $= -0.57 \text{ D}$

The power experienced by the patient when wearing a -8.00 DS polycarbonate lens with a 15-degree pantoscopic tilt is $-8.17 - 0.57 \times 180$.

Appendix A: Entrance and Exit Pupils of Telescopes

In Chapter 12, we learned that an optical system's **entrance pupil** limits the amount of light *entering* the system. The entrance pupil can be a real aperture or an image of one. For a Galilean telescope, there are two possibilities: the objective lens or the image of the eyepiece as seen when looking through the objective. Let's do some calculations to determine which it is.

The first step is to locate the image of the eyepiece as seen through the objective and to determine its size. Figure A-1A shows a Galilean telescope viewed from the objective lens side of the telescope. We'll assume that both the objective and eyepiece have a diameter of 1.5 cm. Since the objective has a power of +10.00 D and eyepiece a power of −25.00 D, when focused for infinity the tube length is 6.0 cm. We can use the vergence relationship to locate the image of the eyepiece as seen through the objective as follows:

$$L' = L + F$$

$$L' = \left(\frac{100}{-6.00 \text{ cm}}\right) + 10.00 \text{ D} = -6.67 \text{ D}$$

$$l' = \frac{n}{L'}$$

$$l' = \frac{100}{-6.67 \text{ D}} = -15.00 \text{ cm}$$

The objective forms a virtual image of the eyepiece that is located 15.00 cm to the left of the objective. What is the size of this image? We calculate magnification as follows:

$$M = \frac{l'}{l}$$

$$M = \frac{-15.00 \text{ cm}}{-6.00 \text{ cm}} = 2.50\times$$

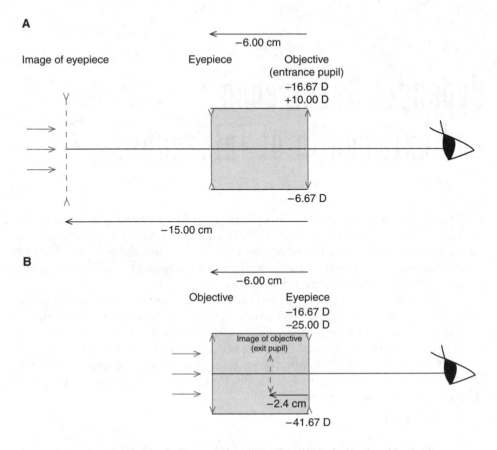

A

−6.00 cm

Image of eyepiece   Eyepiece   Objective
(entrance pupil)
−16.67 D
+10.00 D

−6.67 D

−15.00 cm

B

−6.00 cm

Objective   Eyepiece
−16.67 D
−25.00 D

Image of objective
(exit pupil)

−2.4 cm

−41.67 D

Figure A-1. A. When a Galilean telescope is viewed while facing the objective lens, the observer will see both the objective lens and a virtual image of the eyepiece. Since the objective subtends a smaller angle at the observer's eye, it is the entrance pupil. The three light rays remind us that light is traveling from left to right. **B.** When the same Galilean telescope is viewed while facing the eyepiece, the observer sees the eyepiece and a virtual image of the objective that's within the telescope tube. The image of the objective subtends a smaller angle at the observer's eye, making it the exit pupil.

Since the diameter of the eyepiece is 1.5 cm, the size of its image is

$$(2.50)(1.5 \text{ cm}) = 3.75 \text{ cm}$$

When the telescope is viewed facing the objective lens, does the image of the eyepiece or the objective itself subtend the smallest angle? Let's pick an arbitrary viewing distance of 1.00 m. At this distance, the angle subtended by the objective can be calculated as follows:

$$\tan\theta = \frac{1.5 \text{ cm}}{100 \text{ cm}}$$

$$\theta = 0.9 \text{ degrees}$$

Now, we need to compare this to the angle subtended by the image of the eyepiece, which is

$$\tan\theta = \frac{3.75 \text{ cm}}{115 \text{ cm}}$$

$$\tan\theta = 1.9 \text{ degrees}$$

These calculations tell us that the element subtending the smallest angle when looking at the objective side of the telescope is the objective lens. As we learned in Chapter 12, the objective lens is typically the telescope's entrance pupil.

Next, let's tackle the **exit pupil** of a Galilean telescope, which limits the amount of light *exiting* the system. For these calculations, we view the telescope from the eyepiece side, as illustrated in Figure A-1B. Notice that there are two candidates for the exit pupil: the eyepiece and the image of the objective as seen through the eyepiece. We can locate the objective's image as follows:

$$L' = L + F$$

$$L' = \left(\frac{100}{-6.00 \text{ cm}}\right) + (-25.00 \text{ D}) = -41.67 \text{ D}$$

$$l' = \frac{n}{L'}$$

$$l' = \frac{100}{-41.67 \text{ D}} = -2.4 \text{ cm}$$

To calculate the size of this virtual image, we first calculate the magnification

$$M = \frac{l'}{l}$$

$$M = \frac{-2.4 \text{ cm}}{-6.00 \text{ cm}} = 0.4\times$$

The diameter of the image of the objective is

$$(0.4)(1.5 \text{ cm}) = 0.6 \text{ cm}$$

Since the image of the objective (a virtual image located within the tube) is smaller and farther away than the eyepiece when viewed at a distance of, say, 1.00 m, it must subtend a smaller angle. It serves as the exit pupil for the system.

We can determine the entrance and exit pupils for a Keplerian telescope in much the same way we determined them for a Galilean telescope. Figure A-2A shows a Keplerian telescope viewed from the objective side. The objective and eyepiece

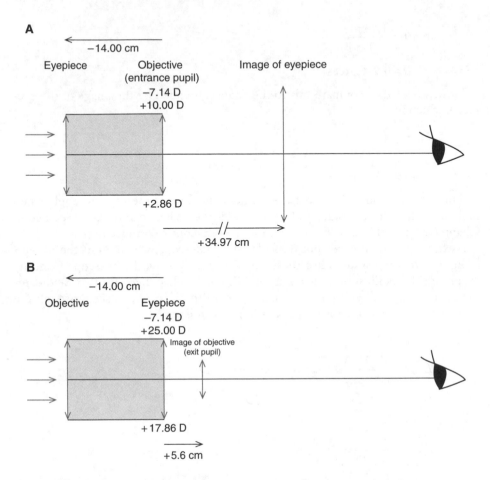

A

−14.00 cm

Eyepiece   Objective   Image of eyepiece
                 (entrance pupil)
                    −7.14 D
                    +10.00 D

                    +2.86 D

                    +34.97 cm

B

−14.00 cm

Objective   Eyepiece
                   −7.14 D
                   +25.00 D
                          Image of objective
                          (exit pupil)

                   +17.86 D

                   +5.6 cm

Figure A-2. A. When a Keplerian telescope is viewed while facing the objective lens, the observer will see both the objective lens and a real image of the eyepiece. Since the objective subtends a smaller angle at the observer's eye, it is the entrance pupil. The three light rays remind us that light is traveling from left to right. **B.** When the same Keplerian telescope is viewed while facing the eyepiece, the observer sees the eyepiece and a real image of the objective that's just outside the telescope tube. The image of the objective subtends a smaller angle at the observer's eye, making it the exit pupil.

powers are, respectively, +10.00 D and +25.00 D and the tube length is 14.00 cm. The entrance pupil is either the objective or the image of the eyepiece as viewed through the objective. The location of this image is

$$L' = L + F$$

$$L' = \left(\frac{100}{-14.00 \text{ cm}} \right) + 10.00 \text{ D} = +2.86 \text{ D}$$

$$l' = \frac{n}{L'}$$

$$l' = \frac{100}{+2.86 \text{ D}} = +34.97 \text{ cm}$$

The image is real and 34.97 cm to the right of the objective. Its magnification and size are

$$M = \frac{l'}{l}$$

$$M = \frac{+34.97 \text{ cm}}{-14.00 \text{ cm}} = -2.5\times$$

$$(-2.5)(1.5 \text{ cm}) = -6.00 \text{ cm}$$

When viewing from the objective side, the objective lens is both smaller and farther away than the image of the eyepiece. Therefore, it subtends a smaller angle and is the entrance pupil.

To determine the exit pupil, we view the telescope from the eyepiece side. As we can see in Figure A-2B, the exit pupil is either the eyepiece or the image of the objective as seen through the eyepiece. The location of this image is

$$L' = L + F$$

$$L' = \left(\frac{100}{-14.00 \text{ cm}}\right) + 25.00 \text{ D} = +17.86 \text{ D}$$

$$l' = \frac{n}{L'}$$

$$l' = \frac{100}{+17.86 \text{ D}} = +5.6 \text{ cm}$$

The image is real and 5.6 cm to the right of the eyepiece. Its magnification and size are

$$M = \frac{l'}{l}$$

$$M = \frac{+5.6 \text{ cm}}{-14.00 \text{ cm}} = -0.4\times$$

$$(-0.4)(1.5 \text{ cm}) = -0.6 \text{ cm}$$

From an arbitrary distance of 1.00 m, the angles subtended by the eyepiece and image of the objective are, respectively,

$$\tan\theta = \frac{1.5 \text{ cm}}{100 \text{ cm}}$$

$$\theta = 0.9 \text{ degrees}$$

and

$$\tan\theta = \frac{0.6 \text{ cm}}{94.4 \text{ cm}}$$

$$\theta = 0.4 \text{ degrees}$$

The image of the objective subtends the smaller angle making it the exit pupil.

Appendix B: Location of Purkinje Image III

Purkinje image III is formed by reflection off the anterior surface of the crystalline lens. Locating this image is a bit complicated because it is formed by rays that are first refracted by the cornea, then reflected off the anterior surface of the crystalline lens, and then refracted once again by the cornea (Fig. B-1). We can simplify the calculations by treating the combined refracting surface and mirror as a single system that we call an **equivalent mirror**.

An equivalent mirror consists of the images of a reflecting surface and its center of curvature as viewed through the *refracting* elements of the system. Purkinje image III is formed by the equivalent mirror that is constituted of the anterior surface of the crystalline lens and its center of curvature *as viewed through the cornea*. To construct this equivalent mirror, we consider the anterior surface of the lens and its center of curvature as objects and the cornea as a refracting element.[1] In Figure B-2A, we've drawn the eye so that the lens is to the left of the cornea. This allows us to use our linear sign convention.

The first step is to calculate the refracting power of the cornea[2]

$$F = \frac{n' - n}{r}$$

$$F = \frac{1.333 - 1.000}{0.0078 \text{ m}}$$

$$F = +42.69 \text{ D}$$

---

1. The cornea both refracts and reflects light. We are now treating it as a refracting element.
2. To determine the refracting power of the cornea, we use 7.80 mm. We do not use the radius of curvature for the reduced eye because this would give us the total refracting power of the eye, combining the powers of both the cornea and unaccommodated lens.

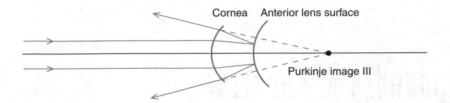

Figure B-1. Purkinje image III is formed by light rays reflected off the anterior crystalline lens surface. In this diagram, light rays originating at infinity are first refracted by the cornea, then reflected off the lens surface and again refracted by the cornea as they leave the eye.

As can be seen in Figure B-2A, the distance from the cornea to the anterior lens surface (the object) is −3.6 mm. The object is located in aqueous, and its vergence is

$$L = \frac{n}{l}$$

$$L = \frac{1.333}{-0.0036 \text{ m}}$$

$$L = -370.28 \text{ D}$$

The vergence relationship is used to locate the image:

$$L' = L + F$$

$$L' = -370.28 \text{ D} + 42.69 \text{ D}$$

$$L' = -327.59 \text{ D}$$

The negative vergence tells us that the image is virtual; a virtual image is located on the same side of the refracting element as the object. Since the rays that form the image are located in air, the image distance is

$$L' = \frac{n'}{l'}$$

or

$$l' = \frac{n'}{L'}$$

$$l' = \frac{(1000)(1.00)}{-327.59 \text{ D}}$$

$$l' = -3.05 \text{ mm}$$

A

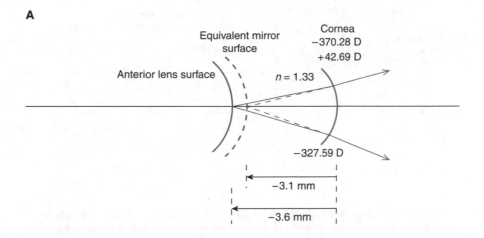

B

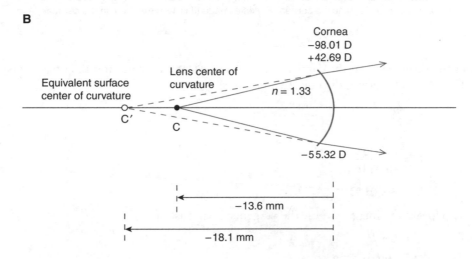

Figure B-2. A. When viewed through the cornea, the anterior lens surface appears to be located 3.1 mm behind the cornea. This image is the surface of the equivalent mirror. This diagram is drawn with the object (lens surface) to the left of the refracting surface (cornea) so that we can use our linear sign convention. As in previous diagrams in this text, object vergence and refracting power are given above the surface and image vergence below. **B.** The anterior lens surface center of curvature is located 13.6 mm to the left of the cornea. After refraction by the cornea, its virtual image is located 18.1 mm to the left of the cornea.

The surface of the equivalent mirror is about 3.1 mm to the left of the cornea.

Next we locate the center of curvature of the equivalent mirror. As can be seen in Figure B-2B, we treat the center of curvature of the crystalline lens anterior surface as the object and the cornea as the refracting element. We haven't discussed this,

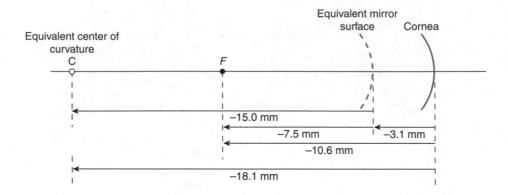

Figure B-3. The corneal surface and equivalent mirror's surface, center of curvature, and focal point are shown. The focal length of the equivalent mirror (7.5 mm) is equal to half of its radius of curvature (15.0 mm). Since the equivalent mirror surface is located 3.1 mm behind the cornea, Purkinje image III is 10.6 mm behind the cornea.

but the distance from the cornea to the anterior lens surface center of curvature is −13.6 mm. Therefore, the object vergence is

$$L = \frac{n}{l}$$

$$L = \frac{1.333}{-0.0136 \text{ m}}$$

$$L = -98.01 \text{ D}$$

To locate the image, we use the vergence relationship

$$L' = L + F$$

$$L' = -98.01 + 42.69 \text{ D}$$

$$L' = -55.32 \text{ D}$$

This negative image vergence tells us that the image is virtual and located on the same side of the cornea as the object. The refracted rays that form the image are located in air:

$$l' = \frac{n'}{L'}$$

$$l' = \frac{(1000)(1.00)}{-55.32 \text{ D}}$$

$$l' = -18.08 \text{ mm}$$

The center of curvature of the equivalent lens is located about 18.1 mm to the left of the corneal surface.

In Figure B-3, we've redrawn the equivalent mirror showing its surface, center of curvature, and focal point. As a reference, we've also included the cornea. We can see that the center of curvature of the equivalent mirror is 15.0 mm to the left of its surface (18.1 – 3.1 mm = 15.0 mm). Therefore the radius of curvature of the equivalent mirror is –15.0 mm. The focal length of the equivalent mirror is –7.5 mm (half of the radius of curvature).[3]

The equivalent mirror can be considered to have the properties of a typical mirror. If the object is located at infinity, the image is located at the focal point of the equivalent mirror, which is 7.5 mm behind the surface of the equivalent mirror. Since the surface of the equivalent mirror is 3.1 behind the corneal surface, the image—Purkinje image III—is 10.6 mm behind the actual corneal surface.

---

3. In deriving the equivalent mirror, it is necessary to first locate the images of the reflecting surface and center of curvature and then to calculate the focal length. *The equivalent focal point cannot be directly determined by locating the image of a surface's focal point.*

Appendix C: Fluid Lenses

The **base curve** of a contact lens is the radius of curvature of its back surface. This value is often converted to diopters using a refractive index of 1.3375, the same index used by the keratometer to convert the corneal surface radius to a dioptric value.

Consider a rigid contact lens with a base curve of 42.00 D that sits on a non-astigmatic cornea. The keratometry readings (often referred to as K readings) are

43.00/090

43.00/180

The patient's prescription when measured at the corneal plane is −3.00 DS. If the power of the contact lens is −2.00 DS, will it correct the patient's ametropia?

The base curve of the contact lens is flatter than the cornea, creating a **fluid lens** composed of tears, which have an index of refraction of about 1.3375. Figure C-1A shows that the front surface of this fluid lens has the same curvature as the contact lens's base curve. Consequently, the front surface of the fluid lens has a power of +42.00 DS. The fluid lens's back surface has the same curvature as the cornea, giving it a power of −43.00 DS. Adding together the front and back surface powers reveals that the fluid lens has a total power of −1.00 DS. The combination of the −2.00 DS contact lens and the −1.00 DS fluid lens fully corrects the 3.00 D of myopia.[1]

What power contact lens is required to correct this patient's myopia if the contact lens has a base curve of 44.00 D?

---

1. These calculations assume the contact lens and fluid lens are in air. In actuality, they are in contact with each other. As demonstrated in Appendix F, when the back surface of the first lens has the same radius as the front surface of the second lens, the combined power of two lenses in air is the same as when they are joined together.

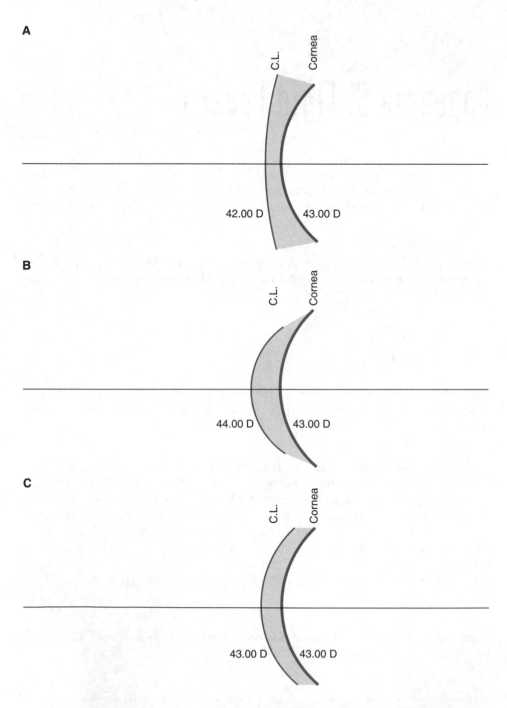

Figure C-1. Fluid lenses formed by rigid contact lenses (CL). **A.** The CL (42.00 D) is flatter than the cornea (43.00 D), creating a –1.00 DS fluid lens. **B.** The CL (44.00 D) is steeper than the cornea (43.00 D), creating a +1.00 DS fluid lens. **C.** The CL (43.00 D) is the same curvature as the cornea (43.00 D), creating a fluid lens of zero power.

Figure C-1B shows that the fluid lens has a power of +1.00 DS. Therefore, to correct the myopia, the contact lens must have a power of −4.00 DS.[2]

What power would be required to correct the myopia if the contact lens has a base curve of 43.00 D?

Since the front and back surfaces of the fluid lens have the same curvature, the fluid lens has no power (Fig. C-1C). Consequently, a −3.00 DS contact lens is required.

Let's consider another example. A patient's eye has the following K readings and refraction as determined in the corneal plane:

44.00/090

43.00/180

−5.00 − 1.00 × 180

Using the terminology of Chapter 9, diagnose the patient's refractive error. If a rigid contact lens with a base curve of 43.00 D is fitted to this cornea, what power is required to correct the patient's ametropia?

The first step, as illustrated in Figure C-2A, is to draw crosses that show the prescription (i.e., the required correction) and patient's corneal powers (i.e., K readings). The former illustrates that both meridians of the eye are myopic and that the vertical meridian is more powerful than the horizontal meridian. The patient has compound myopic with-the-rule astigmatism. The K readings tell us that the cornea is the source of the astigmatism (rather than the crystalline lens). A cornea that has cylindrical power is said to be **toric**.

For a base curve of 43.00 D, what is the power of the fluid lens? From Figure C-2B, we see that fluid lens has a power of −1.00 D in its vertical meridian and no power in its horizontal meridian. Therefore, a −5.00 DS contact lens in combination with the fluid lens will fully correct the refractive error.

If the contact lens has a base curve of 44.00 D, what power is required to correct the ametropia?

---

2. The mnemonic **SAM FAP**, meaning if the lens is **s**teep to **a**dd **m**inus to its power and if **f**lat to **a**dd **p**lus to its power, is handy to memorize.

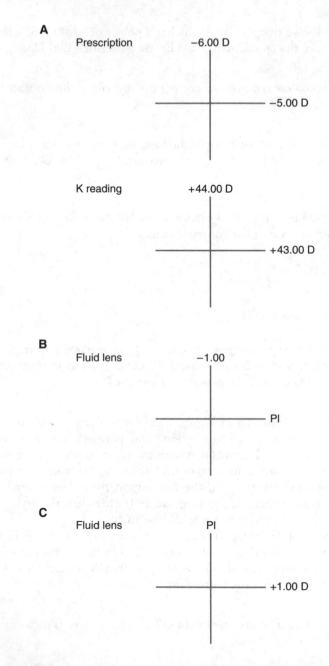

Figure C-2. A. The prescription and corneal power discussed in the text. **B.** Fluid lens when this cornea is fit with a contact lens that has a base curve of 43.00 D. **C.** Fluid lens when this cornea is fit with a contact lens that has a base curve of 44.00 D.

As we can see in Figure C-2C, the fluid lens has powers of zero in the vertical meridian and +1.00 D in the horizontal meridian. Consequently, a −6.00 DS contact lens will correct the ametropia. (A −6.00 DS contact lens combined with a pl + 1.00 × 090 fluid lens results in a correction of −6.00 +1.00 × 090. Transposing this into minus cylinder form, we have −5.00 −1.00 × 180.)

There is much more to learn about the optics of contact lenses. A more detailed and comprehensive discussion of this topic can be found in *Mandell RB. Contact Lens Practice, 4th ed. Springfield, IL: Thomas, 1988.*

Appendix D: Javal's Rule

The cornea and crystalline lens are the primary sources of ocular astigmatism. Corneal toricity can be measured directly with a keratometer or corneal topographer. When the keratometry readings are known, the total amount of ocular astigmatism, as measured in the spectacle plane, can be estimated using Javal's rule:

Est. ocular astig = (corneal astigmatism)(1.25) + (−0.50 × 090)

where Est. ocular astig is the estimated ocular astigmatism in the spectacle plane and corneal astigmatism is the *correction* for corneal toricity in minus cylinder form (as measured in the corneal plane).

What is the rationale for this rule? Corneal astigmatism is multiplied by 1.25 to correct for lens effectivity (Chapter 7). In addition, Javal's rule assumes that the average crystalline lens has a small degree of against-the-rule astigmatism that is correctable with a spectacle lens power of pl − 0.50 × 090.

Let's look at an example. *A patient's K's are as follows:*

> 44.00/090
>
> 43.00/180

Based on Javal's rule, what is the estimated ocular astigmatism in the spectacle plane?

Figure D-1A shows the corneal powers on a lens cross. The required cylindrical correction is also given (in minus cylinder form). While the cornea has 1.00 D of with-the rule-astigmatism, this is partially mitigated by the presumed against-the-rule lenticular astigmatism, resulting in a predicted with-the-rule *ocular* astigmatism of −0.75 D.

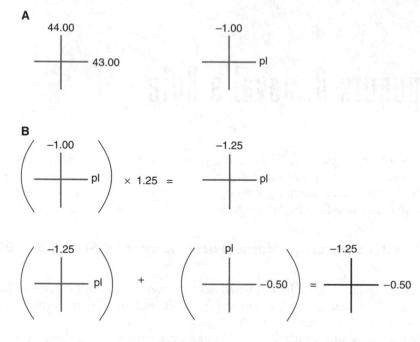

Figure D-1. A. K readings and the required cylindrical correction for the example discussed in the text. **B.** Application of Javal's rule to estimate the amount of ocular astgmatism.

Clinically, Javal's rule is of limited utility because the amount of lenticular astigmatism varies from patient to patient. Although Javal's rule cannot accurately predict the ocular astigmatism for an individual patient, it does reinforce the important point that lenticular astigmatism is often against-the-rule. The amount of against-the-rule astigmatism tends to increase with age due to changes in the crystalline lens.

Appendix E: Derivation of the Paraxial Relationship

Figure E-1 shows a light ray incident upon a spherical refracting surface. According to Snell's law,

$$n \sin\theta = n' \sin\theta'$$

For paraxial rays,[1] we can make the assumption that $\sin\theta = \theta$ (where θ is in radians). Snell's law is then rewritten as

$$n\theta = n'\theta$$

From Figure E-1, we see that

$$\theta = \alpha + \beta$$

and

$$\beta = \theta' + \delta$$

or

$$\theta' = \beta - \delta$$

Substituting into Snell's law, we have

$$n(\alpha + \beta) = n'(\beta - \delta)$$

or

$$n'\delta = -n\alpha + \beta(n' - n)$$

But from Figure E-1, we see that (assuming small angles)

$$\alpha = \frac{b}{-l}$$

$$\beta = \frac{b}{r}$$

---

1. Paraxial rays are close to the optical axis and incident on the central area of the lens; they make sufficiently small angles with the normal that we can assume $\sin\theta = \theta$ (in radians).

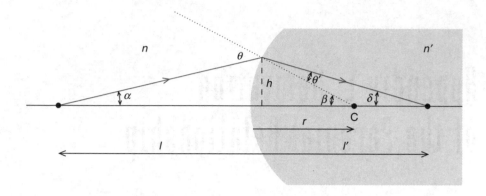

Figure E-1. Assuming small angles, Snell's law can be used to derive the paraxial relationship.

and

$$\delta = \frac{h}{l'}$$

By substitution, we have the paraxial equation

$$\frac{n'}{l'} = \frac{n}{l} + \frac{n' - n}{r}$$

or

$$L' = L + F$$

Appendix F: Correction of Chromatic Aberration

LONGITUDINAL CHROMATIC ABERRATION

While we're usually not concerned with the longitudinal chromatic aberration produced by spectacle lenses, this aberration can be an important consideration in the design of certain optical systems. To minimize longitudinal chromatic aberration, we can combine a lens of a given refractive index with a lens of another index to form an **achromatic doublet**. The component lenses of the doublet are in contact with each other. As illustrated in Figure F-1, one lens has a positive refractive power and the other a negative refractive power. The formulae used to calculate the powers of the component lenses are given below:

$$\frac{F_{Lens1}}{v_{Lens1}} = -\frac{F_{Lens2}}{v_{Lens2}}$$

$$F_{Ach} = F_{Lens1} + F_{Lens2}$$

where F_{Lens1} is the power of the first lens in air, F_{Lens2} is the power of the second lens in air, v_{Lens1} is the constringence of the first lens,[1] v_{Lens2} is the constringence of the second lens, and F_{Ach} is the total power of the achromatic doublet.

Let's apply these formulae. *Using a plus crown glass lens with a constringence of 59.0 and a minus flint glass lens (n = 1.62) with a constringence of 37.0, design a +6.00 D achromatic doublet that minimizes longitudinal chromatic aberration. Specifically, what are the powers of the component lenses?*

---

1. Recall from Chapter 15 that the terms constringence and Abbe value are interchangeable.

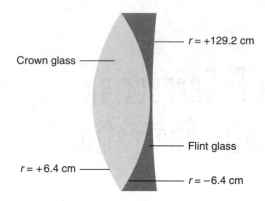

Figure F-1. An achromatic doublet formed by cementing a biconvex crown glass lens to a minus flint glass lens. Radii of curvature are given for the surfaces.

Substituting, we have

$$\frac{F_{Lens1}}{v_{Lens1}} = -\frac{F_{Lens2}}{v_{Lens2}}$$

$$\frac{F_{Lens1}}{59} = -\frac{F_{Lens2}}{37}$$

$$F_{Lens1} = (-1.59)(F_{Lens2})$$

and

$$F_{Ach} = F_{Lens1} + F_{Lens2}$$

$$+6.00\ D = F_{Lens1} + F_{Lens2}$$

Therefore

$$+6.00\ D = -(1.59)(F_{Lens2}) + F_{Lens2}$$

$$F_{Lens2} = -10.17\ D$$

and

$$+6.00\ D = (F_{Lens1}) + (-10.17\ D)$$

$$F_{Lens1} = +16.17\ D$$

These calculations tell us that the power of the crown glass lens in air is +16.17 D and the power of the flint glass lens in air is –10.17 D. To create an achromatic doublet with a combined power of +6.00 D, these two lenses are cemented together.

Assume that the plus crown glass lens is equiconvex. What are the radii of curvature of the four lens surfaces?

Both surfaces of the equiconvex lens have the same power, +8.08 DS. For the front surface,

$$F = \frac{n' - n}{r}$$

$$+8.08 \text{ D} = \frac{1.52 - 1.00}{r}$$

$$r = +0.064 \text{ m}$$

The radius of curvature for the front surface of this equiconvex lens is +6.4 cm and for the back surface, –6.4 cm. From Figure F-1, we see that the front surface of the flint glass lens has the same curvature as the back surface of the crown glass lens. The power of the front surface of the flint glass lens in air is

$$F = \frac{n' - n}{r}$$

$$F = \frac{1.62 - 1.00}{-0.064 \text{ m}}$$

$$F = -9.69 \text{ D}$$

Since the total power of the flint glass lens is –10.17 D, the power of its back surface is –0.48 D. Its radius of curvature is

$$F = \frac{n' - n}{r}$$

$$-0.48 \text{ D} = \frac{1.00 - 1.62}{r}$$

$$r = +1.29 \text{ m}$$

The radii of curvature of all four surfaces of the +6.00 D achromatic doublet are given in Figure F-1.

Although the calculations give the powers of the lenses in air, these lenses are fused to each other. To convince ourselves that the fused doublet has a total power of +6.00 D, let's add together the powers of the three interfaces. For the first interface (air/crown glass) the power is +8.08 D; for the third interface (flint glass/air), the power is –0.48 D. To complete this calculation, we must determine the power at the crown glass/flint glass interface as follows:

$$F = \frac{n' - n}{r}$$

$$F = \frac{1.62 - 1.52}{-0.064}$$

$$F = -1.56 \text{ D}$$

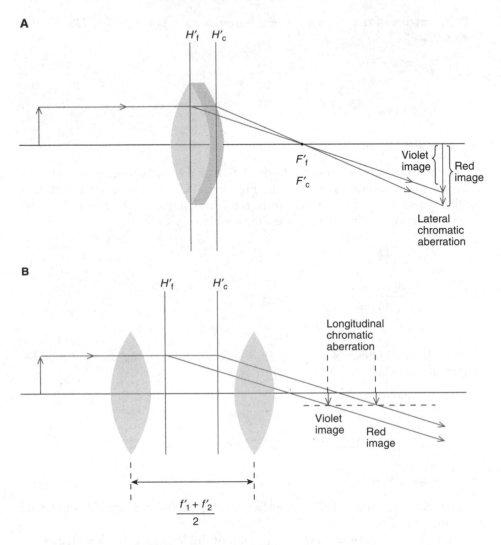

Figure F-2. A. An achromatic doublet has no longitudinal chromatic aberration when the separation of the principal planes for 486 and 656 nm (H'_f and H'_c) results in the focal points for these wavelengths being coincident. When this occurs, however, there is substantial lateral chromatic aberration. **B.** When two lenses are separated by an appropriate distance, lateral chromatic aberration is eliminated. Under these conditions, there may be substantial longitudinal chromatic aberration.

Adding together the powers of the three interfaces, we obtain a total power of approximately +6.00 D. This calculation shows that when the back surface of the first lens has the same radius as the front surface of the second lens, the combined power of two lenses in air is the same as when they are joined together.

LATERAL (TRANSVERSE) CHROMATIC ABERRATION

Lateral chromatic aberration can be a consideration in the design of certain optical systems. Figure F-2A shows a lens that has no *longitudinal* chromatic aberration. The image still suffers from lateral chromatic aberration because each wavelength results in an image of a different size. Consequently, the image has colored fringes.

Lateral chromatic aberration can be minimized with an optical system consisting of two lenses of the same constringence that are separated by the distance *d*, as defined below:

$$d = \frac{f_1' + f_2'}{2}$$

Figure F-2B shows a lens system with minimal lateral chromatic aberration. Note that the amount of longitudinal aberration is substantial. Depending on the intended use of an optical system, it may be a priority either to minimize longitudinal chromatic aberration or to minimize lateral chromatic aberration.

As discussed in Chapter 15, lateral chromatic aberration can reduce image quality when a patient views through a point significantly removed from the optical axis of a spectacle lens that has a low Abbe value (Fig. 15-16). If a lens material with a low Abbe number, such as polycarbonate, is prescribed, it may be important for the optical axis to be in approximate alignment with the patient's pupil, particularly in higher prescriptions.

Practice Examinations[1]

PRACTICE EXAMINATION 1

1. What is the angle of refraction for light incident on ophthalmic plastic (CR39) at an angle of 15.0 degrees? (Chapter 1)

2. As the wavelength increases, the amount of energy per quanta (Chapter 1):
   (a) decreases
   (b) increases
   (c) remains the same

3. What is the vergence at a distance of 40 cm from a point source? (Chapter 1)

4. What is the radius of curvature of a plastic spherical refractive surface whose power is −4.50 D? (Chapter 2)

5. A convex polycarbonate surface has a radius of curvature of 10.00 cm. What is its power? (Chapter 2)

6. A virtual image is: (Chapter 2)
   (a) always erect
   (b) always inverted
   (c) either erect or inverted

7. An object 4.0 mm in height is located 12.0 cm from a +5.00 D CR39 surface. (a) What is the image distance and size? (b) Is the image real or virtual? (c) Is the image erect or inverted? (Chapter 3)

8. A −7.50 D polycarbonate surface forms a virtual image at a distance of 10.0 cm. What is the object distance? (Chapter 3)

9. A penny at the bottom of a pond of water appears to be 2.0 m from its surface. How deep is the pond? (Chapter 3)

---

1. Answers may be found on page 355.

10. A meniscus CR39 lens whose front surface radius of curvature is 16.7 cm has an approximate power of −4.50 D. What is the power of its ocular surface? (Chapter 4)

11. An object 5.0 mm in height is located 6.0 cm from a +12.00 D lens. (a) Locate the image and give its size. (b) Is the image real or virtual? (c) Is the image erect or inverted? (Chapter 4)

12. When an object is situated 7.0 cm from a lens, a virtual image is formed at a distance of 3.0 cm. What is the power of the lens? (Chapter 4)

13. A polycarbonate lens with front and back surface powers of −5.00 and −3.00 D, respectively, has a thickness of 2.5 cm. An object that is 5.0 mm in height is located 25.0 cm from the front surface of the lens. (a) Locate the image with respect to the lens back surface and give its size. (b) Is the image real or virtual? (c) Is the image erect or inverted? (Chapter 5)

14. An object is located 15.0 cm from a 3.5 cm thick CR39 lens that has front and back surface powers of +10.00 and −3.00 D, respectively. (a) Locate the image with respect to the back surface of the lens. (b) If the object's height is 10.0 mm, what is the image's size? (c) Is the image real or virtual? (d) Is the image erect or inverted? (Chapter 5)

15. An object is located 40.0 cm from a +7.50 D thin lens, which is located 25.0 cm from a +10.00 D thin lens. (a) Locate the image with respect to the second lens. (b) If the object's height is 5.0 mm, what is the image's size? (c) Is the image real or virtual? (d) Is the image erect or inverted? (Chapter 5)

16. What is the back vertex power of a high index plastic ($n = 1.74$) lens that is 30.0 mm thick and has front and back surface powers of +8.00 D and −6.00 D, respectively? (Chapter 6)

17. What is the equivalent secondary focal length of a 35.0 mm thick equiconvex polycarbonate lens that has a front surface power of +5.00 D? (Chapter 6)

18. As the thickness of a minus meniscus lens increases, its back vertex power: (Chapter 6)
    (a) decreases in minus power
    (b) increases in minus power
    (c) remains the same

19. A reduced eye with a power of +60.00 D has an axial length of 25.00 mm. Determine the eye's refractive error as measured at the surface of the eye and locate its far point. (Chapter 7)

20. What power spectacle lens is required to correct a reduced eye that has a power of +55.00 D and an axial length of 22.22 mm? Assume a vertex distance of 12.0 mm. (Chapter 7)

21. If a reduced eye is corrected with a −7.50 D lens at a vertex distance of 13.0 mm, what is its axial length if its refractive power is +60.00 D? (Chapter 7)

22. A patient's refractive error as measured in the spectacle plane is +4.50 D. Assuming that the vertex distance is 12.0 mm, how much accommodation is required when the patient views a stimulus located at a distance of 20.00 cm from the eye while wearing contact lenses? (Chapter 8)

23. A patient who has 7.00 D of myopia as measured in the spectacle plane wears her old spectacles, which have a power of −5.00 DS. How much accommodation is required in the corneal plane when the patient views an object 40.00 cm from her eye through her old glasses? (Assume a vertex distance of 13.0 mm.) (Chapter 8)

24. An uncorrected 2.00 D myopic eye (as determined for the corneal plane) exerts half of its accommodation to focus an object at 10.00 cm onto the retina. What is the eye's amplitude of accommodation? (Ignore depth of field.) (Chapter 8)

25. A point source is located 33.33 cm in front of a $+4.00 + 1.00 \times 090$ lens. Describe and locate the images formed by the lens. (Chapter 9)

26. If a cross is situated 25.00 cm from a $+7.50 - 2.00 \times 180$ lens, at what distance from the lens is the horizontal line of the cross focused? (Chapter 9)

27. What is the power in the 60-degree meridian of a $-2.50 - 1.25 \times 090$ lens? (Chapter 9)

28. How much prism is experienced when a −4.00 DS lens is decentered 6.00 mm nasal and 3.00 mm superior to the pupil? (Chapter 10)

29. A patient with an IPD of 60 mm looks through spectacles whose optical centers are separated by 54 mm. If the right lens has a power of −3.00 DS and the left lens a power of −4.00 DS, how much prism does the patient experience? (Chapter 10)

30. When viewing an object located 3.00 m away through a 6.00^Δ prism, how far does the object appear to be displaced from its actual location? (Chapter 10)

31. The true amplitude of accommodation for an emmetropic patient with a hyperfocal distance of 1.00 m is 4.00 D. What is the nearest distance that the patient can see clearly? (Chapter 11)

32. The closest distance that a patient corrected with −2.00 DS contact lenses can see clearly is 10.00 cm. If the patient's true amplitude of accommodation is 9.00 D, what is the farthest distance she can see clearly when she removes her contact lenses? (Chapter 11)

33. Through his add, a patient's range of clear vision is from 100.00 to 25.00 cm. If his total depth of focus is 1.50 D, what is the add power? (Chapter 11)

34. A 70-year-old individual with age-related macular degeneration purchases a magnifier labeled 2.5× from her local pharmacy. If she can read 4 M through her bifocal add at 40 cm, what size print do you expect her to be able to read when looking through the magnifier with her distance prescription? (Assume that the reading material is held at the focal point of the magnifying lens.) (Chapter 12)

35. A patient with 20/400 best-corrected distance visual acuity would like to read 1 M print. What power-magnifying lens should you prescribe? (Chapter 12)

36. You would like to prescribe a 2.5× telemicroscope that enables your 65-year-old patient to read 2 M print. (a) If he can read 6 M print at 40.0 cm, what lens cap power is necessary? (b) What is the working distance? (Chapter 12)

37. What is the spectacle magnification produced by a +10.00 high-index plastic lens ($n = 1.74$) that has a center thickness of 5.00 mm and a front surface power of +3.50 D? (Assume a vertex distance of 13.0 mm.) (Chapter 13)

38. Assuming that it has a positive front surface power, increasing the thickness of a minus lens causes the lens's spectacle magnification to: (Chapter 13)

    (a) decrease

    (b) increase

    (c) remain the same

39. Correction of axial hyperopia with a contact lens causes the image size to: (Chapter 13)

    (a) decrease

    (b) increase

    (c) remain the same

40. An object 4.00 mm in height is located 12.00 cm from a concave mirror whose radius of curvature is 12.0 cm. (a) What is the image distance and size? (b) Is the image real or virtual? (c) Is the image erect or inverted? (Chapter 14)

41. A virtual image is located 10.00 cm from a −7.50 D mirror. Locate the object. (Chapter 14)

42. What percentage of light is transmitted through the front surface of a polycarbonate lens? (Chapter 14)

43. Correction of which of the following aberrations is least important in the design of spectacle lenses? (Chapter 15)
    (a) coma
    (b) curvature of field
    (c) distortion
    (d) oblique astigmatism

44. When a patient wears −6.50 DS polycarbonate spectacles that have a pantoscopic tilt of 25 degrees, what prescription does he experience? (Chapter 15)

45. A hyperopic patient who has had her accommodation paralyzed with a cycloplegic drop views a distant red–green visual acuity chart. Letters on which background are expected to appear clearest? (Chapter 15)
    (a) green
    (b) red
    (c) both will appear equally clear

PRACTICE EXAMINATION 2

1. The angle of refraction for a light ray entering polycarbonate is 10.0 degrees. What is the angle of incidence? (Chapter 1)

2. As the distance from a point source increases, the vergence (absolute value): (Chapter 1)
   (a) decreases
   (b) increases
   (c) remains the same

3. What is the critical angle for light leaving water and entering air? (Chapter 1)

4. As the radius of curvature decreases, the (absolute) power of a surface: (Chapter 2)
   (a) decreases
   (b) increases
   (c) remains the same

5. What is the radius of curvature of a Trivex surface that has a power of +3.00 D? (Chapter 2)

6. A real image is: (Chapter 2)

   (a) always formed by converging rays

   (b) always inverted

   (c) not focusable on a screen

   (d) both "(a)" and "(b)" are correct

   (e) "(a)," "(b)", and "(c)" are correct

7. An object 6 mm in height is located 20.0 cm from a +15.00 D Trivex surface. (a) What is the image distance and size? (b) Is the image real or virtual? (c) Is the image erect or inverted? (Chapter 3)

8. A virtual image is located 6.0 cm from a +20.00 D polycarbonate surface. What is the object distance? (Chapter 3)

9. When a clear pond of water is 1.0 m deep, how deep does it appear to be? (Chapter 3)

10. The ocular surface of a thin +3.00 D polycarbonate meniscus lens has a power of −2.00 D. What is the radius of curvature of its front surface? (Chapter 4)

11. An object 10 mm in height is located 5.0 cm from a −3.00 D lens. (a) Locate the image and determine its size. (b) Is the image real or virtual? (c) Is the image erect or inverted? (Chapter 4)

12. When an object is located 5.0 cm from a lens, a virtual image is formed at a distance of 6.0 cm. What is the power of the lens? (Chapter 4)

13. A CR39 lens with front and back surface powers of −6.00 and +4.00 D, respectively, has a thickness of 3.0 cm. An object that is 6.0 mm in height is located 20.0 cm from the front surface of the lens. (a) Locate the image and give its size. (b) Is the image real or virtual? (c) Is the image erect or inverted? (Chapter 5)

14. An object is located 50.0 cm from a 2.0-cm thick polycarbonate lens that has front and back surface powers of +6.00 and −2.50 D, respectively. (a) Locate the image. (b) If the object's height is 8.0 mm, what is the image's size? (c) Is the image real or virtual? (d) Is the image erect or inverted? (Chapter 5)

15. An object is located 25.0 cm from a +2.00 D thin lens, which is located 15.0 cm from a +5.00 D thin lens. (a) Locate the image. (b) If the object's height is 10.0 mm, what is the image's size? (c) Is the image real or virtual? (d) Is the image erect or inverted? (Chapter 5)

16. Determine the neutralizing power of a 20.0-mm thick CR39 lens that has front and back surface powers of +5.00 D and −3.00 D, respectively. (Chapter 6)

17. As the thickness of a plus meniscus lens increases, its equivalent power: (Chapter 6)

    (a) decreases

    (b) increases

    (c) remains the same

18. What is the back vertex power of an equiconcave Trivex lens that has a thickness of 30.0 mm and a front surface power of −6.50 D? (Chapter 6)

19. When looking through a −3.50 D spectacle lens (vertex distance of 14.0 mm), a patient's far point is 20 cm in front of the spectacle lens. What power contact lens would correct for distance? (Chapter 7)

20. A reduced eye with a power of +60.00 D has an axial length of 20.00 mm. Determine the eye's refractive error as measured at the surface of the eye and locate its far point. (Chapter 7)

21. If a reduced eye is corrected with a +12.50 D lens at a vertex distance of 11.0 mm, what is its axial length if the hyperopia is axial in origin? (Chapter 7)

22. To be fully corrected for distance, a patient requires a +4.50 D contact lens. When viewing an object located at 25.00 cm while wearing a +3.00 D contact lens, how much accommodation is required? (Chapter 8)

23. A 4.00 D myopic eye, as measured in the spectacle plane, views an object through a −5.50 D lens held 5 cm in front of the eye. If the object is 15 cm from the eye, how much accommodation, as measured in the corneal plane, is required for the image to be focused on the retina? (Assume a vertex distance of 1.5 cm.) (Chapter 8)

24. An emmetropic eye's near point of accommodation is 10.00 cm. What power contact lens would allow the eye to view an object located at 15.00 cm while using only half of its amplitude of accommodation? (Ignore depth of field.) (Chapter 8)

25. A point source is located 40.00 cm in front of a +6.00 − 3.00 × 180 lens. Describe and locate the images formed by the lens. (Chapter 9)

26. If a cross is situated 100.00 cm from a +3.00 − 1.00 × 090 lens, at what distance from the lens is the vertical line of the cross focused? (Chapter 9)

27. What is the power in the vertical meridian of a +1.50 − 3.75 × 150 lens? (Chapter 9)

28. When a patient views through a +5.50 DS lens that is decentered 3 mm temporal and 4 mm inferior to the pupil, how much prism is experienced? (Chapter 10)

29. A patient with an IPD of 58 mm has spectacles with optical centers separated by 68 mm. If the right lens has a power of −2.00 + 5.00 × 090 and the left lens has a power of +2.00 DS, how much prism does the patient experience? (Chapter 10)

30. What is the power, in degrees, of a CR39 prism that has an apical angle of 6 degrees? (Chapter 10)

31. What is the nearest distance that can be seen clearly by a 5.00 D corrected hyperopic patient who has a hyperfocal distance of 0.50 m and true amplitude of accommodation of 8.00 D? (Assume that the patient is corrected with a contact lens.) (Chapter 11)

32. The farthest distance that an uncorrected 2.50 D myopic patient can see clearly is 50.00 cm. If the patient's actual amplitude of accommodation is 5.00 D, what is the nearest distance she can see clearly when wearing her distance correction? (Assume that the patient is corrected with a contact lens.) (Chapter 11)

33. When wearing his bifocals, a patient's range of clear vision at near is 50.00 to 25.00 cm. What is the add power if his total depth of focus is 1.00 D? (Chapter 11)

34. A patient views print through a fixed-focus stand magnifier whose height is less than the focal length of its lens. As the patient moves closer to the stand magnifier, magnification will: (Chapter 12)

    (a) decrease

    (b) increase

    (c) remain the same

35. A patient with age-related macular degeneration can read 1 M when looking through a 10.00 D magnifying lens. What do you expect the distance visual acuity to be? (Chapter 12)

36. A patient who can read 8 M print through her add at 40 cm has purchased an electronic handheld magnifier. If the magnifier's maximum magnification is 4×, how close must the patient be to the magnifier to read 1 M print? (Chapter 12)

37. What is the spectacle magnification produced by a −8.75 polycarbonate lens that has a center thickness of 1.75 mm and a front surface power of +4.00 D? (Assume that a vertex distance of 12.0 mm.) (Chapter 13)

38. Increasing the positive power of the front surface of a minus meniscus lens causes the lens's spectacle magnification to: (Chapter 13)

    (a) decrease

    (b) increase

    (c) remain the same

39. Correction of axial hyperopia with a spectacle lens causes the retinal image size to: (Chapter 13)

    (a) decrease

    (b) increase

    (c) remain the same

40. An object 6.00 mm in height is located 20.00 cm from a convex mirror whose radius of curvature is 7.50 cm. (a) What is the image distance and size? (b) Is the image real or virtual? (c) Is the image erect or inverted? (Chapter 14)

41. A virtual image is located 40.00 cm from a +7.50 D mirror. Locate the object. (Chapter 14)

42. To minimize reflections, what should be the refractive index of the antireflective coating applied to a polycarbonate lens? (Chapter 14)

43. Which of the following aberrations may be present for rays that pass through the center of a lens? (Chapter 15)

    (a) coma

    (b) curvature of field

    (c) oblique astigmatism

    (d) spherical aberration

    (e) both "(b)" and "(c)" are correct

44. When a patient wears a −6.00 DS CR-39 lens in a frame with a 20-degree face-form angle, what prescription does the patient experience? (Chapter 15)

45. When prescribing polycarbonate lenses, which of the following is most likely to cause a reduction in visual acuity if the optical centers are not aligned with the patient's pupils? (Chapter 15)

    (a) coma

    (b) lateral chromatic aberration

    (c) longitudinal chromatic aberration

    (d) spherical aberration

Answers to Practice Examinations

PRACTICE EXAMINATION 1

1. 9.9°

2. (a)

3. −2.50 D

4. −11.1 cm

5. +5.86 D

6. (a)

7. (a) Image distance is −45.0 cm and image size is +10 mm; (b) virtual; (c) erect

8. −12.0 cm

9. 2.7 m

10. −7.50 D

11. (a) Image distance is −21.4 cm and image size is +17.9 mm; (b) virtual; (c) erect

12. −19.0 D

13. (a) Image distance is −9.2 cm with respect to the back surface and the image size is +1.6 mm; (b) virtual; (c) erect

14. (a) Image distance is +163.7 cm with respect to the back surface; (b) −118.5 mm; (c) real; (d) inverted

15. (a) Image distance is −10.0 cm with respect to the second lens; (b) −5.0 mm; (c) virtual; (d) inverted

16. +3.28 D

17. +10.58 cm

18. (a)

19. Refractive error is −6.68 D; far point is located 15.0 cm anterior to the eye

20. +4.71 D

21. 25.07 mm

22. 5.00 D

23. 0.49 D

24. 16.00 D

25. A vertical line is formed at +50.00 and a horizontal line at +100.00 cm

26. +66.67 cm

27. −2.81 D

28. 2.4^Δ base out and 1.2^Δ base down

29. 2.1^Δ base out

30. 18 cm

31. 20 cm

32. 100.00 cm

33. 1.75 D

34. 1 M

35. +20 D

36. (a) +3.00 D; (b) 33.3 cm

37. 1.16×

38. (b)

39. (c)

40. (a) The image distance is −12.00 cm and the image size is −4.00 mm; (b) real; (c) inverted

41. −40.00 cm

42. 95%

43. (a)

44. −6.87 − 1.41 × 180

45. Green

PRACTICE EXAMINATION 2

1. 16.0°

2. (a)

3. 48.6°

4. (b)

5. +17.7 cm

6. (d)

7. (a) Image distance is +15.3 cm and image size is −3 mm; (b) real; (c) inverted

8. −2.2 cm

9. 0.8 m

10. +11.7 cm

11. (a) Image distance is −4.3 cm and image size is +8.7 mm; (b) virtual; (c) erect

12. +3.33 D

13. (a) Image distance is −19.9 cm with respect to the back surface and the image size is +4.9 mm; (b) virtual; (c) erect

14. (a) Image distance is +58.4 cm with respect to the back surface; (b) −9.8 mm; (c) real; (d) inverted

15. (a) Image distance is +28.9 cm with respect to the second lens; (b) –8.9 mm; (c) real; (d) inverted

16. +2.12 D

17. (b)

18. –12.26 D

19. –7.60 D

20. The refractive error is +6.65 D and the far point is 15.04 cm posterior to the eye's refractive surface

21. 17.89 mm

22. 5.50 D

23. 4.96 D

24. +1.67 D

25. A vertical line is formed at +28.57 cm and a horizontal line at +200.00 cm

26. +100.00 cm

27. –1.31 D

28. 1.65$^\Delta$ base out and 2.20$^\Delta$ base down

29. 2.5$^\Delta$ base out

30. 3 degrees

31. 10 cm

32. 18.18 cm

33. 2.50 D

34. (b)

35. 20/200

36. 20 cm

37. 0.91×

38. (b)

39. (b)

40. (a) The image distance is +3.16 cm and the image size is +0.95 mm; (b) virtual; (c) erect

41. −10.00 cm

42. 1.26

43. (e)

44. −6.23 − 0.79 × 090

45. (b)

Index

Note: Page numbers followed by *f* indicate figures; those followed by *n* indicate footnotes; those followed by *t* indicate tables.